OPEN SECRET

OPEN

GAY HOLLYWOOD

SECRET

1928 – 2000

David Ehrenstein

Perennial

An Imprint of HarperCollins*Publishers*

A hardcover edition of this book was published in 1998 by
William Morrow and Company, Inc.

OPEN SECRET. Copyright © 1998 by David Ehrenstein. "The Epilogue
Strikes Back" copyright © 2000 by David Ehrenstein. All rights
reserved. Printed in the United States of America. No part of
this book may be used or reproduced in any manner whatsoever
without written permission except in the case of brief quotations
embodied in critical articles and reviews. For information address
HarperCollins Publishers Inc.,
10 East 53rd Street, New York, NY 10022.

HarperCollins books may be purchased for educational, business, or
sales promotional use. For information please write: Special Markets
Department, HarperCollins Publishers Inc., 10 East 53rd Street,
New York, NY 10022.

First Perennial edition published 2000

Designed by Richard Oriolo

The Library of Congress has catalogued the hardcover edition as follows:

Ehrenstein, David.
Open secret : gay Hollywood, 1928–1998 / David Ehrenstein.—1st ed.
p.   cm.
Includes index.
ISBN 0-688-15317-8
1. Homosexuality in motion pictures—United States.   I. Title.
PN1995.9.H55E47   1998   98-35526
791.43'653—21   CIP
ISBN 0-688-17585-6 (pbk.)

00 01 02 03 04 RRD 10 9 8 7 6 5 4 3 2 1

To the memory of
Richard Rouilard

ACKNOWLEDGMENTS

———

I would like to thank Warren Beatty, Jonathan Benair, Steven Bradford, Paul Bresnick, Meredith Brody, Sharon Butler, Tiffany Ann Rose Butler, Michael Caruso, Bob Cohen, Brad Confer, Esther Crayton, Mitchell Fink, Bob Foster, Larry Gross, Alan Helms, Bill Higgins, Robert Hofler, Mark Horowitz, Thomas Pasatieri, Abraham Polonsky, Terry Press, Ben Schafer, Charlotte Sheedy, Julia Sweeney, and all the men and women who granted me interviews.

I would also like to thank the Fray, *Los Angeles* magazine (where a portion of this book first appeared), the Margaret Herrick Library, The Mote *Shake* books, and the staffs of Midway Hospital and the Rancho Los Amigos Medical Center.

And Bill Reed.

C O N T E N T S

—

Contents

PROLOGUE

HYPOTHALAMUS,

MON AMOUR

—

BEGIN AT THE BEGINNING,'' THE KING said to Alice, "and go on till you come to the end: then stop."

It's a perfectly reasonable way to proceed through a place like Lewis

Carroll's Wonderland. But this is a book about Hollywood, which is

to say a place, an industry, and a state of mind. Working in tandem, this tripartite structure is far more bizarre than anything Carroll could ever contrive. Moreover, this is also a book about same-sexuality—a state of mind (and body) coexistent with a history that parallels Hollywood's. For both homosexuality and the movies were invented in the late 1800s. And to return to the scene of this multiple birth, we must begin by means of a detour—to Hungary.

Toward the close of the nineteenth century, a Hungarian journalist named either Károly Benkert or Karl Maria Kertbeny (accounts differ as to which moniker was the pseudonym for the other) coined the term "homosexual" in a pair of pamphlets promoting "sexual freedom," to describe those attracted to members of their own sex. Little is known about Benkert/Kertbeny save for the fact that his pamphlets won the attention of three persons in the then newly developing field of sexual-behavior research: Ernst Jaeger, Karl Ulrichs, and Richard von Krafft-Ebing.[1]

While accounts of same-sex relations can be traced back to the beginnings of recorded time, it is only at this particular juncture when what had been either accepted as natural, rejected as "sinful," or ignored altogether found itself culturally reconfigured as a "perversion" of the "norm" of "heterosexuality." The last-mentioned term was itself newly minted, originating with the aforementioned researchers as a means of identifying those suffering from an *excessive* interest in the opposite sex. But thanks to Benkert/Kertbeny, "homo" quickly gained usage as a means of not only differentiating but *defining* "hetero."

This rhetorical practice intensified in the wake of the publication of Sigmund Freud's *Three Essays on the Theory of Sexuality* in 1905, where, historian Jonathan Ned Katz asserts, "heterosexual and homosexual appeared in public as Siamese twins, the first good, the second bad, bound together for life in unalterable, antagonistic symbiosis." The result, Katz continues, is the formation of a cultural hierarchy in which "heterosexuality is invented in discourse as that which is outside discourse."[2]

That a specified name was sought for an aspect of human sexuality in this particular era was no accident. For as the nineteenth century gave way to the twentieth, a new "middle" class emerged as a cultural buffer between the extremes of rich and poor. Having more social mobility than the latter, yet lacking the divinely ordained authority of the former, this new group quickly found its feet as an arbiter of "proper" behavior in a rapidly expanding public sphere. The meaning of this became clear in 1895 with the imprisonment of Oscar Wilde on "immoral conduct" charges, the climax of a series of legal proceedings that had begun some ten years earlier. While the poet-playwright's sexual orientation was implicitly acknowledged in his work, and well-known within his social circle, the *explicit* testimony of male prostitutes heard in a court of law horrified the new class. "Private" behavior was being being put on "public" display, undermining the value of the middle class's sole social possession: its "good name."

The example of Wilde wasn't lost on his contemporary Marcel Proust, a middle-class aesthete with upper-class social aspirations and like-minded sexuality, who declared in his *Remembrance of Things Past* that the same-sex-oriented constitute

> a race upon which a curse is laid and which must live in falsehood and perjury because it knows that its desire, that which constitutes life's dearest pleasure, is held to be punishable, shameful, an inadmissible thing; which must deny its existence even when Christians, when at the bar of justice they appear and are arraigned, must before Christ and in his name refute as a calumny what is their very life; sons without a mother, to whom they are obliged to lie all her life long and even in the hour when they close her dying eyes; friends without friendships, despite all those which their frequently acknowledged charm inspires and their often generous heart would gladly feel—but can we describe as friendships those relationships which flourish only by virtue of a lie from which the first impulse of trust and sincerity to which they might be tempted to yield would cause them to be rejected with disgust, unless they are dealing with an impartial or perhaps even sympathetic spirit, who

however in that case, misled with regard to them by conventional psychology, will attribute to the vice confessed
the very affection that is most alien to it, just as certain
judges assume and are more inclined to pardon murder
in inverts and treason in Jews for reasons derived from
original sin and racial predestination?[3]

This *sentence* (evoking an amazingly wide range of social circumstance and subjective experience) can be found in *Sodome et
Gomorrhe,* the fourth section of Proust's seven-volume work, rechris-
tened by its English translators C. K. Scott Moncrieff and Terence
Kilmartin as *Cities of the Plain.* This titular alteration typifies the
rhetorical coyness that has surrounded even the most casual discussion of same-sex relations to this very day.

Being the primary, but by no means exclusive, orientation of
the majority, "heterosexuality" has assumed the status of the "normal": a self-evident truth, so universal in scope its name needn't be
mentioned. "Homosexuality," by contrast, has come to be regarded
as embodying the "abnormal," that which must be psychically seg-
regated and socially marginalized at all costs. Consequently, every
appearance of the "homosexual" requires an *explanation*—less from
the party in question than by means of the testimony of a culturally
approved "authority" of one sort or another.

The past half-century has witnessed an endless parade of self-
styled "experts," in such diverse fields as religion, politics, medicine,
psychiatry, and, most recently, genetic science, proudly proclaim one
half-baked idea after another as the "cause" of homosexuality. For
decades a school of psychiatry would have had one believe that a
"distant" father and an "overprotective" mother produced "deviance"
in their offspring. Discredited by the American Psychiatric Association in 1973, this theory's chief exponent, Dr. Charles Socarides, has
continued to ply his familial horror stories to the delight of Christian
fundamentalist ideologues. That his son Richard has become a prominent gay rights advocate, thus revealing the good doctor to be a pro-
moter of the very "neurosis" that he has spent his entire life
attempting to eradicate, has mattered little to Socarides and his fol-

lowers. Others on the religious and ~~~~~ culprit to be "corruption" from an outs~~~~~ O'Hara once described as "a pleasant stranger ~~~~~ the Heaven on Earth Bldg near the Williamsburg Br~~~~~ lis Schlafly and Pat Robertson have not been forthcoming~~~~~ this scenario might have figured in the lives of her son John o~~~~~ speechwriter Mel White.

Most recently, an alleged discrepancy in that part of the brain called the hypothalamus and that "magic bullet" known as DNA (the chlorophyll of the 1990s) have been advanced as *causes du jour* by scientific researcher Simon Le Vay (*The Gay Brain*) and journalist Chandler Burr (*A Separate Creation*). Though same-sex-oriented themselves, both Le Vay and Burr apparently feel the need for personal justification before what writer Christopher Isherwood has so aptly referred to as "the heterosexual dictatorship."[5] Their "I just can't help myself" defense (remindful of the climactic speech delivered by Peter Lorre's murderous pedophile in the film *M*) has little to do with real people and actual lives. But when it comes to the cause-obsessed, *any* excuse will do, just so long as it declines to validate the perfectly reasonable conclusions a sex researcher named Alfred C. Kinsey came to in his 1948 study *Sexual Behavior in the Human Male*: that same-sex attraction is simply a part of human nature, residing to a greater or lesser degree in virtually everyone.

"Actually, there is no such thing as a homosexual person, any more than there is such a thing as a heterosexual person," novelist/essayist/screenwriter Gore Vidal (a participant in Kinsey's study) has noted on more than one occasion. "The words are adjectives describing sexual acts, not people. Those sexual acts are entirely natural; if they were not, no one would be able to perform them."[6] But as logically straightforward as Vidal's words might seem, they don't take into account those only too happy to have homosexual "conduct" added to race, class, religion, and ethnicity as a basis for discrimination. Likewise, Vidal's insistence on "acts" over "persons" fails to speak to those who regard their sexuality in a larger context, as part of a wide variety of emotional and intellectual life experiences. Moreover, it doesn't address the fact that those who've embraced the homosexual done so in order to found a civil rights movement whose relative success has framed one of the most interesting stories in American politics of the last quarter-century.

"Homosexuality shocks less, but continues to be interesting; it is still at that stage of excitation where it provokes what might be called feats of discourse," wrote critic Roland Barthes in 1981 in his preface to Renaud Camus's homoerotic memoir *Tricks*. "Speaking of homosexuality permits those who 'aren't' to show how open, liberal and modern they are; and those who 'are' to bear witness, to assume responsibility, to militate. Everyone gets busy, in different ways, whipping it up." But as attractive as this prospect seems at first, Barthes quickly finds misgivings in that "to proclaim yourself something is always to speak at the behest of a vengeful Other, to enter into his discourse, to argue with him, to seek from him a scrap of identity. What society will not tolerate, is that I should be . . . *nothing*, or to be more exact, that the *something* that I am should be openly expressed as provisional, revocable, insignificant, inessential, in a word: irrelevant. Just say 'I am,' and you will be socially saved."[7]

Still, the act of self-identification is no guarantee against "vengeful Other" attacks, as Barthes's contemporary the philosophical critic Michel Foucault has frequently observed. "I think what most bothers most of those who are not gay about gayness," Foucault claims, "is the gay 'lifestyle,' not the sex acts themselves . . . the common fear that gays will develop relationships that are intense and satisfying even though they do not at all conform to the ideas of relationship held by others. It is the prospect that gays will create as yet unforeseen kinds of relationships that many people cannot tolerate."[8]

The fruits of this intolerance can most clearly be seen with those determined to debunk Kinsey's findings. His famous 1 to 6 scale, indicating a wide range of possible same-sex involvements, has been reduced by the press to an arbitrary 10 percent of alleged exclusivity. This has been further downsized to 1 or 2 percent by those preferring the results of more recent surveys whose participants were asked whether they considered themselves to be homosexual. Kinsey never asked so blunt a question. He simply inquired as to the variety of his subjects' sexual experiences, period. But that won't do in a culture insistent on hard numbers and specified types. As a result, Kinsey biographer James H. Jones brands the good doctor "a homosexual," though everything in Kinsey's life and work would question the validity of such a reflexive labeling.[9]

"The world of sex now turns upside down," Jonathan Ned Katz notes. "Influenced by many social movements, heterosexual and homosexual grow ever more similar. Hence the mass media's mad dash to publicize every new 'scientific' study demonstrating that homosexual desire, and heterosexual, is in the genes, hypothalamus, hormones, or whatever, and never shall the orientations meet. Once again the sure physiological line is drawn. Homosexuals and heterosexuals of biological determinist persuasion sigh with relief: heterosexuals because their feelings are not homosexual, and therefore good, homosexuals because their feelings are natural, and therefore good."[10]

Still, such sexual culture wars rage only for the middle class and the "family values" we're ceaselessly informed they hold so dear. The poor, as always, are ignored. The rich have never had trouble avoiding public view and going their own way, regardless of the impassioned entreaties of "gay liberation" or the rhetorical writhings of the radical right. Those who could afford higher education had easy access to the likes of Proust. Moreover, if they were lucky enough to latch onto a sympathetic philosophy professor, they could engage in lively debates on the meaning of "friendship" as defined in Plato's *Symposium*. The more adventurous might wrestle with the defense of same-sex passion offered by André Gide in *Corydon*. And that's not to mention those academic intrepids alert to the subtext of Oscar Wilde's plays or the main text of Walt Whitman's poetry, or the possible implications of the fact that Shakespeare's sonnets were written to a man.

Such is—and always has been—the life of the mind for the lucky few in the Ivy League.

Everybody else had the movies.

GAY ALL OF A

SUDDEN

—

I FOUND OUT ABOUT ROCK HUDSON IN 1957.
I was ten years old. The girl who told me was nine.

"Do you know what a *ho-mo-sex-u-al* is?"

Susan and I were playing Monopoly on an old card table in her

basement rec room when she lobbed that one at me from out of nowhere. I looked up from Park Place into the biggest cat-that-swallowed-the-canary grin I'd ever seen. Obviously she wasn't expecting a reply.

"There are these *men*," she giggle-gushed excitedly. "They *think* they're girls. But they don't *like* girls." Breaking into peals of laughter, Susan began to wriggle her body about, flip-flopping her hands in the air in a manner I'd later learn was "effeminate."

"*You* know," she said, as if in answer to my stunned silence. "Liberace. Johnnie Ray. Oh, and Rock Hudson! He's one of them too! They're *all over* Hollywood! They all *know* each other! They had this *pajama party*, and the police *raided* it! Tab Hunter was arrested!" And then—after pausing for dramatic effect—the coup de grâce: "It was in *Confidential*!"

Clearly this otherwise ordinary schoolgirl had stumbled on to something big. But what, exactly, was it? Weren't pajama parties for teenage girls only? If these men think they're girls, wouldn't they be wearing nightgowns instead of pajamas? And if you think you're a girl, why wouldn't you *like* girls? I wanted to ask Susan all these questions, but was dumbstruck. I had just begun to discover in myself what the "adult original" paperbacks I'd find at the drugstore a few years later would call "strange twilight urges": I was attracted to other boys. I had no idea what this meant, though it was obvious from everything around me that this wouldn't meet with widespread peer approval. I needed more information. And Susan—of all people—seemed to have it. But in the last analysis she wasn't much help. I *liked* girls. I didn't think that I *was* one. And I had no interest in wearing their clothes or going to pajama parties.

My parents had never said a word to me about "ho-mo-sex-u-als." Neither had any other adult authority or "role model" (that incessant fin-de-siècle buzzword evoking Barbie and G.I. Joe dolls magically rendered life-size and mortal). There was nothing taught about "ho-mo-sex-u-als" in school. The priest never mentioned them in church. There were no programs about them on television. And no one took me to see *Tea and Sympathy*, one of the few films around to deal ever-so-obliquely with the subject. But then, *any* information about sexuality was in scarce supply. The big parent/child "talk"—

that hallowed charade in which the ill-informed lecture the presumed-to-be-ignorant on a subject neither can speak of coherently—was still several years away. And that wouldn't include anything about "ho-mo-sex-u-als" either. Thank the lord we at least had *Confidential!*

If it was in *Confidential,* then it had to be scandalous. And if it was scandalous, then it had to be true. Or at least true enough. "Oh, they make all those things up," my mother would say of the monthly's latest outrage. "That's why they're being sued!" Indeed, the papers that year were filled with tales of *Confidential* editors being hauled into court over something called libel. Never reading much past the headlines, Susan and I had only the vaguest idea of what this meant. All we knew was gossip's unwritten law: where there's smoke, there's fire. We'd long suspected the pristine facades the studios had so carefully constructed around their stars hid darker truths. Occasionally a shade of gray might leak through via the gossip columns of a Hedda Hopper or Louella Parsons. But while they served up plenty of dish on divorce, these decorous sob sisters were near beer next to the hundred-proof Scotch of *Confidential.*

It goes without saying that neither Susan nor I had ever actually read a copy of *Confidential.* Our parents didn't buy it. None of our schoolmates (or their parents) did, either. We knew of only one local newsstand that carried it, and it wasn't about to sell *Confidential* to minors. The best we could manage was to steal a glance at a cover or two when we went to buy our *Mad* magazines. *Confidential* seemed to wink lewdly at us from the overhead rack—like those candy-proffering strangers our parents had warned us so much against. With its stark primary colors, unflatteringly cropped pictures, and lurid headlines promising the "lowdown" on the rich and famous, it seemed a sinister harbinger of a grown-up world we awaited with a mixture of anticipation and dread. The evil twin of the sycophantic *Photoplay, Confidential* countered Hollywood's carefully crafted visions of beautiful clothes, lavish parties, even teeth, and creamy complexions with leeringly detailed accounts of drunken brawls, teenage prostitutes, interracial sex (an especial *Confidential* obsession), and now (gasp! shudder!) *ho-mo-sex-u-als!*

Susan and I had only a passing acquaintance with the so-called facts of life. The nuts-and-bolts on reproduction could be found in any encyclopedia, but you needed a college-level science teacher to make sense of the text. Moreover, it had nothing to say about the physical pleasure we were beginning to learn was part of the package. Back-fence gossip thrived on innuendo, but the neighbors never got around to explaining exactly why they snarled "slut" under their breath every time the garishly dressed woman who lived down the street passed by. More helpful were the teenagers who parked their cars near Susan's home, always prattling about the love lives of celebrities. Though she never said so outright, it was clear these motor-mouthed high-schoolers were her source for learning of Hollywood's pajama-partying ways.

Susan may not have known much about sex, but she was well versed in gender roles. Boys played ball, girls played with dolls. Men liked sports, women liked dresses. Male was strong, female was submissive. Men and women fell in love, married one another, and had children. That was *the law*. Breaking it, as these "ho-mo-sex-u-als" apparently had, suggested that the assigned roles we'd been taught so carefully were in fact arbitrary and subject to change. No wonder Susan surmised these pajama-partyers must "*think* they're girls," yet "don't *like* girls." Still, one of them would have to "be the girl" somehow, to do whatever it was they did, as two sexes were required for every adult activity she knew of outside of sports. But which man would do what? How would he go about being the girl he didn't like? And what was the point of all this, since men couldn't get pregnant or marry one another?

With his toothy grin and conspicuous candelabra, Liberace was too ridiculous for Susan to take seriously—the Richard Simmons of his day. Johnnie Ray's overwrought singing style she likewise found off-putting. By contrast, Tab Hunter's blandly earnest, boy-next-door demeanor were so familiar they seemed downright calculated. Rock Hudson was someone else entirely. Well over six feet tall, wavy-haired, and possessed of the deepest, most mellifluous voice she had ever heard, he seemed an idealized, youthful version of her girlfriends' fathers. What was going on here?

"Homosexual" wasn't part of anyone's everyday vocabulary in

1957. Though Kinsey's wake opened a floodgate of pop-psychology books on "sexual deviance," their conclusions (often as not radically different than those of the doctor who inspired them) hadn't yet impacted on what the Reagan administration would come to refer to as "the general population." "One of *them*" was the favored term for the same-sex-oriented, being euphemistic and therefore *almost* polite. Decidedly impolite were fag and dyke, not so much spoken as wielded, like verbal battering rams. By the time we entered high school, Susan and I would hear "Fag!" and "Dyke!" spat countless times in the faces of any number of hapless parties—myself included. Sexuality needn't be involved at all. If you looked or acted "different," if you declined to conform in any way, you would be certain to "get it" from peers well trained by their elders in the fine art of name-calling and intimidation. The message was clear: fag and dyke were *the worst things in the world*. That too was *the law*, and it would take another two decades before this unwritten statute would find itself facing a fully organized opposition before the Supreme Court of public opinion.

A s I later learned, the pajama-party story wasn't the hot news flash Susan believed it to be. It ran in *Confidential* two years prior to our fateful Monopoly game.[1] Moreover, her informants couldn't have relied on it for their Hudson scoop. The article never mentioned him—only Tab Hunter. (Johnnie Ray and Liberace weren't at the party either, meriting *Confidential* broadsides of their own.) In fact, for all its dirt-digging infamy, the magazine never got around to the "outing" (as the term *Time* magazine coined in 1990 would have it) of Rock Hudson.[2] Yet no one needed to have read *Confidential*, or any of its many imitators (*Rave, Dare, Inside, Exposed, Blast, Whisper, Revealed, Sensation, On the QT, Hush-Hush*), to be "put wise." The truth had been apparent for some time. Rock Hudson's homosexuality was an "open secret" in Hollywood: widely known, and *implicitly* acknowledged by any number of parties from the very beginning of his career.

    " 'Pretty boy Rock Hudson,' they call him now in the gossip

columns," begins an Earl Wilson gossip column in the *New York Post*, dated June 23, 1953. "He's always out with a new movie beauty in the columns—and I happen to believe it's true."[3] What was Wilson talking about? What did he "happen to believe" was true? A former postman and truck driver, born Roy Fitzgerald, Rock Hudson began his acting career under contract to Raoul Walsh, first appearing on-screen in the veteran director's 1948 war drama *Fighter Squadron*. The year of the Wilson column saw Hudson in two other Walsh films—*Gun Fury* and *Sea Devils*—as well as *Seminole, The Golden Blade, Back to God's Country,* and *Taza, Son of Cochise*. These last four were produced by Universal-International, which had by mid-year picked up his contract from Walsh. Hudson's breakthrough film, *Magnificent Obsession*—the biggest hit the studio would enjoy since the heyday of Deanna Durbin—was only a year away. But in 1953 no one could have predicted such a sudden change of fortune for Rock Hudson.

"I remember at one point—this was before we did *The Golden Blade* together—they were going to drop him, because they were just putting him into these things and didn't know what to do with him," Hudson co-star Piper Laurie recalled some forty years later. "I knew about this because a producer with whom I'd done a couple of films told me about it. They claimed they just couldn't find anything for him. I know that what I'm about to tell you may sound self-serving but it's true. I liked working with Rock so much, and I liked *him* so much, that I begged this producer to see if they could do something to help. For whatever reason they kept him on."[4]

Such professional precariousness underscores the fact that the 1953 New York trip (the occasion for Wilson's column) was more than a pro forma exercise in "getting some good publicity." Its starlet-studded dates were clearly the studio's way of testing the waters with the entertainment press, of which Wilson was a prime representative. Was Hudson worth their time and trouble? Or was he just another "pretty boy"—read unserious, read unmasculine, read *homosexual*.

"Robert Taylor was a talented actor who became quite expert, but for a while he was frightened off by being called 'beautiful Bob Taylor,' " director George Cukor recalled in 1972 of the MGM leading man he had directed alongside Greta Garbo in *Camille* in 1936. "In those days," Cukor cautioned, "you had to be very virile or they thought you were degenerate."[5] Cukor, the "woman's director," knew exactly what he was talking about. The pejorative connotation of "pretty boy," like that of "woman's director," was well understood in Hollywood. No one had to spell it out. It was Hollywood slang for "Fag!"

In 1953 "sodomy" statutes were on the books in nearly every state in the union, bolstered by local ordinances that made men and women subject to "disorderly conduct" arrest for even so much as the appearance of same-sex "fraternization." There was no employment protection for any job of any kind. Even the most discreet of citizens in the most mundane of occupations could find themselves subject to firing with impunity, should an unsympathetic boss learn of said employee's "private life." Consequently, any number of otherwise ordinary Americans found themselves in "the closet": a self-imposed regimen of lies, evasions, and distortions designed to hide the fact that they might be anything other than exclusively heterosexual. It is a situation that persists to this very day for the overwhelming majority of the same-sex-oriented in the absence of nationwide, across-the-board job protection, a hit-and-miss patchwork quilt of state and local civil rights ordinances being under constant attack from the "religious" right. In the 1950s, however, potential job loss was far from the worst of it. For, working alongside legal authorities, the medical and psychiatric communities had begun toward the end of World War II to offer those "detained" by the police on "lewd conduct" charges, an alternative to incarceration: electroshock "therapy" and castration as a means of curing their "condition."

Roy Fitzgerald might very well have found himself faced with the prospect of such treatment but that wasn't about to happen to Rock Hudson. True, "moral turpitude" clauses in studio contracts specified that a performer "will not do anything which will tend to degrade him in society or bring him into public disrepute, contempt, scorn or ridicule, or that will tend to shock, insult or offend the community or public morals or decency, or prejudice to the studio or the motion picture industry in general."[6] But Rock Hudson was no expendable day player. He was on the verge of becoming a major investment on the part of Universal-International, and therefore in need of shielding from possible public scorn. For the short term, studio-publicized dates would do. The further insurance of marriage would come later.

Earl Wilson's "and I happen to believe it's true" was a sideways admission of the fact that many others *didn't*. For a columnist like Wilson, the bottom line was Hudson's willingness to be seen "in the columns" with a woman on his arm. Because he played by the rules of compulsory heterosexual display, Wilson felt Hudson was worth the risk. "Like all plain men, we're jealous of pretty boys, and go around sneering at them," the veteran columnist noted. "But Rock's turned out to be the kind who's liked by male reporters half his size and twice his age." For his part, Hudson was surprisingly forthcoming about the role fiction played in the process. "The publicity departments," he told Wilson, "will figure out a story and make the people believe them."[7] Or rather, make the people believe that they *ought* to believe them.

"Why did he wait until he was thirty to find himself a wife when there were so many gals swarming about who aspired for the coveted part of Mrs. Rock Hudson? Why did he rush into matrimony, virtually without warning, after having waited so long?" So screams the subtitle for an article in the December 1957 issue of *TV Scandals*, a short-lived *Confidential* clone.[8] "It was when the gossip columns started calling him 'pretty boy Rock Hudson' that his studio, Universal-International, began to be uneasy," the magazine declares, going on to state that the star's 1955 marriage to Phyllis Gates, secretary to his agent, Henry Willson, was made "on explicit orders from his studio." In short, they *didn't* "believe it was true." But then, neither did anyone else capable of reading between the lines. When all was said and done, the dates and the marriage (which ended in 1958), both bracketed by increasingly inane puff pieces about the ultra-masculine glories of his "bachelor life," made no real impact on Rock Hudson's image, on or off the screen. In fact, in *Pillow Talk,* one of the actor's greatest hits, released one year after the divorce, scriptwriters Stanley Shapiro and Maurice Richlin felt free to incorporate public awareness of the star's sexuality right into the plot. Here was a homosexual actor cast as a heterosexual man *pretending* to be homosexual in order to seduce Doris Day. But in 1959 no one was about to point out the grotesque irony of this situation (as film maker Mark Rappaport would do in his 1992 documentary/essay *Rock Hudson's Home Movies*). All that any member of the fourth estate could manage was to *hint* at the truth—and do so as broadly as possible.

"By the time Hudson got to the third group [of reporters]," wrote *Chicago Today* columnist Johanna Steinmetz of a 1971 press conference, "a question about his 'peculiarities,' which was not intended to be nasty, took on a double edge, bringing strained expressions to the faces of everyone in the room."[9] Hudson held this conference to talk about his new television series, *McMillan and Wife*. But what was on the journalists' minds was his friendship with actor/singer Jim Nabors, which had inspired a widely spread rumor that the two had gotten married in a mock ceremony in Hawaii. The rumor was nothing more than a practical joke making the rounds in show-business circles. Yet many members of the press and public took it seriously—at least up to a point. For whether believed true or not, the Hudson/Nabors marriage allegation provided an opportunity to bring up the star's "peculiarities"—another "polite" way of crying "Fag!"

In the end the imagined marriage to Jim Nabors left *more* of an impression than Hudson's actual betrothal to Phyllis Gates. For as late as 1976, writer Jim Scheetz made oblique reference to it in a *Coronet* magazine piece claiming that long after the joke had run its course, "stories continued to be printed, many of them pure fabrications, some of them stronger than mere implications. Stories that would have led others to quit the business and seek a private life, and even pushed others to suicide."[10] Stories inspiring suicide meant only one thing to someone of Scheetz's generation—homosexuality. Like many other journalists, Scheetz was chomping at the bit to talk about the *real* Hudson. The trouble was, he didn't know how. And neither, had he been so inclined, did Rock Hudson. For while gay liberation may have been been making front-page headlines in 1976, in the entertainment section of the papers "don't ask, don't tell" was the rule. Therefore, it wasn't all that odd to hear so many supposedly seasoned reporters expressing surprise at the "revelation" of "the truth about Rock Hudson" at the time of his death ten years later.

Like Claude Rains in *Casablanca* ("Shocked! Shocked! to hear that gambling has been going on!"), the press, realizing the jig was up, needed a fallback position in order to re-establish its authority. So, rather than admit to concealing the facts, the fourth estate feigned ignorance. As a result Rock Hudson became "The Hunk Who Lived a Lie,"[11] a curious figure winning in death an equal mixture of pity and scorn. In the years that followed, blame for "hiding the truth" was parceled out to his studio; his agent, Henry Willson; and even the moviegoing public, who, it was claimed by one commentator after another, would never "accept" a homosexual movie star. The fact was, they already *had* accepted Rock Hudson—as long as his homosexuality was kept at the discreet distance the press was all too willing to provide. What "the truth about Rock Hudson" really exposed was the fact that in Hollywood "the closet" is less a means of individual self-protection than a press-supported system for keeping the sexual status quo in place.

P eople would always ask what *The Celluloid Closet* was about," activist/historian Vito Russo notes in the introduction to his groundbreaking 1981 book, "and I would always say it was an exploration of gay characters in American film. The response seldom varied. 'Oh, really?' they would ask with a leer. 'Are you using people's real names?' "[12] Naming names wasn't what his book was about, but Russo knew perfectly well that guessing "Who's Gay and Who's Not," as a 1997 headline of the *National Enquirer* so delicately puts it, had long been one of middle-class America's favorite parlor pastimes. In fact, until very recent times, it's been the *only* available avenue for any widespread discussion of the subject.

"People think about Hollywood as being sexually free," says novelist and screenwriter Gavin Lambert. "They half envy it and half think it's wicked. It's part of the attraction, and part of the whole Puritan heritage. Still, I think women are a lot less uptight about this sort of thing than men. That's part of the reason why Rock Hudson was able to go on for as long as he did. Middle-class American men didn't relate to someone like him anyway. They had very strong feelings about the gay next door in the Middle West at that time, however. And the 'heartland' is still a scary place to be gay. That gay man that John Ritter played in *Sling Blade*, living in a small town, was very interesting, and I'm sure it's a true depiction. Whenever you say anything about this country, the opposite is also true, because everything is so polarized. For everybody in that small town who was nice to that gay character, there were just as many who wanted to beat him up."[13]

It has always been easier for middle-class Americans to talk about Hollywood stars rather than Uncle Arthur and his "roommate," Ritchie, or those two women who live down the street who no one has ever seen with a man. It's impolite to stare at the neighbors. But it's virtually *demanded* that we stare at the stars. From morning, afternoon, and late-night talk shows, to worldwide cable news coverage of parties, premieres, and award shows, to "up close and personal" interviews with Barbara Walters or Larry King, the stars always seem to be in our collective faces. Even the tabloids, with their blurry telephoto-lens shots catching the rich and famous in "compromising" positions, only add to the intrigue and the allure.

"When you talk about Hollywood," says novelist James Ellroy, "you're dealing with a bunch of characters whose gifts are erotically derived. They're 'larger than life' 'cause they're forty-foot faces up there on the screen. Their lives are supposed to be our lives. And what's the most interesting thing about people? It's their sexuality. On top of that you've got to remember that these are the people who act out Woody Allen's maxim 'My only regret in life is that I'm not somebody else.' These people spend their whole lives playing somebody else. So you know right away they're schizy. They've got to be out of their minds to one degree or another. That is their gift. That is their *demon*. And generally with actors, the gift is a shallow gift, and the demon is a shallow demon. Ergo, if you're enjoying them—if you're seduced by them for any length of time while they're up there on the screen—you want to deconstruct them."

Ellroy, whose fifties-era Hollywood murder mystery *L.A. Confidential* was turned into a critically lauded 1997 Warner Bros. release, has never disguised his love for tabloid journalism in general, and *Confidential* and its derivatives in particular. In fact, he finds a refreshing honesty to their salaciousness. "I don't give a shit about anything pertaining to the movies," Ellroy says nonchalantly. "All I want to know is who's a homosexual, who's a nymphomaniac, who's a lesbian, who has the biggest dick, and who is the woman who will fuck absolutely anybody—the driver, the car park, the boy who delivers the pizza. That's all!"[14]

In the eyes of the industry, such prurient interest proffers a two-edged sword. On the one hand, sex being a crucial selling point for virtually every picture made or program broadcast, Ellroy's idle musing shouldn't be discouraged. On the other, when you're living in a culture so insistent on the absolute incompatibility of same-sexuality with the heterosexual "majority," Ellroy's words are dangerous. Yet no one would claim his to be a lone voice in the wilderness, for Ellroy echoes countless others who've spoken "off the record" over the years, both within the industry and without.

Homosexuality has always been viewed by the culture that contains it as an *ultimate* piece of knowledge. To know *who's gay* is to "get their number." The trouble is what you've actually got is their area code. Who was Rock Hudson after all? A dreamboat the whole world wanted for a lover; a cornball who adored party games and practical jokes; an alcoholic who courted self-destruction born of deep-seated self-hatred; a manipulative narcissist, bouncing back and forth between older and younger lovers kept waiting at his beck and call; a gracious, if slightly distant, friend to his female co-stars; a true "professional" to the studio's casts and crews; a lonely, terrified AIDS sufferer, whose "soul" Baptist propagandist Shirley Boone claims to have saved at the last moment; or all of the above? And what light does his life shed on Ramon Novarro, or Clifton Webb, or Cesar Romero, or Montgomery Clift, or Anthony Perkins, or any number of others?

Homosexuality doesn't offer the skeleton key to the enigma that is Rock Hudson. Rather, it allows us entry to a room filled to the rafters with *other* keys to *other* rooms. And that's just the "real" Rock

Hudson. There's still the image on the screen to deal with. And that in turn requires facing up to the fact that sexuality is inherently unstable. For while the culture may claim "homo" and "hetero" divisible, the screen finds them occupying the very same space of moviegoing desire. And it is here that the proverbial "Is it a choice?" query resonates the loudest. For Hollywood, however devoted it may be to the "normal," offers us nothing but deviations from that "norm," from one image-consuming moment to the next. This erotic anarchy being too terrifying to contemplate, Hollywood's only recourse has been to pretend that all performers are exclusively heterosexual, and homoerotic imagery is either accidental or inconsequential. That this shallow fiction has stayed in place as long as it has is a tribute to the media's unique ability at catering to the self-delusions of the masses. Whether it has a future, however, is open to question.

"If you're an actor it's very important that you appear to be heterosexual, because that's the majority of this country. That's where the dollars are coming from, and they need to believe in their fantasy world that they can have you. If they think you are totally unobtainable, it won't work." So claims Jill Abrams, a producer for CNN's *Showbiz Today* cable news program.[15] Any number of other industry observers have said much the same thing over the years. The difference is, Abrams counts herself among the ranks of those Hollywood professionals who've declined to treat their sexuality as if it were a state secret. The past two decades have seen a wide variety of producers, directors, writers, agents, executives, and technical personnel join the ranks of the openly gay. Moreover, they've been accompanied by a small but growing number of before-the-camera talents who've sought to challenge the received wisdom on the subject: Tom Hulce, Dan Butler, Amanda Bearse, Scott Thompson, Lea DeLaria, Alexis Arquette, Wilson Cruz, Michael Jeter, Mitchell Anderson, Danny Pintauro, Patrick Bristow, Rupert Everett, and a woman so famous her last name scarcely need be mentioned.

"I am not the first gay person to take a stand, to be basically honest about who I am," Ellen (DeGeneres) told an overflow crowd at the 1997 Human Rights Campaign awards dinner, climaxing a year in which she went from being one in a long line of stand-up-comedians-turned-sitcom-stars to becoming (in her words) "the lesbian formerly known as Ellen."

"I understand there's a greater impact because I'm on television and we place a greater impact on celebrity," she continued. "If I were a gay person who came out at some other job, I might not be standing here—I might have been fired."[16] And that's precisely the point. For in being honest, and coming out as the lesbian all Hollywood (and most of America) knew she was from the start, Ellen was taking a pass on the secrecy privileges extended to others in her profession. Had she chosen silence, the press would have been perfectly willing to look the other way and snicker behind her back, just as it had done with Rock Hudson. Ellen would have had her "privacy," which is to say her managers and publicists would be obliged to scramble to maintain media interest in a performer who couldn't offer heterosexuality as part of her image repertoire. This would have meant her love affair with actress Anne Heche would have had to be hidden from view, a notion the couple had come to find untenable. Moreover, this asexual charade would have flown in the face of the elephant-in-a-bedroom obviousness of her actual sexuality—a fact DeGeneres appears to have felt more keenly than any member of the press or public.

"I just don't understand how people don't *see* it," she told the Human Rights Campaign audience, the logic being that if everyone sees it she doesn't have to say it, as she found herself doing over and over again in the countless articles and interviews about her coming out that flooded the media for over a year and a half. Wasn't she, after all, just the latest in a long line of comediennes like Patsy Kelly, Marjorie Main, Hope Emerson, and Nancy Kulp? Or think of the men: Franklin Pangborn, Clifton Webb, Paul Lynde, or . . . Nathan Lane.

"Look," the *Bird Cage* star finally broke down to *US* magazine after some three years of equivocating about his sexuality in one interview after another. "I'm 40, I'm single and I work in musical theater—You do the math. What do you need, flashcards?"[17] But it's not flashcards that the press requires; it's the *express permission* of the subject it's writing about. For unlike race or gender, religious belief or political persuasion, sexual orientation isn't viewed by the fourth estate as a neutral characteristic. And because of that, Kelly, Main, Emerson, Kulp, Pangborn, Webb, and Lynde never faced the inquiries that are now just beginning to be made about performers' "private lives."

Attributing homosexuality to anyone in print can still, on its face, constitute grounds for a defamation-of-character lawsuit. Few mainstream publications are willing to risk this prospect. But more often than not, such a scenario is foreclosed in advance, by managers and press agents barring the way of journalists likely to ask probing questions of stars whose off-screen activities might be viewed as problematic. As a result, overt recognition of sexual orientation is viewed as permissible in the "legitimate" press only when the party in question insists on stating it formally, publicly, and without equivocation. Once the yep-I'm-gay go-ahead is given, a formal confession of sorts is produced via an interview. This (usually brief) Q&A session is invariably accompanied by the personal testimony of friends, family members, and co-workers, designed to demonstrate that their delicate heterosexual sensibilities haven't been damaged by the presence of those otherwise-oriented in their midst. Following that, the verdict of a hastily assembled kangaroo court of medical, psychoanalytic, and scientific authorities is handed down, assessing the subject's skill in dealing with the personal rejection he or she is sure to face from all and sundry in response to the announcement. Then, as if that weren't enough, polls testifying to the levels of "acceptance" the same-sex-oriented in other walks of life have achieved with the "general public" are brandished in sidebar columns.

For the past decade this elaborate menu of journalistic rituals has been *de rigueur* for even the most casual discussion of celebrity same-sexuality. It is as if the reinvention of the wheel were required for every trip to the store for a quart of milk. No wonder, then, that DeGeneres—after enduring months of such treatment—wondered why it all couldn't have been avoided in advance though the simple recognition of her sexuality at face value. The problem is, the "value" attributed to such a "face" is still a bone of contention in a world that at best regards same-sex affection as a character flaw somewhere between excessive bedwetting and compulsive shoplifting.

"The second issue that drew me to a study of [Dorothy] Arzner," film scholar Judith Mayne notes in her book on the woman who enjoyed a brief directorial career in Hollywood in the 1930s, "came less from her films than the photo graphics I had seen of her. Arzner adopted a persona that can be best described as Butch: She wore tailored, 'masculine' clothing; her short hair was slicked back; she wore no make-up; and she struck poses of confidence and authority. If Arzner was a lesbian I wanted to know how? That is, what it meant to be lesbian or gay in Hollywood during Arzner's time."[18]

If Arzner was a lesbian? No, it's not that academics need flashcards; what haunts Mayne is the negative connotations evoked by drawing attention to "stereotypical" appearance. To say that Dorothy Arzner—or Ellen DeGeneres—"looks like a lesbian" is to tie sexual identity to presentational elements alone. Like "effeminacy" in men, "masculinity" in women can only account for the homosexual status of a limited number of parties, both stopping short in the face of a Raymond Burr or a Spring Byington. Moreover, to want to know "what it meant to be lesbian or gay in Hollywood during Arzner's time" is to enter an arena Mayne herself admits her subject was loath to explore. For honest and open discussion of same-sexuality has only been under way in any widespread way in America within the past ten years. And resistance to the furtherance of this discussion—both organized and ad hoc—has been enormous.

I couldn't care less what people do—as long as they don't do it in public—or—or try to force their ways on the whole damned world." So says Alan, a character in *The Boys in the Band*, a play by Mart Crowley about a group of homosexual New Yorkers first produced in 1968.[19]

"I really don't care if people are born homosexual or not, or whether it is an acquired lifestyle. I do object to having anyone else's lifestyle forced down my throat as an 'accepted lifestyle' by the TV and movie industry on a daily basis." So says Jo Anne Stayton, an actual person, in a letter to *TV Guide* magazine, postmarked Homestead, Florida, in 1997.[20] A lot of things have changed in the twenty-nine years separating Crowley's play from Stayton's letter. But ostentatious feints of indifference to sexual orientation aren't among them.

"I can't tell you how sick I am of this Ellen business," writes another *TV Guide* reader, Marjorie Herder of West Hills, California, of the double-barreled coming out of DeGeneres and Ellen Morgan, the character she played on her ABC television show. "What she is and what she does is her own business. Please stop constantly throwing it in the face of the public."[21]

"A whopping 63 percent of those familiar with the show say they have little or no interest in watching the episode in which Ellen Morgan announces she is gay," claims a *TV Guide* article that ran in advance of the Ellen/*Ellen* event.[22] Yet it would appear these allegedly indifferent televiewers were lying, for over 47 million tuned in on April 25, 1997, to watch "The Episode." And healthy Nielsen numbers were also registered for DeGeneres's appearances on *The Oprah Winfrey Show* and *Primetime Live* around the same time. Still, the size of the ratings hasn't lessened the vehemence of the complainers. Where *Ellen* (and Ellen) hit the wall was in the weeks after the "special episode." For *Ellen* had become a sitcom about a lesbian. And in a culture trained to see coming out as a one-time-only special event, it was well-nigh inconceivable that there be any narrative follow-up. Add to this the overwhelming difficulties involved in maintaining audience interest in a highly competitive audiovisual marketplace and increasingly fragmented culture. Still, despite the eventual loss of her show (partially due to falling ratings, partially as a consequence of network timidity), reverberations from this coming out are still being felt—and will continue to be for a long time to come. For that's where Ellen—the person, not the sitcom—comes in.

"Do I go around saying that I'm straight? Nobody wants to know! Nobody cares!" Carmen Pate of "Concerned Women of America" screamed at DeGeneres on her *Oprah* television appearance, beside herself with horror over the fact that her ten-year-old son saw Ellen's picture on the cover of *Time* and she was forced to "explain" what it meant to him.[23] But her desire for DeGeneres and others like her to stifle themselves has fallen on deaf ears. For well in advance of Ellen's exit from the closet, the media had borne witness to the coming out of pop singers Elton John, Dusty Springfield, Melissa Etheridge, and k. d. lang; tennis pro Martina Navratilova; stage actress Cherry Jones; Olympic diving champion Greg Louganis; ice skater Rudy Galindo; media mogul David Geffen; self-described "right-wing hitman" journalist David Brock; fashion designers Isaac Mizrahi, Todd Oldham, Thierry Mugler, and Jean-Paul Gaultier; celebrity offspring Jason Gould (son of Streisand) and Chastity Bono (daughter of Sonny and Cher); and a host of others in virtually every region, race, religion, class, and walk of life. Moreover, as controversies over gays in the military and "gay marriage" (real, rather than hallucinated à la Hudson/Nabors) give way to page-one coverage of heterosexual military scandals, the rising divorce rate, and marital infidelity, gay and straight seem more culturally intertwined than ever. All the more reason, then, to reconsider the sexual and romantic fantasies Hollywood has constructed over the years, and the people who were part of them. But that requires a willingness to face sexual realities few members of either the press or public have been willing to offer.

W ith *East of Eden*," observed critic Pauline Kael, "film catches up with the cult realities of city parks and Turkish baths; clear meanings or definite values would be too grossly explicit—a vulgar intrusion on the Technicolor night of the soul."[24] She was only stating the obvious. Yet James Dean's homoerotic appeal, not to mention his actual sexual life, has been the most contentious aspect of his posthumous fame, figuring uneasily in every one of the fifty-odd (and still counting) books that have been written about him.

"Whatever sexual aspects Jimmy contained within himself, they were unfissionable parts of his personality, an innate ambiguity which shaded everything he did, revealing and reveiling his intense inner self," writes David Dalton in *James Dean: The Mutant King*,[25] assuming the *noli me tangere* posture taken by most Dean scholars when faced with any other-than-heterosexual information about their beloved.

"Ask almost any James Dean fan what the biggest misconception about him is, and the fan will mention without hesitation 'that he was homosexual,' which they insist he wasn't. And they're right. He was unequivocally bisexual," claims Randal Riese in his encyclopedia of "factoids," *James Dean from A–Z*.[26] One can only wonder which fans Riese was speaking to. For the hectoring insistence of his words only serves to underscore that in press accounts of such celebrities as Elton John, David Geffen, David Bowie, Madonna, Sandra Bernhard, and Andy Dick, bisexuality—presumably constituting a smaller degree of "sin"—has been viewed less as an actual sexual identity than as a public-relations tool for negotiating degrees of homosexual disclosure. But in James Dean's time this wasn't possible, as writer Venable Herndon notes in his *James Dean: A Short Life*, recounting a party the actor once attended with a group of friends. "Toward dawn, one of Jimmy's lovers put him 'up against the wall' about his sexual identity and demanded he 'come out' once and for all, and stop pretending to be sexually interested in women, except, as his accuser put it scornfully, 'for publicity purposes.' "[27] Few Dean scholars have had trouble with such publicity, rhapsodizing about the actor's alleged affairs with Pier Angeli and Ursula Andress. But when it comes to someone like Jack Simmons, who Riese's encyclopedia calls "certainly one of the most mysterious, and therefore interesting, characters involved in the James Dean story," a journalistic brick wall suddenly appears.

"Unfortunately little is known about Jack Simmons or his relationship with Dean," claims Riese of the would-be actor who Dean wanted to play opposite him in *Rebel Without a Cause* instead of Sal Mineo. Simmons, who, Riese notes, "arrived and departed with James Dean" every day of the shoot, was instead given the role of Moose— the gang member who hands Dean the knife in the Griffith Park Observatory fight scene. The picture Riese paints of Simmons silently waiting on Dean hand and foot is scarcely mysterious to those familiar with the master/slave dynamic of the gay leather scene.[28] Likewise, there's nothing obscure about writer Paul Alexander's account in his *Boulevard of Broken Dreams* of Dean's days as the "kept man" of producer Rogers Brackett, who got the actor cast in early bit roles in

Fixed Bayonets and *Has Anybody Seen My Gal?* Yet four decades after his death, the insistence on a heterosexual James Dean is as strong as ever.

"Alexander's inferences about Dean's private life may make for cocktail party chatter, but finally they are irrelevant," writes *Time*'s Richard Corliss,[29] knowing perfectly well it couldn't be more relevant to making sense of both Hollywood's past and its current state as America's moviegoers begin to hover in tremulous anticipation of the prospect of a (gasp!) "openly gay" movie star.

"Thanks to *My Best Friend's Wedding*, people are calling Rupert Everett the gay Cary Grant (if that's not redundant)," says *Newsweek*'s Marc Peyser of the suave British actor, who critics and audiences agree stole the hit 1997 romantic comedy from its star, Julia Roberts.[30] But the real kicker in Peyser's comment is his mention of Cary Grant. For even while those who should know better continue to cling to the fantasy of a straight James Dean, Cary Grant has been casually tossed into homoerotic waters his public image never swam in while he was alive.

"When Katharine Hepburn's Aunt Elizabeth (May Robson) discovers Cary Grant in a lace nightgown," Vito Russo notes of a scene from the screwball classic *Bringing Up Baby*, "she asks him if he dresses like that all the time. Grant leaps into the air and shouts hysterically, 'No! I've just gone gay . . . all of a sudden!' This exchange appears in no version of the published script."[31] It was an extremely rare reference that was also self-referential. For while Grant was married four times, and fathered a daughter late in life, the better part of his youth was spent in the company of other men, the most noteworthy being actor Randolph Scott.

"On and off for a decade, from 1932 to 1942, the two actors shared apartments and houses, a convenient arrangement that was interrupted when one or the other got married, then resumed when both were free, as they most often were, because of separation or divorce," notes writer Gerald Clarke in an article in the April 1996 *Architectural Digest*, [32] illustrated with an extraordinary series of photos of the couple at home.

"Paramount didn't seem to care that the relationship could be interpreted as homosexual," claims biographer Warren G. Harris in his *Cary Grant: A Touch of Elegance*. "In 1933, the average person didn't know what the word meant."[33] But as Kinsey demonstrated, mere word recognition doesn't forgo understanding—save for those who simply *don't wish to understand,* like biographer Graham McCann in his *Cary Grant: A Class Apart*. "In a prim, old-maidish fashion," critic Brendan Gill complains angrily of the book, "McCann cannot bear Grant to be anything but ruggedly heterosexual, and he goes to great lengths to derogate anyone who dares to suggest otherwise."

Gill, for his part, was willing to do a lot more than suggest, for in his review he speaks of Jerome Zerbe, the "strikingly handsome and flirtatious" photographer and socialite who was a lover of both Grant and Scott. "Zerbe," Gill states, "used to tell me of how Grant and he in the nineteen-thirties were obliged to honor the prevailing Hollywood taboos and at the same time generate favorable publicity in movie magazines and among Grant's doting fan clubs. To that end, Grant was reported in the press to be enjoying an impassioned affair with the starlet Betty Furness. Night after night, he took the good-natured Furness out to dinner and returned to her apartment promptly at ten o'clock, after which Zerbe and he and assorted companions went out on the town."

Gill goes on to note that Grant's screen persona finds him "carrying out a bisexual parody that is comical precisely because it is a parody—a genial mocking of the conventional heterosexual relationship. . . . He is nearly always in amused retreat from a woman who, whether consciously or unconsciously, is aggressively pursuing him and is right in supposing that in the end he will prove worthy of her pursuit."

"Poor Cary Grant!" Gill concludes, decrying McCann's heterosexualization. "What about all the men he was attracted to in his youth and with whom he sought to form permanent relationships, always in vain?"[34] Still, the Cary Grant story—which includes a pre–Randolph Scott alliance with designer Orry-Kelly—can't be retro-fitted to James Dean dimensions. For while his marriages to Virginia Cherill, Barbara Hutton, and Betsy Drake might fall along the lines suggested by gay activist Harry Hay, who calls the institution "the casting couch for society,"[35] the same can't necessarily be said of his alliances with Dyan Cannon and Barbara Harris. And that's not to mention the role his experiments with LSD may have played in all this. The important thing to keep in mind—before the inevitable "bisexual" label is whipped out to whisk him away from the scene of the homosexual "crime"—is that the charm, the grace, the sophistication, the *je-ne-sais-quoi*-ness of Cary Grant is plainly and simply *his gayness,* whether Graham McCann likes it or not.

From 1937 to 1938, Jerome Zerbe was the art director for *Bachelor* magazine, a curious, lavishly produced publication that managed to eke out thirteen issues in its brief but vivid life. Society columnist Lucius Beebe was *Bachelor*'s editor. Its director of photography was George Platt Lynes, a portrait specialist who, with Kinsey's encouragement, produced over the next two decades some of the most startlingly explicit homoerotic images ever confected for the private enjoyment of friends and collectors. (They have come to public light only within the last decade, challenging the alleged audaciousness of Robert Mapplethorpe in the process.)

As might be expected, the "bachelors" this trio of gay men were interested in highlighting weren't the sort likely to purchase *Esquire* or *Playboy*. Noël Coward and Cecil Beaton were profiled. "Beefcake" snaps of Errol Flynn and Gary Cooper were featured. This isn't to say that the "fair sex" was banished from *Bachelor*'s pages. "Camp" queens Marlene Dietrich, Garbo Garbo, and Mae West garnered the glamour treatment from the ever-skillful Platt Lynes. In other words, *Bachelor* was the *After Dark* of its day—an implicitly gay magazine tiptoeing toward the edge of the explicit. But there's a major difference between this thirties experiment and its seventies successor. *Bachelor* was a magazine for "walkers"—those gay "extra men" much prized in urban social circles for their ability to squire and entertain wealthy upper-class wives. *After Dark,* hovering on the edge of the gay liberation movement, signaled the end of the "walker" era, whose final curtain came when the AIDS epidemic decimated their ranks.[36] What "walkers" represent historically is the ease with which homosexuality was ensconced in the social life of the moneyed classes. Likewise the Cary Grant–Randolph Scott alliance, hidden in plain sight, speaks of the sort of cultural accommodation Hollywood finessed long before the fateful night of Stonewall supposedly changed the world.

But understanding how this operated, in the midst of a culture that insists on viewing "morality" as a sexual issue alone, is no simple matter. For homosexuality in Hollywood isn't a cultural phenomenon whose history moves in a straight line. It zigs and zags, moving back and forth through times, places, and people—and back and forth again. From the pied-à-terre on North Sweetzer Avenue just off of Santa Monica Boulevard that Grant and Scott once shared, to the leather and motorcycle haunts of Dean, to the offices at the Disney studios today, to the hills above Sunset, the beaches of Malibu, and the deserts of the Coccella Valley, Hollywood (the place, the industry, the fantasy) and homosexuality (the orientation, the "lifestyle," the political "wedge" issue) commingle and collide.

And that's not to mention the rest of America: its "heartland," its urban bulwarks, and its suburbs, where once upon a time in a basement in Queens, Long Island, a pair of elementary-school children played a game of Monopoly so many, many years ago.

TWO

INVISIBLE CITY

———

...a private "club" in the hills up a twisting dirt

road, where men dance with men,

women with women...[1]

I DON'T KNOW WHAT THE NAME OF IT WAS,
or whether it had a name or not," John Rechy recalls, three

decades after mentioning it in passing in his novel *City of Night*. "I

don't know where it *was* exactly, because I didn't have a car when I first lived here, and I would have to"— he pauses, smiles broadly, and chuckles—"surrender to the kindness of strangers."[2]

Rechy has written eight other novels, three plays, and a literary "documentary," *The Sexual Outlaw,* in the years since *City of Night* was first published. But this semiautobiographical novel about the demimonde of male prostitutes plying their trade in New York, New Orleans, and Los Angeles remains a touchstone in American literary, and sexual, history. For the "worm's eye view" of erotic commerce Rechy provides is wide enough to encompass many telling details of life within the same-sex subculture in the years just prior to its uneasy entry to the American "mainstream." The phantom "club," which flourished off and on in the late 1950s and early 1960s, testifies to Rechy's powers of observation.

"I was taken up there by some people I'd met," he recalls nostalgically, sitting in his Los Feliz–area apartment, a stone's throw from the Griffith Park cruising grounds that figure in many of his books. "It was an extraordinary place, that club. And the most extraordinary thing about it was that one didn't consider it extraordinary. We just accepted it. It was almost like going to a foreign country, because you 'passed through customs' to get to the place. There were two people on the road, kind of 'spotting' things, who would check you out. Then you went up and there was this house that had been converted into a dance hall. I remember that they served soft drinks. No liquor. Men danced with men, and women with women. They had a system of flashing lights that warned when the police were on their way. And that was the signal for lesbians to team up with gay men on the dance floor. Everybody of the opposite gender coupled up.

"You must understand, this wasn't an orgy scene or some sort of sex club," Rechy insists. "It was much more *dangerous* than that. A man dancing with another man or a woman dancing with another woman could get arrested back then—just for doing that!"

Rechy is well aware of the fact that the point he's making has to do less with specific laws than the way they're—very selectively— applied. An instructor at an Arthur Murray Dance Studio, obliged to teach a new routine to a member of his or her own sex, would be free to do so without fear of the authorities. Likewise, attendants at a socially approved event, such as a wedding or anniversary celebration, where elderly women often partner one another, could couple up as much as they wished. But unlike such occasions, the dance at the house in the hills was viewed by the police as a prelude to illegal same-sex activity. And the prospect of sex, rather than the presence of dancing, was what brought on a raid.

"I always said no when I was asked to dance," says Rechy, "because at the time I was into masculine role playing. But it was quite a spectacle. The people who went there were largely middle-class, professional types. By that I don't mean presidents of banks—though there might have been. But you did have to have a car to get there. They were educated people. Solid people. I guess a lot from the movies too. Not stars, though. Chorus boys, probably. But it was not *at all* like the bars downtown like the 326.

"We lived on the periphery of arrest. Always. All of us," Rechy says with wry amusement. "A queen walking toward the 326 might enter the way Hedy Lamarr made her entrance in *Ziegfeld Girl*. First the collar would come up. The shirt would turn into a blouse, with a knot here. The pants would become toreador pants. The hair would get fluffed out. Out would come some lipstick, some mascara. It was an extraordinary thing to watch. And then here she comes: John Jones transformed into the lovely Mara. And there would be applause! It was illegal to cross-dress. The police would come and raid it. And talk about the resistance at Stonewall—Jesus Christ, there were *hundreds* of Stonewalls! The squad cars would come. The loudspeaker would say 'Everybody out!' and you filed out while they shoved a light on you. The queens would come out, and believe me they would not go gently into that good wagon. It wasn't like New York, with the Mafia running everything, but there were bars where there were payoffs made. And there were heterosexual bars that were moribund that became gay bars and would thrive."

Rechy knows, of course, that downtown bars and their "outlaw" clientele were worlds away from the "club" in the hills and its well-heeled patrons. But he also knows that the buttoned-down banker and

the flamboyant street queen were as one in the eyes of the law. Moreover, as sexual desire itself levels the playing field, the banker and
the queen may have more in common erotically than they would in
any other social circumstance. And that's not to mention the countless
others whose presentational style and personal tastes ranged from the
obvious to the anonymous. Working as a hustler, as he did in his
youth, gave Rechy the opportunity to witness firsthand the curious
social mobility same-sex orientation provides, with its constant inter-
mingling of "high" and "low" life. Moreover, he's not at all sure that
the strides gays and lesbians have made over the last thirty years have
impacted on their self-image as much as some activists would like to
claim.

　　"This matter of 'Oh, it was all shrouded in guilt' that people
always seem to mention when they talk about the past—that's nonsense," says Rechy. "Yes, you did have all the psychiatrists wanting
to turn people heterosexual back then, but I must say that the vast
majority of the people who did go to the bars, did go to the dance
place in the hills, did cruise the theater balconies and the parks—I
would say that they were guilt-free. I have never felt guilt about my
sexuality. All along I've felt that people who want us to feel guilt are
really stupid. And if you looked at downtown bars like the Waldorf,
the Cellar, the 326—it was so goddamned *open*. It was open even to
the police who would come in, who *knew* some of the queens. This is
one of the things that does not happen now, and I think it's a sign of
repression, not liberation. Those bars were a mixture of extravagant
queens—mean fuckers—very masculine hustlers, and the people
who came for one or the other. So they were mainly hustling bars. But
the sense of exhilaration that was there, I don't find in any of our
somber bars today."

　　The wide open, well-lit, easily accessed night spots of West
Hollywood, Silverlake, and the San Fernando Valley of the 1990s
stand in marked contrast to the world Rechy knew. Though occasionally subject to police harassment (as, for example, in the spate of
disruptions at several Silverlake bars during the summer of 1997,
where owners and patrons were threatened with "lewd conduct" ci-
tations), Los Angeles gay and lesbian nightlife today no longer faces

the constant pressure of LAPD intrusion that typified the past. Undercover entrapment "stings" were common right up through the 1960s, when the bar scene resembled something on the order of a floating crap game as venues opened and closed with dismal regularity.

"The House of Ivy on Cahuenga was very popular in the fifties and sixties," Rechy recalls of one of the more sedate watering holes. "There was also the Lafayette, which was just across the way from it. And then there was the Open Door, which was on the corner of Selma and Ivar where that theater that used to be a strip place is now. I also remember the Cherokee House in Hollywood. Oh, and there was Chee Chee's on Figueroa. Now *that* was a bar! When my editor for *City of Night* said, 'Well, I'd like to see some of the spots,' I didn't quite know what he was looking for—what this impeccable editor might mean by 'spots.' So I took him to Chee Chee's. He peeked in, took one look around, and said, 'Oh, I think I've seen enough!' Just then the police drove up!"

Rechy laughs loudly. "That was one *rough* place. There were some others too, like the Carousel. That was in Venice. It was one of the toughest. A whole scene in *City of Night* is set there."

In his diaries, Christopher Isherwood recalls a decidedly pleasant evening in 1960 he spent at the Carousel with actress Vivien Leigh, "where she was recognized; and it was a pity we got there so late that they were on the point of closing. It was packed. At closing time, the boys were all shouting 'Where's a party?' and then a couple were announced and the addresses given."[3]

At that time "slumming" by a star of Leigh's caliber was relatively rare. But in the 1930s and 1940s it was considered quite chic to drop in at an after-hours "speakeasy" known as Brothers, in the Central Avenue area, near the Hotel Dunbar, where the city's African-American nightlife flourished.

"I used to go there," gay activist Harry Hay recalls. "I used to *dance* there. White boys danced together, and that was okay as far as the management was concerned. But no black man ever danced with a white man—they wouldn't dare. No black man danced with a black man, either. The ones who danced were white boys dancing with white boys. And white girls dancing with white girls—that happened too. But the races didn't mix yet. There was another place too, at East Twenty-seventh Street and Central. It probably had been somebody's apartment. It was sort of a perpetual rent party. I was taken there by somebody I met in Hollywood in '34 or '35. It was the same kind of place."[4]

Brothers was a thoroughly "mixed" affair. Jazz musicians and cabaret performers of every sexual stripe would mingle with the likes of Howard Hughes, George Raft, Humphrey Bogart, and Alan Ladd. This was common in a period that saw any number of gay-and-lesbian-friendly clubs (those that weren't exclusively same-sex-oriented) come and go. Some of them could even boast connections of a sort to the industry. Jane Jones was a Sunset Strip–area club, named after its owner, a singer who can be seen briefly in the 1938 Tyrone Power/Alice Faye vehicle *Alexander's Ragtime Band*. Bruz Fletcher's was another owner-monikered spot, which centered on a singer of "sophisticated" (i.e., slightly risqué) songs. But police crackdowns on his club, coupled with a lack of work opportunities elsewhere, led to Fletcher's suicide in 1941 at the age of thirty-five.[5]

Fletcher tunes like "Nympho-Dipso-Ego Maniac" and "She's My Most Intimate Friend" pushed the edge of the envelope. Ripping it wide open was Rae Bourbon, a legendarily ribald drag *artiste* whose performance at a nameless Cahuenga Avenue club in the 1940s caused the police to close it down. Songs like "I'm a Link in a Daisy Chain" may have provided the incitement for Bourbon's being charged with a "lewd and indecent performance," but the legal glue that made it stick was his cross-dressing, seen as an open-and-shut violation of the law even though he was giving a stage of performance.

Even the *un*raunchy had to mind their p's and q's. The veteran drag performer Julian Eltinge, for example, had to completely rework his act for Los Angeles. Instead of getting into gowns, he had them wheeled out on a rack and then proceeded to *talk* about each of them. The police didn't seem to mind. But then, neither did the public, which stayed away in droves.

The one nightspot that managed for a time to avoid the perils of police pressure and the fickle tastes of Los Angeles's trendier pub crawlers was the Café Gala. Owned by Baroness Catherine Derlanger, a titled Englishwoman with bohemian tastes and the cash to exercise them, the Gala—which sat on the Sunset Strip on the exact spot where Spago stands today—was run by her "constant companion," a gay man named John Walsh. Compact but lavishly decorated, the club featured cabaret acts of all sorts (both Bobby Short and Dorothy Dandridge appeared there), though "male impersonators" were particularly favored. Socially well-connected, Derlanger and Walsh were able to attract the attention of Hollywood stars, and as a result during its ten-year run the Gala managed to acquire a thin veneer of chic. Former MGM publicist Kim Garfield cites it as finding favor with lifelong friends Lana Turner and Judy Garland, who "used to go there just to have a drink and enjoy themselves. The headliner was this lesbian who used to come out in a tuxedo à la Dietrich, and many of the stars would go up to see her perform."[6]

While the Gala's bar area catered to gay men, a well-enforced dress code and other general rules of decorum engineered by Walsh (everyone had to face front, and physical contact beyond a handshake was verboten) kept it from becoming as sexually rowdy as clubs like the Carousel. This low-down-yet-buttoned-up mixture led to an ambience that Christopher Isherwood (who spent the better part of his youth in far wilder circumstances in Berlin) found "camp" in a way most of the Gala's clientele would never have imagined. "I haven't been to a place of this sort in ages," he reports in his *Diaries*, ticking off "the baroque decorations and the cosy red velvet corners, the sharp-faced peroxide pianist with tender memories and a tongue like an adder, the grizzled tomcat tenor, the bitch with a heart of gold, the lame celebrity, the bar mimosa, the public lovers, the amazed millionaire tourist, the garlanded cow, the plumed serpent and the daydream sailor . . . I have loved them all very much and learnt something from each of them. I owe them many of my vividest moments of awareness. But enough is enough. And here we say goodbye."[7]

But before the Gala bid its own adieu, as gay and lesbian nightspots turned increasingly toward the "rough" route Rechy preferred, its lengthy run underscored the fact that bars, nightclubs, and anything else related to the lives of gay Los Angelenos stood a better chance of survival outside the aegis of the LAPD. For the Gala was in West Hollywood, which was patrolled by the far more liberal Sheriff's Department. As the 1950s progressed, it became increasingly clear to all sexual minorities that an untrammeled existence was far more feasible in that part of town.

"You had two guys that were in power then," novelist James Ellroy notes. "Eugene Biscailuz was the chief sheriff of L.A. County. He was this half Anglo, half Spanish Basque. I think he had a little Mexican blood too. He spoke fluent Spanish. He was a sweetheart of a guy, very public relations-minded. His whole thing was the myth of the Wild West; ergo, he had the sheriff's mounted posse, rodeo, annual barbecue. His sheriffs were out there hawking tickets and he would ride there on his palomino stallion, Pal-of-Mine. He came in in 1932 as sheriff, and he was already probably fifty years old. He stayed till about 1958. He was an elected official. Biscailuz was a progressive. The sheriffs were always expanding to various parts of the county and he had to supply to various contract cities.

"For the sheriffs," Ellroy explains, "laws against homosexuality were always too a big a thing to enforce. Besides, it's a preposterous notion that when most of your citizens are of this persuasion you would want to try and do anything about it. The sheriffs have gotten more paramilitary over the years. But there wasn't that hardcore us-versus-them mentality in that department. That came in with William Parker, who became chief of the LAPD in 1950. Parker came out of a tremendous tradition of monetary corruption and incompetence, and he hated it. He was an alcoholic martinet who was given permission to reinstate pre-twentieth-century America.

"It's interesting because it all ties back to Hollywood through the *Dragnet* television show," Ellroy declares. "The dark, dark moment for L.A. law enforcement, and L.A. gays, and L.A. people of color, occurred in the 1950s when Jack Webb met William Parker. They started to market the LAPD's myth nationally. Parker completely dominated Jack Webb and fed off Jack Webb's innate militarism and fixation—and there's a homoerotic aspect to this—with masculine imagery."[8]

Such erotic undertones go some way toward explaining the antipathy the LAPD has always held toward the city's gay and lesbian citizens. The atmosphere it produced is best recalled by an anecdote publicist Harry Clein loves to tell, which was related to him by an older gentleman at a gay "consciousness raising" meeting he attended in New York in the mid-seventies.

"There was a man from Los Angeles there, and he told a story about a bar that was at the corner of La Brea and Wilshire—or maybe it was one block south. I even remember it, because it had become a cabaret at one point, and they used to do shows there. Not gay shows—straight ones. Anyway, he said that in the 1940s everybody wore ties and jackets and hats, even if you went on a picnic. You look at old movies, and you can see that's true—ties and jackets and hats all the time. He said that at this bar nobody *ever* checked their hat, because if it were raided, you had to be able to make a fast exit. So you kept your hat on!"[9]

Things changed by the 1970s, for not only had hats gone out of fashion, but the rise of the activist movement brought a militant mood to the bar scene. With the election of gay officials on the city council from the 1980s on, the LAPD's confrontational stance has become largely moot. Moreover, the police in Los Angeles have never held the sort of sway over the lives of sexual minorities common to the authorities in other major American cities. In fact, the town's disorderly sprawl makes widespread, well-organized police control of any sort nearly inconceivable—a fact made all too clear by the riots of 1992.

In many ways Los Angeles is less a city than an enormous suburb broken into a series of tiny hamlets (Hollywood, West Hollywood, South Central, Watts, Beverly Hills, Brentwood, Silverlake, et al.) with mini-centers of their own. This bizarre, pretzel-like structure took shape partially as a consequence of specific planning (making de facto racial segregation systemic in a way atypical of other U.S. cities). But the town's al fresco social organization also came about in response to the vagaries of where its wealthier citizens chose to settle at any given moment (Hancock Park, Beverly Hills, Bel Air, Brentwood, Malibu).

Still, the most important factor in Los Angeles's curious socio-geographic distribution was born of the rise of the motion-picture industry. The founding moguls, being Jewish, would have had no end of trouble getting in the *back* door of New York or Chicago society. In Los Angeles they could rule a social landscape of their own devising, aping European nobility, as Louis B. Mayer did in his lavish mansion, with no one to object. Likewise, William Randolph Hearst would have found it next to impossible to carry on his affair with actress Marion Davies in any context other than the one provided by Hollywood. For while San Simeon was well outside Los Angeles, its doors were open to any number of the town's stars, few of whom were likely to take exception to the Hearst-Davies alliance. In much the same manner, the xenophobia that gripped so much of American culture had little chance of taking root in Hollywood, which from earliest days welcomed any number of European writers, directors, and performers to its ranks, including the widely imitated (and discreetly same-sex-oriented) F. W. Murnau. It was no surprise, then, that Los Angeles became a refuge for the rarefied likes of novelist Thomas Mann, composer Arnold Schoenberg, and playwright Bertolt Brecht in the wake of Hitler's rise.

Yet for all of this, the upper hand the industry's "enlightened" elements have always held has been a tenuous one in terms of the rest of the town. "Los Angeles," writes architecture critic Reyner Banham, "is the Middle West raised to flash-point, the authoritarian dogmas of the Bible Belt and the perennial revolt against them colliding at critical mass under the palm trees. Out of it comes a cultural situation where only the extreme is normal, and the Middle Way is just the unused reservation down the centre of the Freeway."[10] The seismic social upheavals of the 1990s certainly bear this out in full, with racial animosity toward Asians and Latinos, as well as African-Americans, running unchecked. Yet within this chaos, calm has always been possible—even for the whose live their lives on the sociosexual edge.

"California in my mind was a sunny land of movie studios and beautifully naked people," notes painter David Hockney in his autobiography.[11] Living in darkest—wettest—England, the future visual poet laureate of Los Angeles was first lured to the city by the films of Laurel and Hardy. Noticing the shadows the classic clowns cast on the ground, Hockney realized they were shot in a place where the sun shone all the time. He found himself spurred to go there even more by *Physique Pictorial,* the Los Angeles–based periodical that offered soft-core homoerotica in the guise of a "physical culture" monthly promoting "bodybuilding." On his arrival in the early 1960s, Hockney made a beeline to the magazine's headquarters "in a very seedy area of downtown Los Angeles," meeting its manager, photographer Bob Mizer, "a wonderful complete madman." There the painter discovered, to his delight, an unconscious parody of a movie studio, featuring "a tacky swimming pool surrounded by Hollywood Greek plaster statues. It was marvelous!" What Hockney had in fact found was a world linked directly to John Rechy, whose *City of Night* he greatly admired. "I love downtown Los Angeles—marvelous gay bars full of mad Mexican queens, all tacky and everything," he enthuses, noting that most of Mizer's "models" were youths just off the bus from Anytown U.S.A. and available for rent.

"I'd begun to be interested in America from a sexual point of view," he declares. "The art I didn't care about." But the work he produced proved otherwise. For in his canvases of the late 1960s, Hockney rendered Los Angeles a paradise of palm trees and swimming pools, usually inhabited by beautiful young men. It was a vision of homoerotic splendor underscoring that Los Angeles, unlike most major American cities, offered the prospect of sexual pleasure to be enjoyed in full, at leisure, and—most important of all—in private. For these sixties-era canvases speak of a longstanding gay L.A. tradition of gracious living and boy-filled pools going back to the silent era. And the linchpin of that era, the very thing that made such sybaritic pleasures possible, was the *demand* for exoticism Hollywood engendered in the mass audience it served, partially through the films themselves, but far more pervasively by means of the carefully engineered spectacle of public relations. For whatever the stars' "real lives" may have been like, it was always fantasy that was put on public display.

"Sublime, eccentric, they build themselves pseudo-feudal cha-

teaus, houses copied from Roman antique temples, with marble swimming pools, menageries, private railroads," notes sociologist Edgar
Morin of the stars of the silent era. "They live at a distance, far beyond
all mortals. They consume their lives in caprice. They love each other,
destroy each other, and their confused passions are as fatal in life as
in the movies. They are unaware of marriage except to princes and
aristocrats. Pola Negri gives her hand to Count Eugene Domski, then
to Prince Serge Mdivani."[12]

   And so Theodosia Goodman of Cincinnati, Ohio, became Theda
Bara of Goodness-knows-where, Arabia. Likewise, a standard-issue
cosmetics heiress named Winifred Hudnut transformed herself into
Natacha Rambova, who—despite a fondness for members of her own
sex—married Rudolph Valentino, an Italian ballroom-dancing gigolo,
and turned him into a leading man, famous the world over for playing
(you guessed it) Arabians.

   "I think Nazimova really started the exotic thing," says Gavin
Lambert, biographer of one of Hudnut/Rambova's most famous lovers,
whose 1923 film of Oscar Wilde's *Salome* is one of the great curios-
ities of the silent era. "She was the prototype of them all. Garbo and
Dietrich came later. Part of the change came with the talkies, because
most of the exotic silent stars couldn't speak English very well. Anna
Sten, Vilma Banky, Olga Baclanova—there was a whole slew of them
that vanished because nobody could understand a word of what they
were saying. Garbo and Dietrich survived. The other thing . . . it
wasn't just the talkies and it wasn't just the thirties that brought about
this change, the Depression had a lot to do with it. The Depression
brought people down to earth. In the twenties the country was at a
peak of prosperity. And Hollywood was created by foreigners. The
studios did, in a way, pretend to speak for middle-class values. And
nobody could speak up for them more strongly than Louis B. Mayer.
In the early days people could get away with things in the movies and
in their personal lives. But so many things happened at the end of
the twenties to bring in censorship—which was very important.

   "A story I'm inclined to believe," Lambert continues, "was that
the whole censorship thing started with Hearst and Mae West. Mae
West had apparently said something derogatory about Marion Davies

to Louella Parsons, and Louella Parsons reported this to Hearst, who said, 'We're gonna get Mae West.' And it certainly happened that they ran a campaign against her—that she was obscene, indecent, and un-American. Of course things did get out of hand with the death of Wallace Reid, and the murder of William Desmond Taylor, and the Fatty Arbuckle scandal. But a number of things were happening to make changes unavoidable. It was a mixture of personal, social, and economic things all eventually coinciding to create this new point of view in which you had to be, on the surface, 'respectable.' "

Lambert feels that Hearst's establishment of Louella Parsons as the town's premier gossip purveyor was engineered to some extent as a preemptive strike against those few brave souls who might raise a journalistic eyebrow over his liaison with Davies. "But it was also a very smart move in general, because his readers lapped it up. It started Malibu Colony! The stars started building houses out there to be out of the range of Parsons's spies, who didn't get much beyond Romanoff's. So those stars would drive twenty-five miles to be able to fuck in peace."[13]

Still, there were those who dared to move against the socio-sexual tide, betting that their exotic images held more sway than the disapproving words of any self-appointed "moral" arbiter. "One very prominent lady star," Motion Picture Production Code administrator Joseph Breen wrote to his boss Will Hays in 1931, *told a group of correspondents who were interviewing her* [emphasis his] that she is a lesbian."[14] It doesn't take the proverbial rocket scientist to guess that the lady in question was in all likelihood Marlene Dietrich, who throughout her career did little to disguise her numerous affairs with persons of either sex, counting on the press itself to supply the "discretion" to which she was indifferent. No one else of that era was anxious to follow her example.

Yet just beyond the confines of the studios, Los Angeles—particularly in the period immediately following World War II—was fast becoming a hotbed of sexual radicalism. For it was here, not at New York's Stonewall, that the first shots were fired in the gay and lesbian rights movement that would explode in the 1970s. In the early 1950s, a loose network of clandestine discussion groups, which would eventually grow into the Mattachine Society, the One Institute, and the Daughters of Bilitis, began to question the sexual status quo. Many members of these groups came to the aide of Dr. Evelyn Hooker, a psychologist who, spurred by Kinsey's findings, began to engineer a set of experiments with standardized tests that would prove that same-sex orientation wasn't, in and of itself, the psychologically crippling syndrome that many of her generation believed it to be. Opposition to Hooker's research was considerable, as Christopher Isherwood, who became a close friend of hers, notes in a June 26, 1960, diary entry: "Evelyn told us how a perfectly serious psychologist asked her: 'Is there anything in homosexuality which corresponds to falling in love?'!!"[15]

Isherwood was one of the few within the industry to pay Hooker, or anyone else interested in challenging the sexual establishment, any attention. For while the sounds of protest may have been rising in the rest of Los Angeles, in fifties-era Hollywood they fall on exceedingly deaf ears.

There was never dialogue of any sort between Hollywood and the gay and lesbian movement. *Never*," activist Harry Hay declares emphatically. "And anybody who tried to create a dialogue immediately lost their connections with Hollywood. You were *out*."

Anyone meeting the eighty-six-year-old activist for the first time might think he was going out of his way to make a point. But as those who have known Hay over the years, and seen his activism grow to encompass everything from anthropology to Native American religious practices to the founding of the Radical Faeries movement, knows, he is not a man to waffle when making a point—and he's not shy about making points on any subject. Sitting in the book-and-manuscript-filled West Hollywood apartment he shares with John Burnside, his lover of the last three decades, Hay is as combative as ever, whether speaking of the past or of the present.

"In Hollywood in the studio days, important stars were protected," Hay recalls sardonically. "They were *all* protected in a sense. But they had to protect themselves also, because the industry felt that families in, say, Iowa would not buy Hollywood movies if it were known in any way that these people were 'tainted.' So from '34 on, as far as Hollywood was *officially* concerned, anyone gay or lesbian would be fired. That's why Louella Parsons and Hedda Hopper, who came along a bit later, were so important. They watched very carefully anything that happened with anyone in Hollywood. They operated out of two or three famous restaurants right across the street from the studios—RKO, Paramount, 20th Century-Fox, and MGM in Culver City. They had hundreds of stringers out there listening to see if they could pick up any dirt. Whether you had a contract at a high level or a low level, unless you were seen at certain places—like the Trocadero or Ciro's—or unless you were seen at a party with an 'important' person at least once a week, you were *reported* to Parsons or Hopper. Then you were called on the carpet by the studio and told 'We can't have this kind of thing going on.' Unless you showed yourself as a 'respectable person' you'd lose your contract."

Born in England in 1912, Hay came with his family to settle in Los Angeles in 1916 by way of Chile, where his father had worked in a copper mine. Discovering his sexuality in the late 1920s, Hay entered Stanford University in 1930, where he excelled at theater and music. In the years that followed, he came to know a number of important artists who shared his sexual orientation, including composer John Cage and choreographer Lester Horton. But for Hay personally, a more crucial figure of this period was actor Will Geer, with whom he began an affair in 1934. Geer (known to millions of 1970s televiewers as Grandpa of *The Waltons*) and Hay worked together in agitprop theater, union organizing, and other left-wing political activities, including Communist Party membership. At the same time, Hay became involved with Jungian psychotherapy, which—like the party—insisted on heterosexual unions. Hay married in 1938, as did Geer around that time. By the late 1940s, however, Hay dropped any form of heterosexual pretense, and in 1950 he began an affair with a then little-known fashion designer, Rudi Gernreich. Gernreich, whose "topless" bathing suit would become a defining artifact of the "Swinging Sixties," lent considerable financial support—though not his name—to Hay's efforts, which as the years rolled on saw him quickly

move to a leadership role in what by the 1970s had become a nationwide gay and lesbian civil rights movement.

"Any cop on the corner of any small town west of the Mississippi," says Hay of the world he grew up in, "could tell you who a
homosexual was: he was a hetero that had gone perverted. He was a
hetero who had become 'degenerate.' He was someone who had been
misled by either family or social mentors, but he was a hetero. That
was true right on up through when I began to push the fact that we
were a cultural minority, about 1948. The people who came into the
movement around '51 or '52 wanted no part of the idea of a cultural
minority. All they wanted to do was be exactly the same as everybody
else. All they wanted to do was get the movement to change the laws,
just a little *teeny* bit, to make it possible for same-sex relations to be
legal. By the time of Stonewall, everybody assumed that we'd always
thought we were a cultural minority. A 180-degree change in nineteen
years.

"In 1948, the negative image we all had of ourselves was so
intense. We had no information to go with otherwise. We had to change
the image of ourselves from a negative one to a positive one. So we
changed our name from 'homosexual' to 'homophile.' Whenever we
got picked up in an entrapment case, or got blackmailed or whatever
else, when we were taken into court we insisted on being called 'ho-
mophiles.' The cops and the judge and the lawyers didn't know what
the word meant, so they had to ask us. And that's how we got to define
ourselves as we wished. By '64 or '65 you'd hear the judge instruct
the jury, 'A homophile is a person who loves his own sex.' You notice
they didn't say 'her' at that point. It was always 'he.'

"The 1950s were terribly difficult, awful times. We were trying
to get people to understand that we loved each other. Then comes the
sixties, and everybody's moving toward different kinds of sexual liberation. So at the end of that period, all of a sudden Stonewall erupts.
Out here in Los Angeles in May of 1969 we worked to recall a re-
calcitrant, homophobic city council member, whose name was Paul
Langfort—and we achieved it. He was replaced by a man named
Edward Stevenson, who died in office. His wife, Peggy Stevenson,
took over, and she was councilperson for Hollywood for the next

twelve to fifteen years. So when Stonewall came along we said, 'What do you know? New York's catching up!' Because by that time, between San Francisco and L.A., we had done all kinds of things. In 1966 we had a motorcade here in Los Angeles—an open motorcade of fifteen cars with gay rights signs on top. But same-sex protection legislation doesn't show up until the mid-eighties. So you see we were fighting all kinds of things over the years.

"The thing you must remember is, when we started in 1948," Hay explains, "hundreds of groups had already come together and gone, from 1920 on. Say, for example, you and I would get together and get in touch with half a dozen other people. We liked it so much, we'd all of us pledge to each bring one more friend. So the second time we had a meeting our membership doubled. Everybody felt this was a wonderful way to cruise and meet a whole bunch of people you'd never met in your life before. And so the third meeting would be double again. But about the fourth or fifth meeting people began to drop off, so by the sixth meeting we'd be back to the original six people. This would go on over and over and over again.

"It was my brilliant idea to use the Kinsey report as an organizing tool for discussion groups. Most people were afraid of even doing that. All the Kinsey report did was note that *at least* 10 percent of American males had had homosexual experiences. In other words, we found out that there weren't hundreds in Los Angeles, there were *thousands*. But this was just a statistic. So in order to get groups started to talk about what it meant, we had to have important people to sponsor them. And to get the important people was a hard job."

What happened to the groups, Hay feels, was that they quickly discovered that conversations inevitably led to a call for action. And for most group members, who had to marshal all their courage just to attend a privately held talk, taking action of any sort was no simple task.

"Christopher Isherwood, for example, chaperoned Dr. Evelyn Hooker to a Mattachine meeting at my mother's house in May of 1952," Hay recalls. "She wanted to request permission to use one of our groups as the basis for her study. He came to that meeting with her and ran us up one side and down the other. He said, 'You're

calling on the wrong people. You should get to the people of privilege.
You should get to the people with money. You should curry favor with
the people who are important.' But he never did *anything*. Never. We
never got any help from anybody. We never even saw a check."[16]

Isherwood may have been no stranger to sexual daring in his
youth. But by 1952 he was moved to temper protest with caution, his
call for people of "privilege" invoking the safe harbor upper-middle-
class "deviants" could always claim. For Isherwood had been given
a peek at what lay just beyond the "respectable" curtain in December
of 1949, when he and a friend, Jim Charlton, were arrested in a raid
at a Santa Monica bar called the Variety. Questioned at the police
station, the pair denied being homosexual—and were released. "I
ought to have called their bluff, insisted on being locked up, hired a
lawyer, taken the case to the Supreme Court, started a nationwide
stink," Isherwood wrote of the incident. "Why didn't I? Because I'm
cowardly, slack, weak, compromised. My life at present is such a
mess."[17]

Isherwood wasn't ready to risk involvement in the sort of activism that led Hay and his allies to challenge police entrapment pro-
cedures in 1952 when Mattachine Society member Dale Jennings was
arrested.

"I was a well-known Marxist teacher in that period," Hay recalls, "and one of the people I knew was a lawyer who worked for
waterfront unions. I thought he would be an excellent lawyer for us.
He said, 'Sure, I'll take the case, but you guys are going to have to
come down to my office and tell me what it means to be a homosexual.'
And so we came out to each other and came out to him."

Jennings won his case simply by doing what no one who had
been arrested for "lewd conduct" before had dared—forcing the police to prove their charges. They couldn't. Yet so little serious attention was paid to gay and lesbian life that this important early victory
barely registered in the press. As a consequence, activists learned
that the social "discretion" that had helped so many in the past was
a hindrance to achieving the political ends the Jennings case had
won.

"Before this 'outing' period began, we only had one security—

silence. My security was your silence. That was understood. Always,"
Hay explains. "If you gained someone's friendship and trust, that was
a very sacred thing. You didn't give him away. If you did, it would
become known that you were someone who would *talk*. Because of
that, there was an enormous amount of difficulty in gay people just
getting to know one another. You never knew who you were talking
to, so you were very, very careful. How did I know, talking to you
right now, that you wouldn't call me up in an hour or so and say,
'You'd better come up with five hundred dollars or I'll turn your name
in to the *Times*'? For years the lower-left-hand corner of the Metro
section of the *Los Angeles Times* had a box with information about
bars that had been raided and people who had been apprehended,
and your name and address would appear in that little box. And if it
did, you automatically lost your job, you automatically lost your insurance, and you probably lost your lodgings too. You were wiped
out! That went on *every day*. That's why the blackmailer asked for
five hundred bucks. That was a lot in that period. Wages have changed
immensely. Up until about 1960, most people who had low-level jobs
didn't live in apartments. They lived in boardinghouses. You might
be lucky and find an open slot at a boardinghouse where there was
one other person like yourself. Most of the kids I knew who lived in
boardinghouses didn't know anybody else there with who was gay. I
lived in New York from about '36 to '42. Cruising up Fifth Avenue,
you might meet people who would know each other, but they never
lived on the same block. You were very careful *not* to know anybody
who lived on your block. You lived a very buttoned-up life. If your
family knew about you, they threw you out. If your church knew about
you, they threw you out. So the thick wall between the outside world
and your own inner world was enormous. Once you met other people
like yourself you felt safe. Most people, if they were lucky, found a
little niche of twenty or thirty others like themselves. That was a
wonderful place to be. But there were stories about us in the papers
every day. We were called degenerates. We were called perverts. So
if you had that image of yourself, and all the people around you, you
believed.

  "We had signals to communicate with each other," Hay says

with amusement. "Not very many people knew that—that was a very 'underground' thing. We all wore handkerchiefs in our coat pocket. If I wore a scarlet handkerchief, you could suspect I *might* be homosexual. But you'd have to go through a whole lot of conversation— at least ten or fifteen minutes—before you got to that point. I would find a way to engage you in a desultory conversation—not giving anything else away—and I'd wait for a signal from you. You'd usually ask me for a match. We'd go through these protocols and I'd be satisfied that you were trustworthy, or one of us would back off and I'd have no information about you and you'd have no information about me. And don't think this stopped after 1965!

"The most famous cruising ground of the 1930s was Hollywood Boulevard—Hollywood and Vine. The Bentleys and the Bugattis— and the Rolls-Royces, for the 'poorer' people—used to ride up and down the boulevard. Someone would catch your eye, and you'd saunter around the corner to the Plaza Hotel parking lot. If you liked the look of the guy, and he with you, you'd get into the car with him and have desultory conversation for about three blocks while you sized each other up. You had to be careful if you decided you wanted to get out of the car, because there would be cops hanging around all the time watching, and not in unmarked cars. If I'm picking you up, you don't know whether or not I'm going to turn you in. And I don't know you're not going to turn me in, either. We've got a lot of things to go through first. Because in that period if you resisted, and the police saw you resisting, it would come under the heading of 'lewd and lascivious behavior.' You could be tried for that and get six months in the county jail. If you got arrested the second time, you were automatically sent to Atascadero. And at Atascadero they gave you your choice of 'cures'—either lobotomy or castration. It was very common. We all knew this. There are a lot of people still walking around town who had this done to them."

But that was the fate of those unlucky enough to live outside the industry's confines, Hay explains. "Most people in Hollywood who were gay knew how to get handsome young men into their beds. But not here in Hollywood. They would go to Big Bear or Laguna or Lake Tahoe, or Palm Springs, and later on Laquita, which was beyond Palm

Springs. They were all 'getaways' for a time, but some of them—like Palm Springs—became too obvious."

Fashions in getaways come and go. But for Hay, the emphasis has always been on the problems that must be faced once the weekend is over. And while he has few regrets, he's well aware that he's paid a price for his militancy in a town where private life always has had a very public dimension.

"Ever since we started the movement I have been an open gay person," Hay says evenly. "I've been shunned as a pariah by the heteros I knew before I came out. It's very difficult to live in a city where you know an awful lot of people who, when they see you coming along the block, will cross the street. I went through that for twenty years. The people who now speak to me remember there was a time when we didn't speak. And they're very embarrassed. It's difficult for them to face up to that even now. And I have been *honored* by those people at public events. You can't change your personality. You can't change your character. It would never have been in my heart to have done that to them, back then. There's always an uncomfortable silence. Even in the middle of a renewed friendship. There's always that spot. You can't get rid of it. But you see, that's because the self-loathing has still not been removed."[18]

I n the sixties I used to go to a bar called the Red Raven that used to show movies," publicist Harry Clein recalls. "It's a chicken-wing place now. Just east of La Brea on Melrose. Someone must have told me about it, because it was the only bar I knew of then. Later I discovered the Gallery Room. Actually, a *straight* man first took me to dinner there with several other people. It's now Chef's Ming's Chinese restaurant. It's on the southwest corner of Crescent Heights and Santa Monica. It was a great bar. I started going there probably in '68 and on till sometime into the seventies. We would all meet there—everybody I knew of in the business. It was very much of a show-biz hangout. They had hamburgers and things, so people would go there for dinner. It was, in a sense, a pub. 'I'll meet you at the Gallery Room,' we'd say. It was the *nicest* place I'd ever been to. It was like a gay *Cheers*. You could go in there for conversation, or just hang out. If I was lonely it was a place to go. Everyone was welcome. Even women would come. Several really close friends came out just through my meeting them at the bar. I miss having a place like it today. It wasn't a place that anyone felt ashamed to be at—although I never used the front entrance. I always used the back."[19]

In other words, for all the advances that had been made from the days when gays kept their hats on, a soupçon of self-loathing remained. In more recent times, however, the days when the closet was still in full force are being regarded, by a new generation, with a curiously amused nostalgia. And nowhere is this more evident than at Numbers, a hustler bar still operating as if gay liberation had never happened. To those who go there in earnest, it never has. But a new crowd has started to show up—to watch the "old" crowd.

"I love it. It's totally silly," says comedienne Lea DeLaria, who like so many others on the gay L.A. "cutting edge" took to dropping in at Numbers for a drink—after catching a film at the Sunset 5 complex across the street—and reveling in the retro atmosphere. "It's just so slutty. There are still guys who go there Friday and Saturday nights to eat prime rib—and buy a hustler!"[20]

"That place always reminds me of a Ross Hunter movie," says actor/publicist Mickey Cottrell, another Numbers enthusiast. "I remember talking to the bartender who has been there the longest— from the day they opened in 1979. I said to him, 'Tell me where everybody sat.' And he said, 'Tennessee Williams always sat *there*. Truman Capote sat in the booth next to him. Sometimes they spoke to each other and sometimes they didn't. Gore Vidal always sat at the bar. He came in about twice a year.' He pointed out all the different places. It was just great.

"What's happened to Numbers, becoming popular with people who aren't into the hustler scene, is part of the changes that have been taking place in all of gay culture," Cottrell claims. "Now there's a chicness to these kinds of places. When Bruce La Bruce had his opening-night part for his movie *Hustler White*, he had it at the Spotlight, that Hollywood hustler bar. I'm sure it was the first opening-night party for *anything* ever conducted there. We also had a surprise birthday party for that Mapplethorpe model Robert—the bald-headed drag queen—at Numbers. It was great. Tony, the guy who runs the place, just loved it."21

Perhaps as a result of the tensions created between its serious-minded clientele and the casual interlopers from the Sunset 5, the spring of 1998 saw Numbers move from its original Sunset Boulevard locale to the more traditional West Hollywood setting of Santa Monica Boulevard.

That John Rechy's outlaw world has become a camp artifact could scarcely have been foreseen by those who lived through the up-heavals gay and lesbian Los Angeles has gone through over the past half-century. But that doesn't mean the danger Rechy wrote of has vanished from the scene completely. It has just taken on a new form.

"My nephew has been gay from the day he was born!" says writer-director Bill Condon. "He's *obsessed* with *The Sound of Music*. He begged for Maria's bonnet at age four! We gave it to him as a Christmas present. He opened the box, took it out, and said, 'Maria would never wear this!' He's totally into musicals. So he comes to L.A. to visit his 'Auntie Bill.' Suddenly he's sixteen and sort of coming into his own. He's sort of coy about whether he's done anything or not. But I went to a friend's party one weekend, so we went along to that. There was a group of about five of us. We walk into that house about eleven-thirty for a nine o'clock party. It was sort of at its height. There were all sorts of people there, but just making your way from the front door to the backyard there were about a hundred and fifty young men. About a hundred are twentysomething, and thirty or so are under twenty. It was interesting to be in this place with my nephew, who's sort of unsophisticated compared to these guys. But he's got a real sophisticated veneer. The thing is, he looks like he's thirteen, and he was being hit on by the chicken hawks, who in this case were twenty-two! It's an interesting phenomenon—this really strange thing going on with Generation X people, maybe because they missed out because of AIDS. But there's this whole X/Y phenomenon of really being obsessed with teenagers—and there's no taboo involved at all. It's an ancient, classic *Death in Venice* gay model. The Abbey phenomenon in West Hollywood is part of this. Because it's a coffee house, all those kids who can't legally drink hang out there till two o'clock. Combined with what's going on with people meeting each other on the Internet, it's the next big story that's going to break. Watch out."[22]

THREE

NOBODY SAID

ANYTHING

—

L UMBERING ACROSS A BARREN LANDSCAPE, storm clouds and lightning bolts flashing on the horizon be-hind him, comes a strange yet oddly familiar figure: a tall man in a black suit, two sizes too small, with heavy back platform shoes on his feet. There's no mistaking his identity—it's the Frankenstein monster. Still, some of the details are missing. Instead of the usual chalk-white pallor, with jagged facial scars and metal bolts on either side of the neck, this "monster's" look is clean, smooth—almost handsome. Only the high forehead suggests the character being played—or rather, evoked. For on this balmy evening in July of 1997 on a set at the Realart Studios in the Echo Park area of Los Angeles, actor Brendan Fraser isn't going through the usual paces as the world's umpteenth Boris Karloff imitator. Rather, he's performing in a half-dream, half-reverie set on the battlefields of World War I—the symbolic birthplace of the patchwork zombie Karloff embodied over half a century before.

This eerie evocation forms the opening shot of *Gods and Monsters*, a film not about the 1931 horror film and its 1935 sequel but about their maker, James Whale. Adapted by writer-director Bill Condon from Christopher Bram's novel *Father of Frankenstein*, *Gods and Monsters* stars Ian McKellen as Whale, with Fraser cast in the fictional role of Clayton Boone, a gardener who strikes up a quasi-friendship with the director in the days before the latter's death. Though Condon's previous credits include directing *Candyman: Farewell to the Flesh* and the scripts of *Strange Behavior* and *Strange Invaders*—and modern horror maestro Clive Barker is the executive co-producer— *Gods and Monsters* is in no sense a horror movie. Budgeted at $3.5 million, it's a low-key "art house" item with "crossover" potential of several different kinds.

As a "gay" film, with "carriage trade" ambience (courtesy of its star Ian McKellen), *Gods and Monsters* is aimed chiefly at sophisticated urban audiences. As it centers on the creator of some of the most famous films ever made, buffs young and old are sure to be interested. In addition, it stands a chance of attracting more general audiences, for co-star Fraser's latest vehicle, *George of the Jungle*, opened to favorable reviews and major box-office returns. Though it's a filmmaking world away from the knockabout comedy of *George*, *Gods* is in many ways a perfect follow-up film for Fraser, who like so many actors of his generation knows that nothing looks better on a résumé than a healthy mix of "commercial" and "serious" items. Though Fraser's buff physique, so successfully displayed in *George*, is on view here too (complemented in one shot by a fetching artificial appendectomy scar), it's utilized for a far different purpose. McKellen's Whale is sexually attracted to and at the same time terrified of (hence the *Frankenstein* reverie) the naive young gardener, who both inspires the dying director à la *Death in Venice* and serves as a hostile interloper much in the manner of William Holden's screenwriter, Joe Gillis, in *Sunset Boulevard*. This itself is an ironic notion, in that no small number of Hollywood citizens saw in Whale's death an uncanny real-life echo of the climax of Billy Wilder's 1950 masterpiece.

"James Whale, who died in the Gothic circumstances so dear to his own heroes—he was found after a mysterious fall into his swimming pool one night in 1957—still remains something of an enigma," critic Tom Milne wrote in 1973. "His name is revered in the history of horror movies for his work on *Frankenstein* (1931), *The Old Dark House* (1932), *The Invisible Man* (1933) and *The Bride of Frankenstein* (1935), yet the other seventeen films he directed seem to have entirely escaped the history books."[1]

Part of this enigma proceeds from the fact that Whale rose so high in Hollywood in the early thirties only to fall so precipitously as that decade came to an end. Though the horror features secured his place in film history, Whale also produced and directed the well-regarded 1936 version of *Show Boat* starring Irene Dunne and Paul Robeson; a pair of highly stylish and sophisticated comedies, *Remember Last Night?* (1935) and *The Great Garrick* (1937); and several sharply crafted melodramas, including *Waterloo Bridge* (1930), *The Kiss Before the Mirror* (1933), *One More River* (1934), and *The Man in the Iron Mask* (1939). An artist, actor, and theatrical designer, Whale first won notice in Britain for his direction of the R. C. Sheriff play *Journey's End*, a drama of World War I, which he filmed in 1930 shortly after shooting dialogue scenes for Howard Hughes's *Hell's Angels* (which had originally gone into production as a silent).

The Road Back, Whale's 1937 film of Erich Maria Remarque's sequel to *All Quiet on the Western Front,* would have brought him to the scene of the "Great War" once again. Moreover, coming on the heels of *Show Boat*, it was expected to secure his growing reputation as one of Hollywood's most important A-list directors. But the Laemmle family, who had given Whale creative carte blanche in the past, had lost control of Universal by the time production on *The Road Back* began. When the Nazi government objected to the film's allegedly anti-German elements, and threatened a trans-European boycott of all Universal product, the studio's new owners were easily cowed. Whale was thrown off the project, and "comic relief" scenes featuring actor Andy Devine, shot by another director, were inserted to tone down the elements the Nazis disapproved of. *The Road Back* was a critical and commercial disaster. Unable to establish a foothold at other studios, Whale eventually found himself working out his Universal contract with second-rate material like *Wives Under Suspicion* (1938), a vastly inferior semi-remake of *The Kiss Before the Mirror*, and the misbegotten jungle-set melodrama *Green Hell* (1940). In frustration, he walked off the set of his last contracted Universal film, *They Dare Not Love* (1940); and outside of an unreleased independently produced 1949 short feature, *Hello Out There* (based on the William Saroyan play), never directed a motion picture again.

Fortunately, Whale had invested the money he'd earned during his A-list days wisely and was able to retire in great comfort, returning to his first love, painting. In fact, in many ways Whale was well on his way to living "happily ever after" until a series of strokes left him both physically and spiritually depleted and led him to commit suicide. This fact was made clear in the note Whale left behind. But this wasn't made known to the public at the time of his death, appearing in full only in James Curtis's biography, published in 1982.[2] This, coupled with the fact that a revival of interest in his horror films was still several years away, led to the general impression in 1957 that Whale was merely a Hollywood has-been. This sad scenario took on a *Hollywood Babylon* aura as reports of Whale's sexuality—never the subject of scandal or any sort of public discussion during his lifetime—suddenly came to light. Was Whale's death the result of foul play? A murderous hustler perhaps? Calling Kenneth Anger!

"Jimmy Whale was the first guy who was blackballed because he refused to stay in the closet," director Robert Aldrich told activist/

historian Vito Russo in the early 1980s. "Mitchell Leisen and all those other guys played it straight, and they were on board, but Whale said, 'fuck it, I'm a great director and I don't have to put up with this bullshit'—and he *was* a great director, not just a company director. And he was just unemployed after that—never worked again."[3]

Ironically, Realart Studios, where much of *Gods and Monsters* is being shot, once belonged to Robert Aldrich. In fact, two of his most famous Hollywood-set melodramas, *Whatever Happened to Baby Jane* and *The Legend of Lylah Clare*, were filmed there. But none of the gay men involved in the making of *Gods and Monsters*, who in addition to McKellen, Condon, and Barker include associate producer Sam Irvin and project advisors film historian David J. Skal and director Curtis Harrington, share Aldrich's view of Whale's decline.

"I think the temptation is to make him into some sort of hero or victim because he was gay, and I suspect that's exaggerated," says McKellen, who, resplendent in a white wig, bears an uncanny resemblance to Whale. "The rumor was for years that he'd lost his career because he was relatively open. That doesn't seem to have been the case."

To McKellen, rather than evoking any sort of failure, Whale represents a great success. The actor is particularly struck by the fact that while coming from a lower-middle-class background, Whale had a chance in Hollywood to rise, both in life and in work, to a level that he never would have achieved in his homeland. "Imagine what his father would have thought of his son; by his early fifties being able to say 'I've got enough money. I can retire.' It was a dream—like winning the lottery. Essentially, Whale had done that. He had a life he enjoyed, away from the constraints of England." Moreover, McKellen isn't entirely convinced that Whale wasn't enjoying himself even in the professional decline of his last studio days. "Isn't it *Green Hell* where you have George Sanders and Vincent Price in the middle of the jungle in very tight-fitting military outfits, rather perky hats, shaved and coiffured—with Douglas Fairbanks Jr., who's not gay but is very cute? Does it not look like three queens on safari, getting away from it all? There must have been a lot of laughing on that set."[4]

Novelist Christopher Bram, who unlike so many others in his

profession is perfectly delighted by the film that's being made of his work, agrees with McKellen—pointing to Whale's long, and within Hollywood circles quite well-known, relationship with producer David Lewis as proof of the fact that sexuality played no real role in the director's rise and fall.

"The usual story is that Whale was a gay filmmaker and his career was destroyed by being 'openly' gay," says Bram, who is well aware that "openness" as a concept is of recent vintage, with no resonance in the world Whale knew. "It wasn't because of homosexuality that Whale's career came to an end. For one thing, Hollywood then was a small town. People knew who was gay and who wasn't. There were no secrets about Whale and David Lewis. But nobody said anything about it, either."[5] Bram feels that, outside of the usual petty sniping, the town would have had little to "say" about a couple who lived rather circumspect lives, away from the usual social circuit, where they enjoyed the friendship of a small, mainly British, circle.

Lewis, in Bram's view, is every bit as interesting as his lover. Part of the "brain trust" of advisors that worked under legendary MGM production chief Irving Thalberg, he rose to the rank of producer of such classics as Greta Garbo's *Camille*. Moving to Warner Bros. toward the close of the thirties, Lewis went on to produce such notable Bette Davis vehicles as *Dark Victory* (1939) and *All This and Heaven Too* (1940) as well as Ronald Reagan's most memorable acting turn, *King's Row* (1942). While at MGM in the early thirties, Lewis tried to borrow his lover from Universal in order to direct *Goodbye, Mr. Chips,* a film whose setting and emotional tone would have been ideal for Whale. It was not to be, but Whale was loaned to that studio in 1938—the year before Sam Wood's film of *Goodbye, Mr. Chips* was released—for *Port of the Seven Seas*. A version of Marcel Pagnol's *Fanny* trilogy, scripted by (of all people) Preston Sturges, and designed as a vehicle for Wallace Beery, it met with neither critical nor public approval.

Whale and Lewis were still close friends at the time of the director's death, though their love affair (which began in 1929) had faded. In the early 1950s, Whale took up with Pierre Foegel, a Frenchman working as his chauffeur. But at the time of his death that affair too had run its course. Both Lewis and Foegel were notified when Whale's body was discovered at the bottom of his pool in May of 1957, which as circumstance would have it was an already disastrous year for Lewis. He was producing *Raintree County,* a lavish adaptation of Ross Lockridge's Civil War novel that MGM hoped would be its next *Gone With the Wind.* Those hopes were dashed when the film's star, Montgomery Clift, sustained injuries in a traffic accident that greatly disfigured his once breathtakingly handsome face. Stitched back together, the alcoholic and emotionally erratic Clift completed work on *Raintree County.* But the production, already troubled by his behavior prior to the accident, never recovered in its wake—and neither did Clift. One of the biggest critical and financial flops of its era, *Raintree County* was David Lewis's last film. He died of pneumonia in 1987 in greatly reduced—and, as with Whale, somewhat mysterious—circumstances. According to newspaper accounts of the time, traces of cocaine and methadone, origin unknown, were found in Lewis's blood.[6] That, plus rumors of foul play, led to a police inquiry—which led nowhere.

Wandering through the sound stages at Realart, where the battlefield set stands next to a recreation of Frankenstein's laboratory, Christopher Bram is grinning from ear to ear. "I've always loved Whale's movies," says the novelist (whose books include two other dips into the gay past: *Hold Tight* and *Almost History*), pleased at seeing his work come to life. "I've been fascinated by them, in fact. I also knew that he was gay and had heard that his career came to an end because he was that. But then it wasn't until one night a friend of mine who is a documentary filmmaker was telling me he wanted to do a film for the BBC about James Whale that I thought about writing about him myself. There's no footage of Whale at work, and no interview footage of him, either. My friend knew he was going to have to use a fictional framework, so he asked if I had any ideas. As soon as he said that my mind started clicking. He knew a couple of things about Whale I didn't know. I knew some things he didn't know. I came up with the title *Father of Frankenstein* that night, and with the opening of the novel—a dark and stormy night on a hillside on Amalfi Drive. I did a little research, made a few notes. Then I happened to be in L.A. on an author's tour, and a friend said, 'Let's see if we can find the site of James Whale's house.' I didn't know it still existed. So we had the address and found the house. It's still there. The back-yard has been terraced, and the area where he had his artist's studio and the pool had been is now an apartment building. But the house is still recognizable. It was being renovated and nobody was living there, so we could snoop around. I looked in, saw it had the old pegged oak floors, and said to myself, This is it! But it wasn't until I got back to New York and started writing up my notes I realized I had to write a novel. I decided that I wanted to explore fictionally what little has been known or published about Whale. At this time there were three biographies of him, of varying degrees of trustworthiness—the best being by James Curtis. There were big gaps about Whale's private life, but that gave me more room as a novelist to explore it. If Curtis had filled in those gaps, it would have killed all my desire to write the novel.

"One of the things that first drew me to Whale," Bram contin-ues, "was that he did serve in the First World War. It made his career in a way. He was a poor working-class boy. He did not go to college. He went to art school. But when the war came he enlisted. He became an officer very early, and he started mixing with a different class of people. When he was in prisoner-of-war camp he started doing both his sketching for theater and cartoon work, and he began to direct plays and act a little. He was a provincial player for several years. He met Ernest Thesiger at that time, who had also been in the war. Later he met Charles Laughton and Elsa Lanchester. He played Laughton's son in a play called *The Man with Red Hair*. He designed several sets. But then there was this play *Journey's End* by R. C. Sherriff. Nobody wanted to direct it. Nobody thought it would come to anything, and it was a huge hit. It was the first play Whale directed. It made his career, and it made Colin Clive's career—he played the lead. It would have made Laurence Olivier's career too, at the time, if he hadn't dropped out of it early in the run. So the war made Whale. It destroyed the nineteenth century and was the beginning of the twentieth century—and it made James Whale. It gave a whole new color to his horror movies. They were not vague horrors. They were horrors built on history."

As for the end of Whale's career, Bram agrees with McKellen that it might not have been ignominious after all. "The story is that when he walked off *They Dare Not Love*—a bad picture with an awful title—he said, 'I've been saving up my berries. I don't need to do this anymore.' He was perfectly justified in retiring. He wanted to get back to his painting. Maybe there was a Norma Desmond side of him that wanted to go back to pictures, but we just don't know."

There was, of course, a very Norma Desmond side to his death. For as Bram well knows, reality has a way of being trumped by the movies, and never more so than in the case of Whale. "In my book I explain that he was at the *bottom* of the pool. People say, 'Well, wouldn't he be floating?' I try to explain to them no; the body has to decompose before it rises to the surface, and that takes time. 'Well, what about *Sunset Boulevard*?' Well, it's biologically impossible, but it's such a great shot, who's going to criticize it?"[7]

Writer-director Bill Condon, who after a series of genre movies is breaking new ground with *Gods and Monsters,* regards Whale as one of his personal "gods." Even while setting up a shot, he finds himself talking about the great director, almost by force of habit. "The thing to remember about Whale," Condon declares, "is that he had that amazing position—that even a director like George Cukor didn't have—of being the 'favorite son' to a mogul that *didn't interfere*. Whale actually got to make the movies the way he wanted to for the better part of his career. He was so spoiled by that—so spoiled that when it disappeared, he lost interest in making films."

"One thing I fought for was to make the film in wide screen," Condon continues, "because I wanted to make it visually like a fifties movie. It would show that Whale, in 1957, was really someone who was out of his time. In that way it's more the young Boone character's movie than it is his. Whale keeps having these flashbacks to times that were more expressionist—the 1930s, and before that World War I. The styles kind of meet at the end of the film, when you can't tell the difference between the real world and the dream world he lives in. Basically Whale's life is a movie that can't get made, so he's always commenting on it. In real life Whale had these two people working for him—a maid and a housekeeper, Anna and Johanna. We turned them into this one character, Hanna. It's a bit of a stock character, but the way Lynn Redgrave plays her, there's this slight sense of irony, of Una O'Connor, who played the maid in the *Frankenstein* films and *The Invisible Man*. That's what excited me about this project. It can be so rich as a movie—which is rare.

"What I saw in the book that I felt was so wonderful was that incredibly specific point of view that is all over Whale's movies," Condon continues. "It was possible to try to make a movie that had some of that. I wouldn't define it as 'camp,' but there's some kind of delicate irony going on all the time. I saw that in the novel, but putting it on screen there's so much more of it—incredible shifts of mood and tone. It's mostly comic, even though it's a story about the end of this man's life. Ian, everything about him, is attuned to that. It's a novel that covers a lot of ground about Whale and about Hollywood, and without taking too much out of it I wanted to be able to sort of condense it into the running time of a movie.

"There are a lot of gay movies being made today, but because it was about a guy who ultimately committed suicide, and that Ian would be in this sort of traditional role of an older man interested in a younger one, there were *so* many gay people who said no to it. They wanted me to make a movie about how Whale was a wonderful '*out*' person. They didn't want the rest. It's sort of like what black movies were in the Sidney Poitier days. All the gay movies are supposed to have these upbeat, positive images. It was actually a battle to do something that has these sides to it that are pretty dark. So it wasn't the gay subject matter that some people found objectionable, but the fact that it was being treated in a 'traditional' way. Still, I think people will be surprised by it. We have this scene where it's like this memory of a pool party and a guy says, 'Jimmy, come watch me dive.' He's naked, and there's this amazingly beatific smile on Ian's face. I've never seen the admission that gay sexuality is anything more than beautiful and pleasurable in a movie before. I think Ian and every-thing he's going to bring to it is going to make up for any of those PC concerns. It's unembarrassed. It's acknowledging a phenomenon, not apologizing for it."[8]

"It's not by accident that you make such a classic as *Frankenstein*," says director Curtis Harrington, who met Whale in 1948 at a time when the California-born teenager was making a series of experimental shorts. "Most directors' best films are the most personal, and *The Old Dark House* is a very personal film," says Harrington, who helped restore it in the 1980s as a stipulation of the contract he had signed with Whale's old studio, Universal.

"James Whale was a truly kind and generous person," says Harrington, whose many independent features, including *Night Tide* (1962), *What's the Matter With Helen?* (1971), and *The Killing Kind* (1973), are often highlighted by traces of Whale's influence. "He was very kind to me as a young admirer. I remember particularly when I went to Europe in the fifties, I'd sent him a postcard, so when he decided to take a vacation and come to Europe too he got in touch with me. I was living in the cheapest Left Bank hotel you could find. He wasn't staying at the Ritz, but a very nice place called the Hôtel Royale. I remember one night he took me to dinner and when we parted company that evening he said, 'Curtis, I admire you so much for your courage, the fact that you've done this on your own, coming to Europe.' And he pulled out a 1,000-franc note and said, 'If this will help you a little, I want you to have it.' That was probably only a hundred dollars, but in my position it was tremendous lot. And it was such a sweet, spontaneous gesture. That's the kind of person he was. The thing I was able to do for him later was when I'd gone over to London, Gavin Lambert and I arranged a special screening of *The Old Dark House* at the British Film Institute. I think that was one of the first times anyone had done anything like that. Tributes and homages weren't done much in those days. Whale was so touched. He was just like a little kid. He got huge applause—the audience response was so positive.

"When I first met Whale, he and Lewis were still living together in the house in Pacific Palisades, but I think the intimacy of their relationship had already pretty much come to an end. They were really just friends at that point. I went to Europe, and by the time I got back

David had his own place. Bill Condon and the production people arranged for Ian McKellen and I to visit the Amalfi Drive house together so that I could reminisce. It's not the same. At some point Goldie Hawn and Kurt Russell lived there, and she completely remodeled the whole thing, so it was very hard for me to evoke in my mind the original house. The interior had changed so much. It was certainly far more Goldie Hawn than James Whale by the time Ian and I visited there. The thing I tried to convey to Ian, to give him clues to how to portray James Whale as accurately as possible, was that the most outstanding quality of his personality was his sense of humor. He was just bursting with humor—this very personal, very sophisticated view of everything. Some people might call it camp. I don't see it that way, because it's very genuine. It's not spurious or silly. It's a really special sense of humor—dark but not cynical. It's filled with enormous goodwill and charm.

"David Lewis was a man of immense personal style," Harrington recalls sadly. "He dressed beautifully. He was bright and charming. He was an enormously sympathetic person. It upset me terribly, what happened to him. When he was first on his own he would have parties that I would go to. Lovely dinner parties. He had a modern house with a pool off of Laurel Canyon, up by Woodrow Wilson Drive. He was in that for quite a long while. He had a French lover too, for a while, who finally left him. It seems to have been a terrible blow to him psychologically. And then the next thing I knew he was in a still very elegant apartment—more modest. I visited him there two or three times. And then it was just downhill all the way.

"His last film, *Raintree County,* was a total disaster. He had a magnificent office at MGM, and I remember thinking, He seems to have nothing to do. The desk didn't have any papers on it. There was a little pad he could doodle on. That was it. And he made a terrible choice of director. Eddie Dmytryk was the wrong man for a film like *Raintree County*. It needed someone like Cukor. David Lewis ended up in a *tiny* flat in West Hollywood. All the elegance was gone. It was just pathetic. I didn't really even want to see him at that point. It was just so sad. I have no idea why he lost all his money. Jimmy lived in great splendor until he died. I never understood what happened to David financially. I still don't.

"As for Whale, after he came back from Europe I rarely saw him again. Not that we had any sort of relationship, but I'd got the feeling that Pierre really didn't want him to have his own friends around. Other than one party I never went to his house. And to be quite honest, I didn't like Pierre at all. He was a terrible snob. He wasn't worthy of Whale. He was just a hustler on the make, and he *made it*. I know James was happy with him, because once in Paris he said, 'He makes me feel young.' So what more could you ask?"[9]

Were Whale still alive, besides this film tribute, he probably couldn't ask for anything more than the unexpected revival of the career of Gloria Stuart. The star of three Whale classics—*The Old Dark House, The Kiss Before the Mirror*, and *The Invisible Man*—has become a star all over again in James Cameron's *Titanic*, playing the key role of a 101-year-old survivor of the fabled ocean disaster. Delighted at her newfound fame, Stuart—doing publicity chores for the megabudgeted spectacular—is just as enthusiastic about Whale, and the new generation that has come to appreciate his work.

"After I'd had my career," says the eighty-six-year-old actress, who retired from the screen in the mid-1940s, "I went to live in England for a while. When I came back to Hollywood—not as an actress, just to live—I couldn't believe that James had disappeared as a persona. It didn't seem possible. What happened? Why? This brilliant, brilliant man. He never had his due. Maybe he will get his due now. I remember once going to a story conference with a producer who said, 'I want a story with *statue*!' So maybe James will gain the rightful 'statue' he deserves!

"James contributed a great many of the wonderful touches *personally*," Stuart recalls. "For example, in *The Old Dark House*, when Ernest Thesiger takes the flowers out of the vase and throws them into the fireplace—that was not in the script. That was James's idea. Or when he holds his fork up with a potato on it and he says, 'Have a po-tay-to!' *That* was James. [Thesiger] started to do the scene and James said, 'Wait a minute—hold it up, Ernest—"Have a po-tay-to!" ' So he was really creative as a writer as well as a director. That scene where I did those little silhouettes I did with my hands on the walls? James. And so was that other scene where I'm walking through the hall in that white gown with Karloff coming after me. I said to him, 'I don't understand. Everybody else is wet and muddy, and hasn't changed for dinner, and I come in in a Jean Harlow bias-cut silk gown with earrings and pearls. What is this? Doesn't make sense.' And he said, 'Oh yes. When Boris chases you through the halls and into the living room I want you to appear like a white flame!' Okay, James. It was ridiculous, but for the tone of that film it was just right."

On a more personal level, Stuart's memories of Whale are remindful of the discretion that was the watchcry of stylish gay men of his time. "I remember James took me to the theater to see Lunt and Fontanne and Jane Cowl, Katharine Cornell—and I think a couple of times David Lewis was along. But that was the only contact I ever had with him. James came over to see me when I played in *Peer Gynt* and *Romeo and Juliet* in Pasadena. That was when I was still making nine films a year. Oh God, the young are strong! But I don't remember David coming along with him then. That was in 1932 or '33. I don't know whether they were seeing each other then or not. But later on I do remember David being around with James. The three of us would go to the opera or the ballet together. That was always on James's instigation. He liked me very much, and I thought he was wonderful because he was my savior professionally. He was giving me wonderful parts to play. He was witty. I appreciate that kind of wit—with a knife. Oh, boy—slice right through you."

Stuart smiles; then her face darkens slightly and she asks, with all due sincerity: "Tell me, do *you* think he killed himself?"[10]

Jimmy Whale said, 'You will love it here in Hollywood, Charles. I'm pouring the gold through my hair and enjoying every minute of it.' Charles was horrified by that. But Jimmy did love money," notes Elsa Lanchester in her autobiography. Going on about what "a wonderful tango dancer" Whale was, Lanchester notes that the painter and costume designer Doris Zinkheisen was Whale's most frequent tango partner, and that they were once engaged to be married, "but at some point around the time when he was directing the play *Journey's End*, they parted. I don't think James Whale ever got over it."[11]

Whale was, however, sufficiently composed to offer Zinkheisen the plum assignment of designing the costumes for *Show Boat* seven years later. If Whale truly contemplated marrying Zinkheisen, it would have been a marriage of the so-called New York variety—in which a gay man and a straight woman forge an alliance for social purposes, with full knowledge of sexual realities. If Whale contemplated one with Zinkheisen, he changed his mind on meeting David Lewis, opting for the truth, which, as horror-film historian David Skal points out, was "not an easy thing [then], and not an easy thing now."[12]

Still, it appears to have been considerably easier than what Lanchester and Laughton settled for, which, she confesses semifrankly, resulted in his sneaking around behind her back, and risking arrest in the process. Detailing the aftermath of Laughton's incarceration for soliciting a male hustler in London early in their marriage, she claims, "It was only *afterward*, in later years, that the boy episode proved to grow into a great wall—never mentioned but distinctly *there*. I can think of no indication whatsoever that Charles liked young men prior to that time. Obviously, he needed secret and degrading episodes. I would say that he only began to 'love' young men when he reached the age of about forty. It was his change of life. Then I was relieved. It was so safe."[13]

"Oh, they were just *vicious* to each other!" says artist Don Bachardy. "She was one of those women who affected 'surprise.' A sofa where she discovered him having sex with a young man, she burned! She saw herself as a victim. She was just deluding herself on purpose."

Bachardy recalls how Laughton would seek refuge at his and his lover Christopher Isherwood's Santa Monica Canyon home when the acting couple would fight. "She was always attracted to queer men. She was just that kind of masochist who made up her mind to go after people she couldn't have. She pretended not to know that Charles was queer! She even pretended not to know what homosexuality was!"

Bachardy laughs. "She got what she was after," he says dryly.[14]

*   *   *

"Cukor didn't approve of James Whale," Gavin Lambert recalls. "I remember his talking about that. He thought Whale asked for it by flaunting it. Whale took David Lewis with him to parties. George would never have gone to a party with another guy. That was the problem for directors or anyone of note in Hollywood if they were gay. They had to lead more or less hidden lives, so it became almost impossible for them to have a continuing relationship with another person. James Whale and David Lewis were the exception. Cukor *never* had anyone. Irving Rapper? I don't think so. They were almost sort of *steered* to hustlers and call boys."[15]

With a list of credits that includes *Dinner at Eight, Little Women, Camille, The Women, The Philadelphia Story, Gaslight, Adam's Rib, Born Yesterday, A Star Is Born* (1954), and *My Fair Lady*, George Cukor embodied the A-list director like no one else in Hollywood history. That he held that position so long, helming his last feature, *Rich and Famous*, at the age of eighty-one, is a testament not only to Cukor's talent but his tenacity in remaining at both the top of his profession and the tip of everyone's lips. Cukor "networked" constantly, exchanging favors, offering advice (suggesting Gloria Swanson when Billy Wilder was searching for a star for *Sunset Boulevard*), and charming the wives of studio bosses whose "macho" demeanor scarcely meshed with his own. Ever mindful of appearances, Cukor wouldn't dream of attending a social gathering without a woman to accompany him as "beard," even though everyone in town knew the truth of his sexual life.

Everyone outside of town was put "in the know" as well when his Sunday-afternoon pool parties, where Cukor and his intimates relaxed with their boyfriends *du jour*, were described in telling detail in *City of Night:* "A swimming pool dominates one level of the garden, bordered by marble benches. . . . The director makes his entrance, emerging out of the white walls of the house in slacks and sport shirt: a tiny, skinny, wiry old man with alert, determined eyes. He looks at Skipper appraisingly. 'You're much better-looking than your photographs, young man,' he says, 'and I might add you look good in clothes.' "[16]

"Beyond that circle of his friends, Cukor was incredibly closeted," Rechy declares. "Of course, everybody *knew*. But that was another kind of closetry, because he kept the two worlds so separate. I know from having experienced one aspect of it—the parties for the boys. Not for Vivien Leigh. I had stew. And I know he didn't serve Vivien Leigh stew. Most people didn't know what a sonofabitch he was. Oh, what the fuck—he *exploited* people. But those he exploited were *not* innocent. There was no innocence. Nobody was brought from a cove of innocence into a lair of corruption. We were looking to *get there*. That's a very important thing to remember. But the power that Cukor had was a lasting power: the power of fame and money.

"I don't think any of the people he picked up ended up famous," the writer continues, squelching rumors that some of Cukor's better-looking leading men may have had offscreen duties. "The people I was writing about all lasted very briefly and were replaced rather cruelly. I saw that. It happened with two people I knew. In *City of Night* I made them into a composite of one person. They went from Cukor to be passed on to other members of his group. A lot of people courted his favor, including that photographer Bob Mizer. In fact, I did some photographs for the gentleman myself.

"Ironically, Cukor was once interviewed and said, 'I take my inspiration for my films ranging from Dostoyevsky to John Rechy'— obviously not even remembering at the time that I'd met him. He was very campy, but he had a cruel streak, and not only toward the 'boys.' I saw him once do a brutal imitation of Lana Turner testifying in that very ugly Johnny Stompanato murder case. He 'did' her on the stand, posing and posturing, and denying she'd committed a certain sexual act. It was very, very cruel. And this is one of the things I picked up on that I mentioned to Gavin. He said, 'I never saw that part of George.' He wouldn't have. Cukor knew Gavin was a writer. He didn't know I was, too. I saw only that 'boys' night' aspect of him. It was dinner for 'the boys,' and the men who brought 'the boys' to him, and a swimming party. But it wasn't a sex party. No. Not like that at all. I would say it was more like an *audition*."[17]

Cukor's inner circle included director Jack Gage (whose Rosalind Russell vehicle, *The Velvet Touch*, is a prime piece of late-forties camp), noted photographer and art director George Hoyningen-Huene, and several actors of varying degrees of obscurity: Andy Lawler, John Darrow, Richard Cromwell, and Lon McAllister. But the name that carries most resonance today is William Haines. As an actor in the mid-to-late 1920s, Haines played boyish leading men—carefree prankster types who by the last reel have been chastened enough to mend their mildly irresponsible ways. One of ten MGM stars to get above-the-title billing in 1927, and the first to test for the "talkies,"[18] Haines is seen at his best in King Vidor's *Show People* (1928), a satire of Hollywood starring Marion Davies—who was also a personal friend. In fact, Haines could count a number of stars as close personal friends, including Joan Crawford and Carole Lombard. Such friendships proved important when, according to writer Anita Loos, Louis B. Mayer called him on the carpet as "vague hints of misdemeanor were cropping up in Louella Parsons's column. . . . 'I'm going to give you a choice,' said L.B. 'You're either to give up that boyfriend of yours or I'll cancel your contract!' Without even a moment's hesitation, Bill opted for love and told L.B. to tear up his contract."[19] Many years later Haines and his lover, Jimmy Shields, sent Mayer an anniversary card reading "And you said it wouldn't last!"

Haines's sexuality was scarcely news to Mayer, or anyone else in Hollywood. In her memoirs, Louise Brooks recounts a weekend she, her friend Pepi Lederer (Marion Davies's lesbian niece), Haines, and several other "younger degenerates" spent at San Simeon—cavorting beneath the disapproving but coolly tolerant eye of William Randolph Hearst. "Exactly ten minutes before dinner was announced, cocktails were served in the assembly hall. Anyone who dared to gulp down two in this time span was treated to an unforgettably frosty stare from Mr. Hearst, who did his best to curb Marion's drinking."[20]

Mayer's stare was clearly frostier than Hearst's, but this didn't bother Haines, who remarked years later, " 'I could sort of see the career was petering out."[21] He was right: Cary Grant was waiting in the wings. Haines was a popular personality for several years, but he was coming to the end of his run. In fact, even before Mayer pulled the plug, "the oldest college boy in North America"[22] had made plans to change careers. Haines became an interior decorator. Crawford and Lombard were his first clients. They were shortly followed by Claudette Colbert, Joan Bennett, Lionel Barrymore, Jack Warner, and Nunnally Johnson. In addition to the over four hundred homes he decorated over the years, Haines designed the Mocambo nightclub, and in 1969 he designed Winfield House, the London residence of the then-ambassador to Great Britain, Walter Annenberg.

"Scandal touched Bill only once, in 1939," industry scribe Ezra Goodman claimed in a 1949 *New York Times* profile. "Jimmy Shields and he were living in Manhattan Beach, a town they had made fashionable for beach living. A neighbor accused one of Haines's house guests of propositioning his son, went to the police, and it made the local papers. It was quashed, but Bill and Shields quickly moved to Malibu."[22] But according to Cukor biographers Patrick McGilligan and Emmanuel Levy, that was merely the first time a scandal that touched Haines had *made the papers,* for at the time of *Camille* Haines and Cukor were briefly held by the authorities on a solicitation charge.[23] But Cukor, unlike Haines, was so valuable to the studio that the incident—which was kept out of the papers—never threatened his career. What exactly happened has never been made clear, and isn't likely to be.

"If it's a misdemeanor that old, you're never going to find it in the computer," claims novelist and police buff James Ellroy. "They purge personal documents like that. When I investigated my mother's murder case, I found it was tough turning up stuff even on my own criminal record 'cause it was just misdemeanor convictions, and my last one was twenty years ago. Anything more than that is tough to find. And if Cukor kept a California driver's license, once he died it went right out of the system."[24]

That the reckless Haines and the cautious Cukor maintained a long—if occasionally edgy—friendship is one of gay Hollywood's most interesting sidelights. In the cache of Cukor correspondences on file at the Academy of Motion Picture Arts and Sciences Library, an exchange at the time *My Fair Lady* was nominated for the Oscar indicates that Cukor and Haines were patching things up after an estrangement of some sort. "Sire all is forgiven. Please return to the Palace," Haines writes. "The knock you hear at the Palace gates will be me," Cukor replies.[25]

In recent years the claim that an intemperate remark made either by or about Haines, to the effect that Clark Gable may have once "tricked" with him, has surfaced as an explanation as to why Cukor was fired from *Gone With the Wind*. This doesn't seem likely in light of the fact that Haines, being such a close friend of Gable's wife, Carole Lombard, had crossed paths with Gable any number of times before. Cukor's far less publicized clashes with producer David O. Selznick were far more likely the inspiration for the exit, the director and the producer both being strong-willed, take-charge personalities. In the end, the claim that Gable was fearful that a "woman's director" wouldn't attend to his needs finessed the situation for publicity purposes. It increased Gable's profile with a public that was blissfully unaware of the term's real meaning. In Hollywood it was understood otherwise: Clark Gable didn't like "fags"—or at least this *particular* one.

I am one of untold scores of people for whom George was such an extraordinary and important mentor," says *Los Angeles Times* film critic Kevin Thomas. "Scarcely a day goes by without my thinking about him. I met a lot of people through George. One of them is one of my closest friends to this day. It really wasn't always such a friendly atmosphere out there. We all lived in the real world as well as the movies. And George moved at the top levels of high society.

"George was a delightful contradiction," Thomas recalls. "In larger straight society he was capable of being one of the great snobs, and I say that as lovingly as I know how. What is not sometimes understood is that in gay society he was a remarkable democrat. He reached out to gay men in every aspect of the business. You would go to dinner at George's and you might meet a world-famous director or producer or an associate producer, or an editor, or a set decorator— or Christopher Isherwood and Don Bachardy. I remember once there was this very rotund elderly guy who had been Cary Grant's secretary. He was a rather seedy character, and you'd hardly think of George Cukor having somebody's *secretary* to dinner, but he was a regular. As long as a person was presentable, and could hold up a conversation, they were *in*. He liked conversation to be buoyant and upbeat. It was almost never about sex per se. And it was not overly gossipy. If some gay issue came up, it came up, but it was in the context of the world at large. It wasn't like who's-doing-what-with-whoever. Sometimes with some of the people he knew or had known, some wonderful stories from the past would emerge. He loved to talk about Vivien Leigh, for example. Occasionally he would say, 'I told Kate this the other day,' or 'Kate's coming in next week,' but it was just *lively*. He usually loved to have four people every night for dinner.

"Now, as we know, George could be very volatile, and he could be very protective," Thomas continues, evoking a Cukor quite different than the one Rechy knew. "George must have upset Ted Morgan when he went to do his really quite good book on Somerset Maugham, because when I got to the end of that book and I was checking a footnote, the whole book was destroyed for me, because he had a really nasty footnote in the back about George. George must have told him, 'No, I'm not going to talk about Maugham.' That must have provoked Morgan, for it was one of the most petty and distorted acts from a serious writer I've ever seen. One of the things that was really outrageous was he said George would entertain his straight friends and the leftovers would be given to the hustlers. Well, I'm here to tell you that if there was a socially acceptable hustler, with nice table manners, occasionally he would be at the table too with all the rest of them all equal under the sight of God.

"One of the funniest moments of my whole friendship with George was when one such gentleman said, 'Oh, hi, Kevin, how are you?' before George had a chance to introduce us. George was vastly amused. But George was very loving. He didn't want people to dump their personal problems on them. He didn't want to hear a lot of gloom and doom and that kind of stuff. But current events, new movies, new plays, personalities—he kept up very well.

"He could alienate people. George was very quick to judge. If

he decided he liked you, he liked you, and if he didn't, he didn't. But
he was certainly a very big focal point for dozens of us—for generations, I'm sure. Now, you couldn't get away with being as bitchy as
George was. You had to be careful not to emulate that too much. You
couldn't *be* George Cukor. And there were times in his life when *he*
couldn't be George Cukor, either. But those of us who were part of
his circle of gay friends were also included on other occasions. There
were a couple of events I was invited to that were perfectly heterosexual occasions. Now I don't think a hustler ever sat down with Kate
Hepburn or Ethel Barrymore, but in regards to gay people of his time
and place he did extend a hand. And everybody was encouraged never
to feel sorry for themselves: 'Press on' and 'Stand up' and 'You deserve
better treatment than that.' "[26]

Thomas takes particular amusement at the letters in the Motion
Picture Academy file that Cukor wrote to Alan Searle, the secretary
(and lover) of novelist Somerset Maugham. Cukor took a special interest in Searle in the 1970s, when poor health and poorer spirits laid
him low. Encouraging "the Earl of Searle" to come visit him in Hollywood, Cukor enumerates the mutual friends, "Searle enthusiasts,"
anxiously awaiting him. "Then there is another category of enthusiast.
There are the body-builders . . . models . . . masseurs . . . actors in
porno pictures and other related (?) activities."[27]

"Oh, Alan was absolutely outrageous!" Thomas says, laughing.
"He may have been the most decadent person I've ever known. When
he came for his annual stay, he would make full use of a certain male
madam in West Hollywood, the famous Scottie, who certainly did have
a lot of clientele. George once said to me, 'You know, I really *must*
take him to lunch. It would be the *nice* thing to do!' The prime numbers of the day were always around when Alan was in town—Colt
models and the like. Then Alan would want to go to a certain restaurant in the Marina because the waiters were particularly cute. He
really was an unapologetic dirty old man. He'd say, 'Oh, in Monte
Carlo they don't have boys like you have here!'"

Still, for all the pleasures he may have enjoyed in separating
public life from private, Cukor, Thomas feels, paid a high price
for it.

"Henry Hathaway once said, 'George is married to the industry.' Because of that, I think, friends were very important to him. But love was difficult for George. He did experience it a couple of times, I know, but . . . it doesn't always work out for all of us, you know? I think anybody as romantic as he was found love difficult. He did not have a Don Bachardy. Now it's very true that for his generation, for men of his time, he could not have had this major career and taken a male lover to all those premieres at the Carthay Circle. That would just never have worked. But I get very resentful when I read accounts that label George as closeted. I don't think it's fair. I think the one word George would have used, and it's not such a terrible thing to be even today, is 'discreet.' I don't think he thought he was fooling anybody. Actually, considering his stature, and the vulnerability that that brought, he was pretty good about living his private life.

" 'Tough' was George's favorite word," Thomas continues. "He used 'tough' in a different way, not just 'hard' but 'tough' in the sense of being resilient. If he said of someone—a woman or a man—who had some challenge facing them, 'He's tough,' that was a great compliment. But he had a very good antenna for what would fly and what wouldn't in any given situation. He never would have survived if he didn't. I know that some people were offended by him and didn't feel too kindly for one reason or another.

"You see all these articles about 'role models,' and sometimes it gets a little bit repetitive and heavy-handed, but when I think about George it's in this way. For a gay man of my generation he was certainly—my God, he was ten years older than my parents! Few of us thought we could attain that stature and reputation. But you could do something for yourself even if you were—heaven forbid—gay. 'Don't feel sorry for yourself. Just go out and do it the best you can and stand your ground.' This is what his gift was to other gay men: an example.

"I remember standing by the pool with George once, talking, and him saying, 'I just can't come out. I'm just too old.' I understand that. He knew very well about the whole issue of memoirs, and he finally realized it was an impossibility for him. Everything has to be seen in context of the era. You cannot expect people to have done certain things at certain times when it wasn't viable. I remember sometime in the 1970s being at George's house for dinner with Christopher Isherwood and Don Bachardy. And Christopher Isherwood was really 'We all have to be out!' Well, here was George at the end of this fabulous career. It was harder and harder for him to get pictures, as anybody would know. I remember that I was really teed off because I had read enough about Isherwood to know that although he had lived very modestly in a bohemian way, he always had some small stipend from the family that kept the wolf from the door. He was a writer. He was a free agent. Here I was at the *Los Angeles Times*, which was not a congenial place to be out in the 1970s. I make no apologies about being discreet—as if I had anything much to be discreet about! But, on the other hand, here was George in his seventies and still wanting to sustain a glorious career. I really resented that on the part of Isherwood. That's so easy for you to say. You're a world-famous novelist. You don't have to go to the office and work. You don't have to try to get a contract with some studio. George didn't make movies for gay audiences. But he had enough talent and skill to make them very personal experiences. I think George's films are marked by a very bemused compassion. And they are filled with romantic longing."[28]

When I arrived at Fox," recalls Gavin Lambert, who came to the studio to work with director Nicholas Ray in 1956, "one of the first things that struck me was Nick Ray sat me down and gave me a little lecture: 'Don't let people think that you're gay.' Now the head of public relations at Fox back then was Frank McCarthy. He was an ex–four-star general, and he was gay. And his lover was a guy called Rupert Allen, who was a publicist. They lived in the same house, but they went to parties in separate cars with 'beards,' and left the parties with their 'beards.' It was so absurd because everyone *knew*. Frank was a very important guy, but this was playing the game. It was a charade that was insisted upon. To a certain extent it was stopping a bit in the sixties, because there were a lot of changes going on then. I had a few movie-star friends—Natalie Wood, Leslie Caron, Rita Hayworth. They knew about me. I had a lover at that time, it was quite open, and they would invite him and me to parties. So for certain people—the best people—it was already beginning to change in the sixties."[29]

Lambert came to know Ray when his favorable review of the director's first film, *They Live by Night* (1950), spurred its European release. Meeting in London sometime afterward, the novelist and the director "hit it off very quickly." Hired as Ray's personal assistant, Lambert did some uncredited rewrites on Ray's *Bigger Than Life* and *The True Story of Jesse James,* but gained full screen credit for *Bitter Victory.*

"I don't know whether I thought about coming to Hollywood in terms of social life," the writer recalls. "I just knew I had to get out of England. I wanted to live in California. And of course all my ideas about living in America, and living in California, came from the movies. When I got here it was the last gasp of the studio system. The walls were still standing, but there were quite a few cracks in them. But it was all still here in place, so in that way it was exactly what I thought it was. Of course, until you have experience of it, you can't quite imagine the ruthlessness of studio power. That I had to learn."

Lambert also learned about the real Hollywood—both inside and outside the studio walls. He describes it quite tellingly in *The Slide Area, The Goodbye People,* and *Inside Daisy Clover*—which was filmed by Robert Mulligan from a script written by Lambert himself in 1966. This semicautionary tale of a teenage singing star, and her unhappy marriage to a leading man whose alcoholism hides his true sexual nature, is a touchstone in any discussion of gay Hollywood of the studio era.

"None of the characters were meant to be specific people," the novelist explains. "There's a touch of Judy Garland in Daisy, but she's not Judy Garland. Wade Lewis is not Monty Clift, but there's an element of Monty Clift—the unhappy bisexual who can't make up his mind what to do about it."

Onscreen talents may have had offscreen troubles, but for other gays and lesbians, Hollywood—much like the legitimate theater—was something a refuge. The Arthur Freed unit at MGM, responsible for the studio's most famous and celebrated musicals (*Meet Me in St.*

Louis, Easter Parade, Singin' in the Rain, The Band Wagon, and *An American in Paris*), was so gay-friendly that its members were commonly referred to in the industry as "Freed's Fairies," whether deserving the label or not. (Freed himself was straight.)

"I don't know whether you will understand what I say," remarks Freed's chief assistant, Lela Simone, in her oral history of the unit, "but Vincente Minnelli worked like a homosexual. I don't mean that nastily."[30] Producer Hank Moonjean (*The Great Gatsby, Dangerous Liaisons*), who began his career as an assistant director at MGM, knows exactly what Simone is referring to. "At the time I knew him, Minnelli was carrying on affairs with several women. But still he was the most *effeminate* man I have ever known!"[31]

An equally important "Freed Fairy," who was indeed gay, was Roger Edens. A songwriter and vocal coach, Edens first gained wide public attention for the "special material" he created for films, such as the "Dear Mr. Gable" arrangement of "You Made Me Love You" for *Broadway Melody of 1938*, which helped to jump-start Judy Garland's career. The innocence Garland projected in this number stands in marked contrast to the extreme sophistication of another song Edens and his chief collaborator, Kay Thompson, wrote for the singer—the "Great Lady Gives an Interview" sequence from *Ziegfeld Follies* (1944). Known among her gay fans as "The National Anthem," this spoof of Greer Garson's personal tics goes a long way toward explaining Garland's cult appeal. But such numbers only scratch the surface of Edens's contributions as an associate producer.

"Roger Edens *was* the Freed unit," Simone declares. "Roger was not, in essence, a modest fellow. He was a well-mannered person who would express his negative opinion about something in a high-class manner." And like all gay men of his era, Edens had to toe a careful line. In fact, Simone claims, one of his chief collaborators, writer Leonard Gershe, "was anonymous" in terms of his work with Edens. "I have a feeling that that was partly Lennie's wish. He did not want, under any circumstances, to be the protégé of a man who was more or less known as a homosexual."[32] Still, Gershe had no problems working with the producer-musician on *Funny Face,* a film that saw the chief members of Freed unit working, for one time only, at Paramount.

"Roger was married to someone, but I only saw her once. She was not around," claims Kay Thompson.[33] Hank Moonjean also recalls an Edens spouse. But Don Bachardy, who could see Edens's home from the window of his own house on the other side of Santa Monica Canyon, remembers no Mrs. Edens, and none was listed in Edens's 1970 obituary—making this questionably the quietest "New York" marriage on record.

Charles Walters, another "Freed Fairy" of note, never took the marriage route. Graceful and good-looking, this dancer and director (who can be seen partnering Garland in the "Embraceable You" number in *Girl Crazy* and the "Broadway Rhythm" finale of *Presenting Lily Mars*) became one of MGM's most reliable craftsmen. His best-remembered films—*Good News, Easter Parade,* and *High Society*—were enormous box-office hits. But outside of the offbeat Leslie Caron vehicle *Lili,* he never acquired the patina of "prestige" worn by Freed-unit directors like Minnelli or Stanley Donen, though his contributions to the genre are in many ways just as crucial. It was Walters who staged the song numbers for *Meet Me in St. Louis,* and when Freed was displeased with some sequences of Minnelli's *Gigi,* he turned to Walters to reshoot "The Night They Invented Champagne" and "Yes, I Remember It Well." In addition to his musicals, Walters directed several successful comedies, including *The Tender Trap* with Frank Sinatra and Debbie Reynolds and the early Shirley MacLaine vehicle *Ask Any Girl.*

On a more personal level, a note in the Cukor letters file finds the musical veteran complimenting the "prestige" project expert on *Les Girls,* a sophisticated musical made with considerable difficulty due to the director's dislike of his leading lady Mitzi Gaynor and frequent clashes with star Gene Kelly. Assuring Cukor that it was all worth it in the end, Walters signs his note "Madeleine Carroll."[34] That signature is in all likelihood the only example of a "gay subtext" to be found in all of Walters. And the same can be said of other similar talents of the studio era.

Mitchell Leisen, who began his career as a costume designer, was responsible for directing a number of graceful comedies and dramas, including *Midnight* (1939) and *Swing High, Swing Low* (1937). Like William Haines, he was great pal of Carole Lombard's. But he earned the undying enmity of Billy Wilder, who felt the director showed more concern for Claudette Colbert's hemlines than the lines Wilder had given her to speak in *Arise, My Love* (1940).[35] Irving Rapper, a "woman's director" par excellence, was another steady studio hand. Guiding Bette Davis through *Now, Voyager* (1942), *Deception* (1946), and *The Corn Is Green* (1945), he ended his career with two of the strangest independent projects ever made: *The Christine Jorgensen Story* (1970) and *Born Again* (1978), the tale of the alleged spiritual "redemption" of chief Nixon aide and Watergate "plumber" Charles Colson.

Dorothy Arzner was for a while a cause célèbre among feminist film scholars. But to a large degree, their embrace was not unlike that of the studios, who saw a "woman director" as an exploitable novelty and nothing more. While her work is not without interest, particularly her version of George Kelly's *Craig's Wife* (1936) and the Lucille Ball–starred *Dance, Girl, Dance* (1940), the downward course of her career can best be explained by the simple fact that she never recovered after the failure of the Joan Crawford vehicle *The Bride Wore Red* (1937). (*Dance, Girl, Dance* pleased neither critics nor audiences at the time of its release.)

Far more interesting, in terms of more active gay influence, was writer John Van Druten. His adaptation of his play *The Voice of the Turtle* (1947, directed by Irving Rapper) touched ever-so-carefully on promiscuity (thanks to the strictures of the Production Code), evoking much of the sexual freedom of the 1940s that came as a result of the war. While he is most famous for *I Am a Camera*, his 1954 adaptation of Isherwood's *Berlin Stories*, which in turn became the basis for the musical *Cabaret*, his gayest work is unquestionably *Bell, Book and Candle* (1958). No one with any degree of familiarity with post–World War II Greenwich Village life will have any trouble seeing the "witches" and "warlocks" of this romantic fantasy for the gays and lesbians they really are, even in the midst of a purely heterosexual main plot.

But in many ways the most significant gay talent of the studio era wasn't a director, a writer, or an actor, but a choreographer. In the entire history of the studio era, nothing is more blatantly homoerotic than Jack Cole's "Is There Anyone Here for Love" in *Gentlemen Prefer Blondes*. Placing Jane Russell amidst a bevy of musclemen who seem to have stepped right out of a Quaintance drawing, it remains a high-water mark of gay Hollywood outrageousness. Still, this number doesn't represent Cole at his most audacious. That's to be found in his *heterosexual* work. It was Cole who created Rita Hayworth's "Put the Blame on Mame" in *Gilda*, carefully framing and choreographing the simplest gestures so that the removal of one glove has the erotic impact of a full striptease routine. He did similar duties for Marilyn Monroe, not only in her legendary "Heat Wave" number from *There's No Business Like Show Business* but even offering advice for her nonmusical films. In fact, it might be argued that Cole, who won the complete trust and confidence of the emotionally fragile love goddess, was far more important to her work than any of her acting coaches. They could talk "the Method" till the cows came home, but when it came to getting Marilyn to get up from a chair, cross a room, and open a door, Jack Cole was the man to call.[36]

Cole's nonverbal power sits oddly alongside the difficulties verbally dextrous gays have had in Hollywood. While Gore Vidal has had any number of witty and insightful things to say about the movies in his novels *Myra Breckinridge* and *Myron*, his film credits are a mixed bag. His adaptations of works by Paddy Chayevsky (*The Catered Affair*) and Tennessee Williams (*Suddenly, Last Summer*) were first-rate, and his play *The Best Man* (whose plot involves a presidential candidate's gay indiscretion) was transferred to the screen to his liking. The same can't be said of Arthur Penn's 1958 rendition of Vidal's Billy the Kid saga, *The Left-Handed Gun* (which was remade for cable television in 1989 as *Gore Vidal's Billy the Kid*), or such cinematic debacles as the Michael Sarne–directed *Myra Breckinridge* (1970) or the Bob Guccione–confected *Caligula* (1980).

"There were several bungalows around the pool," Vidal writes in his memoirs of his stay at the Beverly Hills Hotel. "Nick Ray lived in one, preparing *Rebel Without a Cause* and rather openly having an affair with the adolescent Sal Mineo, while the sallow Jimmy Dean skulked in and out, unrecognizable behind thick glasses that distorted myopic eyes."[37] It's a passage that leaves one longing for the Hollywood film Vidal might have made.

"Gore was so determined to prove that directors are meaningless, and the writer is the key figure," says Gavin Lambert. "He's not a very good scriptwriter. His books about the movies, *Myra Breckinridge* and *Myron*, are dazzling. But Gore basically despises movies. He's a fan, but he thinks they're inferior. And I don't think you can write a good movie if you think that. I think you've really got to care about the movies to write good ones."

Moreover, in Lambert's view, Christopher Isherwood had the same problem. "I don't think Isherwood is in that way a typical Hollywood figure. He always lived his own life. He was always Christopher Isherwood. He was *occasionally* a screenwriter. I think he was chagrined that he never became a great Hollywood screenwriter, because he wanted to be, but it never happened. His one original was disastrously miscast, with a bad director—*Diane*. The script was probably a lot better than it seemed to be, but what appeared on the screen was pretty dreadful."[38]

Isherwood in all likelihood agreed, particularly in light of the struggle he had to get this historical romance about fabled courtesan Diane de Poitiers up on screen in spite of the Breen office, which claimed the film condoned adultery. "Although the office representative kept protesting that they were only explaining the workings of the code," Isherwood complains in his *Diaries*, "you could fairly smell their black pornographic Catholic spite. If they had it their way, adultery would be punished by stoning, and homosexuality by being burned alive." Still, he couldn't have been entirely surprised by industry attitudes in 1955, for in 1942 he recounts a conversation he had with screenwriter Lesser Samuels, who complained that a producer had called a scene he had written "faggoty" just because it depicted an older man giving counsel to a college youth.[39]

Arthur Laurents, by contrast, had a smoother overall career. This was partly due to the fact that the bulk of his fame rested on such theatrical triumphs as *Gypsy* and *West Side Story*, but also due to the fact that most of his Hollywood films were made as independent productions. Laurents (who served alongside George Cukor in the Signal Corps, where he wrote and Cukor directed a short entitled *Resistance and Ohm's Law*) first gained notice for the Max Ophuls film *Caught* (1948), the sharpest film à clef ever made about Howard Hughes. Laurents's play about wartime anti-Semitism, *Home of the Brave*, was successfully reconfigured in 1949 by Carl Foreman as one of Hollywood's first serious explorations of antiblack racism. David Lean's *Summertime* (1955), a film of Laurents's play about a lonely spinster, *Time of the Cuckoo*, was likewise memorable, thanks to its star Katharine Hepburn. In fact, Laurents's most conventional film of the studio era might be said to be *Anastasia* (1955), which brought Ingrid Bergman back to Hollywood after the "disgrace" of her alliance with Roberto Rossellini—the biggest heterosexual scandal the town had ever known. As if that weren't enough to fill out a résumé, Laurents hit the jackpot yet again in the 1970s with his scripts for *The Way We Were* (1973) and *The Turning Point* (1977). But in gay terms, these all pale next to *Rope*, his greatly revamped version of Patrick Hamilton's play, directed by Alfred Hitchcock in 1948.

Inspired by the Leopold and Loeb murder case, this story of two New York sophisticates who murder a friend for the sheer thrill of it has been talked about more for its mobile camera technique than for its content—which isn't surprising, considering how explosive that content is. The dialogue clearly indicates a complex series of gay relationships, with women assuming the role of "beards." As might be expected of any such film made during this period, same-sexuality never became a topic of discussion among the filmmakers or the principal players—even though John Dall was gay, and Farley Granger was having an affair with Laurents at the time. *Rope* captures the atmosphere of the city's upper-crust gay world in a way that wouldn't be seen again until *The Boys in the Band*. And *Boys*, when brought to the screen in 1971, was an independent, off-Hollywood production.

"In 1962 I sold a script to Fox," *Boys* author Mart Crowley recalls. "I had read a novel that had been sent to my friend Natalie Wood to see if she were interested in it so a deal could be set up at a studio. It was called *Cassandra at the Wedding* by Dorothy Baker.

I sat down and wrote the script from that novel and never even told Natalie about it. Dorothy Baker was most famous for *Young Man with a Horn*. Even though she was married and had children, she was obviously a woman who had some sexual conflicts that were reflected in her writing—namely the Lauren Bacall character in *Young Man with a Horn*, who couldn't decide whether she liked men or women. Baker had written a play called *Trio* which was a homosexual/heterosexual triangle. It was one of the first things that Richard Widmark starred in—in 1947, on Broadway, for about ten minutes. It was fairly shocking. It was two women and one man, of course, not two men and one woman. But that's what Dorothy Baker was interested in: women. So there was this novel, *Cassandra at the Wedding*, which again was about a triangle. This time it was two girls who were identical twins and one man that one girl falls in love with and gets engaged to and is about to marry and her sister who identifies so strongly that she's about to go berserk because her sister is "leaving" her, abandoning her by marrying this man. And she tries to break up the wedding and comes to realize in the process that she's a lesbian. The last scene of it takes place on the Golden Gate bridge, in which I think she sees a sort of male-identified woman who's been appearing throughout the story who is a painter. She runs into her and it's like Alice Adams walking up those stairs to typing school at the end of that novel. You don't know whether she's going to jump off the bridge or go find this girl and get real. So had it been made, it would have had two Natalie Woods—one of them a gay Natalie Wood. That would have been something for that time. In fact, when they were thinking of doing it, every overt reference as to what was really going on with that character was constantly excised from the script. We had a not too subtle phrase: dykeism . . . 'You gotta get rid of the dykeisms in this scene.' And we would roar with laughter even then, Martin Manulis, the producer, and I. I don't know who first called it 'the dykeisms.' Maybe Darryl Zanuck."[40]

But that was the sixties. In the years soon to come, the "dykeisms" could no longer be ignored.

F O U R

IT'S A SCANDAL!

———

TRANSCRIPT OF DOCKET (CRIMINAL) CASE NO. C-9848. Defendant in Court having been duly arraigned for judgement and there being no legal cause why sentence should not be pronounced. Whereupon it is so ordered and adjudged by the Court this 2-6-51 that for said offense of Violation of Section 415, Penal Code, the said ARTHUR ANDREW GELIEN be imprisoned in the County Jail of the Court of Los Angeles for the term of 30 days and the said defendant be discharged at the expiration of said term. It is further ordered that the ex-

ecution of sentence be suspended and that the defendant
be placed on summary probation for 1 year subject to the
following terms of probation. Pay $50.00 through Court.
Stay granted until 2-7-51, 4 PM. Obey all laws for period
of probation. See C-8063.

So reads the document reproduced at the bottom of page 18 of
the September 1955 issue of *Confidential* magazine. In a way this
transcript, with its skillfully "torn" edge, is an illustration, much like
the photograph that accompanies it of the defendant in question,
known to the world then as now as Tab Hunter. But this excerpt from
a legal filing is more important than any "paparazzi" snapshot, and
far more telling than the article itself. For while *Confidential* made
its name by turning its back on Hollywood PR *politesse* and running
with whatever it could unearth about stars and celebrities—the more
"outrageous," the better—it relied for the most part on sources viewed
by traditional journalists as "unverifiable": waiters, hat-check girls,
bouncers, bellhops, private eyes, and prostitutes of both sexes. This
was very different. For gossip, however juicy, is as nothing compared
to an actual legal filing certifying that an arrest had been made and
a judgment rendered on a performer whose wholesome appearance
was being flashed across every media outlet then in operation.

"Disorderly Conduct Charge Against Tab Hunter" relates in
Confidential's inimitably smarmy style "the real lowdown" that the
"build-up boys thought was safely locked in the records of the Los
Angeles County vice squad confidential file Z-84254. It is the racy
story of a night in October, 1950, when the husky Hunter kid landed
in jail, along with some 26 other good-looking young men, after the
cops broke up a pajama party they staged—strictly for the boys."
Going on to detail how an LAPD vice officer, while "drifting in and
out of Hollywood's gay bars . . . looking and listening for tips on the
newest notions of the limp-wristed lads," learned from "a couple of
lispers" about "a big binge that very evening, at 2501 Hope Street in
Walnut Park, a suburb of Los Angeles," the piece makes special note
that "there was only one dashing requirement—bring pajamas." It
then goes on to disclose how the police detective "and his pals" ar-

rived at the party around ten-thirty that evening, and "after watching the strange goings-on" for about a half an hour, said officer walked to a window, "quietly signaled outside and a few minutes later the whole party was under arrest."

The charge was violating California's Penal Code, Section 647.5, which calls for the incarceration of "idle, lewd or dissolute persons or associates of known thieves." In other words, as the partygoers weren't caught *in flagrante delicto,* "sodomy" charges were out of the question. So they were booked on the next-best thing: the "idle, lewd or dissolute" statute, which dealt with outward appearance and its implied intent to commit an illegal sexual act. Vaguer than any sodomy statute, it's no wonder that this charge was knocked down to simple "disorderly conduct." And as Gelien had no previous criminal record, a fifty-dollar wrist-slapping was about as far as any reasonable judicial authority would be willing to go. *Confidential,* however, could go the distance, journalistically speaking. For while in 1950 "there were no big names in the catch, so far as the cops could tell," the magazine knew in 1955 that Gelien was a major haul. For as Tab Hunter, Arthur Andrew Gelien was in the midst of publicizing *Battle Cry*—a World War II drama in which same-sex "pajama parties" play no part. As the events of 1950–51 were a matter of public record, the magazine had a perfect right to print them. In fact, so emboldened was it by this state of affairs that *Confidential* felt free not only to provide colorfully confected details of the "bust," but also Gelien/Hunter's age, birthdate, and Social Security number.[1]

This wasn't Louella Parsons raising a decorous eyebrow over William Haines's offscreen obstreperousness. It wasn't Earl Wilson signaling between the lines that he knew perfectly well that Rock Hudson's "dates" were for display purposes only. It wasn't even *Confidential*'s usual sort of sneering at the effeminacy of Johnnie Ray, Noël Coward, or Liberace. Tab Hunter wasn't a soigné sophisticate; he was the boy-next-door. And, according to conventional wisdom, the revelation that the boy-next-door desired the company of other boys-next-door should have brought about the immediate cessation of the young actor's career. That did not happen. Tab Hunter continued to work at Warner Bros., appearing in "A"-quality releases for that studio and others, including *Lafayette Escadrille, Damn Yankees, That Kind of Woman, They Came to Cordura,* and *The Pleasure of His Company*. By the mid-1960s, Hunter's teen-idol days, and his Warner Bros. contract, had come to an end. But the "pajama party" can't be said to have played a role in bringing about their conclusion. He'd had his run, and that was that.

Like most performers of his era and acting caliber, Hunter has continued to work intermittently in film, television, and theater. Unlike most others, however, Hunter has found a niche of sorts in independent film, appearing to considerable comic effect in John Waters's *Polyester* (1981) and Paul Bartel's *Lust in the Dust* (1985), co-starring on both occasions with the transvestite comedian Divine. He has never discussed his sexuality, and outside of a 1974 profile by Warhol acolyte Brigid Berlin for *Interview* magazine, he has allowed the "pajama party" episode to vanish into the ozone of Hollywood lore.

"Do you want to hear the true story on that?" Hunter asks Berlin.

> I was getting kicked out of the service for being under age. A friend of mine asked me if I wanted to go to a party, and I said "fine." So we drove to the party and I walk in and I thought, Oh shit! It's a bunch of *frrruitas* [sic] doing their number. When I say doing their number I mean—they were dancing but there were more than two women dressed in mannish attire. There were guys and gals and they were dancing and you know . . . and I thought what a bore! Smoke filled rooms—and I'd seen all that when I was fourteen years old. So I really didn't care to see it. So I walked to the refrigerator and opened it up because I was always hungry. And I started to fix myself a peanut butter sandwich and in walked the cops. But there was nothing wrong. I mean there wasn't a pajama party. There wasn't any of that shit.

In other words, it was just a dance party—much along the lines of the one John Rechy attended in the Hollywood Hills. Consequently, there was a level at which it wasn't all that difficult to deal with from a public-relations standpoint. *Nothing happened.* It was nothing at all like pop star George Michael's arrest for "lewd conduct" in a Beverly Hills restroom forty-eight years later. But an arrest is still an arrest. And when same-sex relations are involved, it's quite a bit more than that. Hunter, however, had Warner Bros. on his side.

"Actually, two nice things happened from that magazine," Hunter recalls in his *Interview* interview:

> One, I met Harry Weiss who was an attorney out on the West Coast. Really a delightful man. The second thing was when I won the "Audience Award" for being the most popular piece of crap since I don't know when. We were all standing there. *Time* and *Look*'s light bulbs were flashing like mad, and one guy said 'Smile pretty Tab, this is for *Confidential*!' I said 'Oh shit!' and I threw up my arms and started to turn around and the nicest thing Jack Warner ever said to me as he threw his arms around me, he said 'That's ok! Today's headlines, tomorrow's toilet paper.' People live in all kinds of . . . you know—they try to put in their own inferences, you know—to say this and that—and it's boring.[2]

But one would be hard-pressed to find anything *less* boring than Tab Hunter being arrested at a gay house party, be it 1951, 1955, 1974, or even now in the wake of George Michael. To Berlin, Hunter manages to convey an aura of world-weariness with no small amount of skill ("I'd seen all that when I was 14 years old") while at the same time cleverly conflating his publicity chores for *Battle Cry* ("Smile pretty Tab") with what happened on the night of the arrest, where no cameras were present (the shot of Hunter used to illustrate the *Confidential* article was a typical freelance publicity snap). His mention of lawyer Harry Weiss and studio head Jack Warner in practically the same breath speaks to the behind-the-scenes maneuvering that was going on at the time. The decision was that Warner Bros. would say nothing and ride out the storm. It was the only logical choice.

By the time *Battle Cry* was released, the studio had already invested an enormous amount of time and money in making a star of Tab Hunter. It was in no mood to simply kiss it all goodbye. Hunter wasn't a featured or supporting player like Sheila James Kuehl, whose success as Zelda Gilroy on the *Many Loves of Dobie Gillis* television series inspired plans for a show of her own, which were scotched when the network brass found her "just a little too butch."[3] He wasn't a marginal performer on the cusp of a break, like Tucker Smith, whose turn as Ice in *West Side Story* was expected to jump-start a larger career had his "private life" (exposed in a columnist's "blind item") not supplied casting directors with a reason to give him the go-by.

Tab Hunter was well past all that. More important, he was more than willing to hold up his end of the deal. His dates with women were a well-established publicity spectacle, and he obviously wasn't about to RSVP to any future "pajama party" invitations. The "legitimate" press was no threat. Fear of losing favor with the studio—and thereby access to any number of stars—kept it from launching a similar investigation into Hunter's past, or making note of anything less than conventional about his situation circa 1955. Consequently, for all its sensational potential, the actual impact of *Confidential*'s "pajama party" story was minimal.

"The thing you've got to remember about *Confidential*," Gavin Lambert notes today, "is that it was quite different from Parsons and Hopper in that it wasn't read by nearly so many people. The 'pajama party' story *became* famous later on, but at the time it appeared *Confidential* wasn't part of the national press. It was really a local rag. Warner Bros. probably said the story was unfortunate, but it's not *The New York Times* or a Hearst paper. Say nothing and let it cool off. And this was because it wasn't seen as breaking on a national level. That would be the acid test now. If the equivalent of that story were blasted across the papers and was on the TV news it would be different. Nowadays gay bars aren't raided that much. Supposing a few years back a major star had been caught in a gay bar raid. Well, all the newspapers across the land could report that he was in that bar."[4]

Whether they *would*, even today, is open to question. And it's doubtful that any current journal would run with such a story as aggressively as *Confidential*. After all, the Walnut Park "pajama party" didn't take place at a gay bar, but rather at a private home. Exactly how "private" it really was, in police terms, can be gauged from the fact that all it took to incite an arrest was for one partygoer to show the slightest sign of affection toward another of the same sex. So how did pajamas fit into the picture? *Confidential* had to work a sex angle in there somewhere.

"He hasn't a steady girl friend, and he claims he has no preferences in girls. ('I like blondes, brunettes, red-heads, and in-between shades.') He used to date Marilyn Erskine and Debbie Reynolds. Now he dates Lori Nelson and Dorothy Malone," says Hollywood scribe Sidney Skolsky in a column that appeared the same year as the *Confidential* broadside.[5] Starlets Mary Ann Mobley and Venetia Stevenson were also cited as Hunter escorts in profiles that ran around the same time. So effective were these heterosexual dates, they helped provide cover for an affair with Anthony Perkins that took place around the same period.[6]

The only cloud on the horizon appeared—once again—courtesy of *Confidential*. During the magazine's 1957 trial for conspiracy to publish libel and obscenities, Arthur Crowley, attorney for *Confidential*'s "West Coast representatives," Fred and Marjorie Mead, subpoenaed Hunter in order to ask "the blond-haired actor-idol of teenagers . . . whether the article about him was true."[7] Hunter was never called. Had he been, the trial could have opened his "private life" to full public view. But by 1957 it was *Confidential*, not Tab Hunter, that was on the ropes and fighting for its life. Why it had managed to flourish so brightly—if briefly—sheds more light on Hollywood itself than on the motley crew of tabloid journalists, disgruntled press agents, and unscrupulous private eyes that made it all possible.

"The Hollywood press hacks have been doing the dirty work

for the big boys for years and, as the scavengers and jackals of Hollywood, have been happy to feed on the leavings. In a multi-million dollar racket, the pathetic press has been content to be purchased for pennies," veteran entertainment reporter Ezra Goodman claims in his 1961 analysis of the *Confidential* era. Noting that "MGM once forbade mentioning that Norma Shearer had two children and that Robert Montgomery was a father," Goodman describes the Hollywood of the mid-fifties as being both fearful of, yet not-so-secretly delighted by a publication that, while scarcely a beacon of truth, was refreshingly resistant to the carloads of lies the "legitimate" press was required to peddle.[8] In his biography of gossip monger Walter Winchell, film historian Neal Gabler claims that by the mid-thirties "studio chiefs issued an informal edict compelling writers to submit their stories to the studios for approval. Newspapers and magazines complied on a threat of losing movie advertising."[9] But as any journalist who has worked the entertainment beat of any era is well aware, no studio-enforced "edict" is required to keep the press in line. It functions solely at the discretion of the stars' managers, publicists, and press agents, who are capable of denying informational access at a moment's notice.

In 1935, when Loretta Young became pregnant by Clark Gable during the shooting of *Call of the Wild,* she had no end of assistance in finessing the situation. "Only a few have long known that one of the sweet, pure and demure mothered a child out of wedlock and later went through the motions of publically adopting the infant," wrote Louella Parsons as a "blind item" in her memoirs several decades afterward.[10] But the great gossip maven was exaggerating, for as the daughter in question discovered when *she* learned the truth (from her husband on their wedding night, no less), most of Hollywood had known for years—and said nothing.[11]

In protecting Loretta, Hollywood was protecting itself. Like several other actresses whose careers first blossomed in the 1930s (Barbara Stanwyck among them), Young had gone from sensational sex melodramas like *Employees' Entrance* to more demure romantic fare. And as Hollywood had learned from the scandals at the end of the silent era, onscreen images worked best when matched to offscreen ones. It's an attitude that Young would come to adopt with a vengeance. But the simple fact for her, or any star of her caliber, was that there was no way in 1935 for an out-of-wedlock pregnancy to be viewed as anything less than a career disaster. For that very reason, MGM had an abortion provider on staff. Known within industry circles, this fact was never noted even by the "scandal" press.[12] Still, Hollywood "tolerance" had its limits. For in 1949, when, during the shooting of the film *Stromboli,* Ingrid Bergman became pregnant by director Roberto Rossellini—while still legally married to estranged husband Petter Lindstrom—it caused a nationwide uproar.

"Oh, I can't tell you how big that was," journalist Kevin Thomas recalls. "It's hard today to imagine all that now, but she was a world-famous movie star. It was devastating. It was like a nuclear bomb to American society. It's very hard to convey to today's world the impact of that scandal. She was denounced on the floor of Congress. People could never get that upset today."[12] Indeed, with Madonna siring a child by a fitness trainer with whom she's no longer romantically involved; Michael Jackson arranging the impregnation of his plastic surgeon's office assistant prior to marrying her, while continuing to "date" his ex-wife, Lisa Marie Presley; actors Uma Thurman and Ethan Hawke formally announcing their expectation of issue, prior to marriage; and the not only unmarried but heterosexually unlinked Jodie Foster disclosing her pregnancy while pointedly declining to discuss "the father, the method or anything of that nature,"[13] the landscape of "scandal" has changed radically, at least as far as childbirth is concerned.

In a way, Ingrid Bergman wasn't "punished" for getting pregnant out of wedlock but rather for doing so outside the aegis of Hollywood. By making a low-budget independent film with a foreign director at the height of her career, she had broken with the studios—and the Loretta Young–styled protection they might have provided—in a highly dramatic way. Her films with Rossellini, while inspiring a new generation of European writer-directors that included Michelangelo Antonioni, Jean-Luc Godard, and Eric Rohmer, were dismissed as technically incompetent by an American press in thrall to Hollywood. No better example of this can be found than in *Daily*

Variety taking the unprecedented step of first proclaiming *Stromboli* "a peak in artistic triumphs," only to reverse itself one month later by declaring that it "reflects no credit on [Rossellini] from a creative or any other point of view."[14] Bergman's subsequent films with the director, whom she had by then married, were likewise dismissed in America. When she "came to heel"—divorcing Rossellini, returning to Hollywood, and making the thoroughly conventional romantic melodrama *Anastasia*—Bergman was "forgiven" by the fourth estate with laudatory reviews, and by the industry with an Academy Award. Clearly her "crime" wasn't against public "morality" but against Hollywood hegemony. The "scandal" of Bergman's pregnancy, breathlessly broadcast by Louella Parsons as an "exclusive," had, in fact, nothing "exclusive" about it. For as any truly conscientious reader knew, the French and Italian papers had made note of Bergman's pregnancy months in advance. Yet so culturally powerful was the U.S. press at the time that only the acknowledgement of an "official" American source could make this simple fact a reality.

"Parsons could have gotten the story anywhere," says Gavin Lambert, "but she was apparently encouraged by Howard Hughes to run with it the way she did because of the contract that Bergman had signed. Hughes put up money for *Stromboli* on condition that she would do a project for him. So when she did *Stromboli* and it bombed, he said, 'You owe me this picture.' She said, 'I can't make it, I'm pregnant.' And *that's* when he said to Parsons, 'Get her.' The fact that Rossellini was a foreigner was very important to the way that story was played."[15]

Indeed, American xenophobia was exploited by the "scandal"— even though the star in question was Swedish. The image of the sexually rapacious foreigner had been a mainstay of Hollywood ever since DeMille's 1914 potboiler *The Cheat*, in which a soigné Sessue Hayakawa tempted a coquettish Fannie Ward. At the time of the Bergman affair, international "playboys," particularly those of Latin American extraction, had begun to make for sensational copy once again, as Paris and Rome provided a new stage for "outrageous" behavior for the entertainment of an allegedly "moral" American middle class. In the end, Bergman and Rossellini unwittingly opened a crack in a door that Hollywood press agentry had long thought sealed shut. It was only a matter of time before someone would try to push that crack wide open. And that, in fact, was *Confidential*'s mandate.

First appearing in 1952, *Confidential* was in many ways an inevitable offshoot of post–World War II crime magazines, whose lurid coverage of sex and violence went verbally beyond the visual excesses of the urban tabloid press. Its publisher, Robert Harrison, got his start writing for motion-picture trade papers before moving on to the likes of *Wink*, *Titter*, and *Flirt*, while the magazine's editor, Al Covoni, began his career at *True Detective*. Together they provided an irresistible combination of pseudosophistication and cheap thrills. Supposedly inspired by the Kefauver hearings on organized crime, *Confidential* strove to provide common gossip with the patina of serious investigative reporting.[16] At the same time, it tried to create the sense that it was part of the established Hollywood community. That was accomplished through those "West Coast representatives," Fred and Marjorie Mead—a couple who, according to Ezra Goodman, "lived conspicuously in a lavish Beverly Hills home and were *persona grata* at many a movietown gathering." While the Meads smoothed the way socially, *Confidential* went about behind the scenes, scooping up the "dirt" from the expected sources, and even a few unexpected ones, including (according to Goodman), "one of the leading 'male' gossipists in Hollywood," pumped for information by means of "an unpublished story about this columnist's amorous activities [the magazine held] as a journalistic sword over his head." In fact, the entire magazine was a quasi-blackmail operation. Like a bargain-basement private eye working to "get the goods" on a spouse in a divorce case, *Confidential* would set about putting together a dossier on a carefully targeted star. Once it was assembled, part of the story might be run— with the rest held back in the hopes of monetary reward. In some cases the studio was approached at the start—and would cooperate.

"Twentieth Century–Fox," Goodman claims, "funneled a yarn about Marilyn Monroe, with whom it was then at odds, to *Rave* [a *Confidential* rival] in order to get that magazine to drop a story about a sensational triangle involving one of the studio's top executives. *Confidential* ran a story about Universal-International actor Rory Calhoun's jail record for robbery, conveniently provided by the studio, in exchange for the magazine's eliminating a story about the homosexual activities of a more important U-I star."[17]

Still, "Rory Calhoun: But for the Grace of God, Still a Convict," which ran in *Confidential*'s May 1955 issue, was small potatoes compared to what might have been run about Rock Hudson, had *Confidential* felt free to run it. Consequently, if the Calhoun story constituted a trade-off, it was scarcely an even one. Another legend about the magazine's editorial silence on Rock has it that a Hudson exposé was put aside in favor of one about his (purely platonic) friend George Nader. But Nader, whose career never rose to Hudsonian levels, wasn't broadsided by *Confidential*. A formal blackmail payment would be the only logical explanation for the magazine holding back on Hudson. But most of those connected with either *Confidential* or Universal-International have long passed from the scene, and those who remain are as loath to comment on anything pertaining to same-sexuality as any onscreen performer of that era.

In the end *Confidential* was brought down by legal means—a series of increasingly expensive lawsuits. Actress Dorothy Dandridge was the first to fight back, winning an out-of-court settlement of $10,000 over an article in the May 1957 issue, purporting to tell what she "did in the woods" with men of various races.[18] Liberace did even better, garnering $40,000 in a suit over a July 1957 piece, "Why Liberace's Theme Song Should Be 'Mad About the Boy,' " by proving he wasn't in Dallas, Texas, at the time the actions in the story purportedly took place—and cleverly avoiding pointed questions about the truth of his sexual life in the process.[19] The grand finale came in October 1957 in a more broadly based claim brought by the state of California charging conspiracy to commit libel and distribute pornography. After what Ezra Goodman described as "two months of blaring headlines, more than 2,000 pages of lurid testimony and a record fourteen days of jury deadlock," charges were dropped, and *Confidential* "announced that it would adopt a new editorial format minus stories about the private lives of celebrities."[20] It died a quick death shortly afterwards.

Overall, the record of *Confidential* and its imitators on dealing with gay Hollywood is a curious one. Like Tab Hunter, singer Johnnie Ray became an easy target because of his vice arrest records.[21] Noël Coward earned sneering broadsides ("Noel Coward: Las Vegas' Queerest Hit," *Revealed*, November 1955; "When Johnnie Ray Was Noel Coward's Houseguest," *Top Secret*, August 1957) for being foreign, effete, and distanced from the middle classes. Likewise, the sapphic dalliances of Marlene Dietrich ("The Untold Story of Marlene Dietrich," *Confidential*, July 1955) and Greta Garbo ("Greta Garbo's Gay Love Life," *Uncensored*, May 1956) scarcely upset "front porch" America. But one would look long and hard to find stories suggesting a top star like Tyrone Power or Barbara Stanwyck was other than heterosexual. And even the stories run on the far-from-"mainstream" Montgomery Clift centered on his personal quirks and obsessive friendship with singer Libby Holman ("Montgomery Clift's Odd Sex Secret," *Exclusive*, November 1955; "Monty Clift's Strange Obsession," *Inside*, February 1957; "Montgomery Clift's Weird Compulsions," *Suppressed*, June 1957), rather than his affair with actor Jack Larson, who at the time was playing Jimmie Olsen on the *Superman* television series.[22] In fact, for all their supposed sophistication, the "scandal" rags were painfully naive when it came to same-sex matters, running such decidedly unshocking stuff as "Whoops! Why Those Gay Boys Just Love Bette, Joan, Tallulah and Judy!" in the July 1964 issue of *Inside Story*, and " 'I'm No Pansy' Says Warren Beatty," in the May 1962 issue of *Whisper*.

In 1964, the same publication ran a roundup piece on "Homosexuality in Hollywood" in its November issue. Declaring that "the gay guys and dolls have become the real rulers of this make-believe empire," *Whisper* stage-whispered that "the queer coup was so swift and silent that hardly anyone outside the industry realized what was happening." Feigning editorial seriousness, the magazine claimed it "decided to withhold names—not to protect the Purple-People-Eaters involved—but to give the motion picture industry a chance to take a good hard look at the situation as it is today." In other words, in light of the *Confidential* fiasco, "blind items" would be the rule of the day.

The "tall dark and handsome [actor] with broad shoulders and a dimpled chin" the article identifies as "Case A" was obviously Rock

Hudson. But "Case C," who "prefers sweatshirts and jeans to suits and ties," could be any number of performers in the James Dean/ Marlon Brando mode. Likewise, generic were remarks pertaining to an actor whose studio "had doubts about his manhood" and consequently lived "in constant fear that a certain photo will achieve widespread circulation. . . . This candid snapshot shows the world-famous star performing an intimate act—with another male." Tales of a husband-and-wife team who shared the favors of a male "Hollywood newcomer" and a "perennial girl-next-door-type" could fill several bills. But "Case H," a "former movie villain who became the hero of a long-running TV series, this portly actor," was plainly Raymond Burr.[23]

If anyone objected to any of this, they kept it to themselves. Nineteen sixty-four marked a relatively quiet period on the "scandal" front. The likes of *Whisper* were not long for this world. The use of blind items for mentions of "shocking" same-sex activity was standard practice by then for columnists in supposedly "respectable" journals. The Stonewall uprising, and the re-emergence of the gay and lesbian civil rights movement that came in its wake, was a full five years away, and its effect on Hollywood, and the rest of the country, unfelt for at least another seven or so after that. Yet the impact of what the "scandal" press did in its heyday—and the contrast it made with the rest of the press—is still recalled every time same-sex issues are put in the spotlight.

"You know the Robert Mitchum story where he's hanging out with Charles Laughton and Laughton's boyfriend, and he's bombed out of his mind?" asks James Ellroy, a devoted scandal-rag aficionado. "This is '54, '55, when they're doing *Night of the Hunter*. It's a lunch break, and Mitchum pours ketchup on his dick and says, 'Which one of you fags wants to eat this?' The way it got written up was with him being at a party throwing ketchup on himself and saying 'I'm a hamburger.' It's not quite the same thing."

Ellroy learned the true story of Mitchum's prank from Fred Otash, the man who served as *Confidential*'s "private eye" on the sex lives of the stars, and who was both the inspiration and information source for any number of aspects of Ellroy novels of the "scandal" era, *L.A. Confidential*, and *Hollywood Nocturnes*. "Freddie was this Lebanese guy who was a leg breaker for the LAPD from '45 to '55. He was a marine drill sergeant during World War II, and came on the LAPD right after the war," recalls Ellroy, whose outward appearance suggests a mild-mannered certified public accountant, but whose language is redolent of the "hardboiled" detectives and "cynical" journalists of the 1940s.

"When William Wharton took over stewardship of the LAPD prior to William Parker taking over in 1950, he formed a goon squad of ex-marines to take care of organized crime figures: take 'em off the bus, airplane, train, beat the shit out of 'em, and put 'em back on. Otash was one of those guys. He was Anita Ekberg's boyfriend in the early 1950s, before she got fat. He was a big, good-looking guy— swarthy, dark-haired. Some people wanted to make him a movie star. But he was *so* homophobic—so convinced that everyone in Hollywood, all the producers, all the directors, were 'homos'—that he wouldn't go for it, despite the promises of big money.

"At some point, and it's ambiguous—Freddie and I were working around to the topic when he died—he started doing favors for people in Hollywood. You needed to get your girlfriend an abortion? Freddie's the guy. You needed to get a drunk-and-disorderly charge dropped? Freddie's the guy. You needed to break up a squeeze on a gay actor? Freddie's the guy. Now, Freddie was a big homophobe— an outrageous homophobe. This is my Freddie Otash: 'Rah, rah, rah, rah, rah, fags, niggers, Jews, rah, rah, rah, rah, rah.' 'Hey, Freddie, tell me about Ava Gardner.' 'Rah, rah, rah, I fucked her. She said I was the best, rah, rah, rah, rah, rah, fags, niggers, Jews.' 'Hey, Freddie, tell me about Jayne Mansfield.' 'Rah, rah, rah, rah, I fucked her. She said I was the best, rah, rah, rah, rah, fags, niggers, Jews.' 'Hey, Freddie, what about Marilyn Monroe?' 'Rah, rah, rah, I didn't fuck her. She must have been a dyke!'

"I know that Freddie was involved in a shakedown during a strike," Ellroy continues. "One of Universal's biggest stars was getting fifty thousand dollars a week, and they wanted to violate his contract. Essentially Freddie was supposed to put him in bed with an actress who he'd wanted to ram for a long time. The actress ratted Freddie off to the star. That's the kind of thing Freddie did. Freddie was the guy you went to if you wanted a picture of Rock Hudson with a dick in his mouth."[24]

Rock Hudson, in point of fact, makes an appearance in Otash's 1976 memoir, *Investigation: Hollywood,* as an unidentified "Mr. Star," whose wife is upset that he has returned from a European film shoot with a male lover in tow. The dialogue of the chapter, coyly entitled "Homosexuals Are Also Movie Stars," can be found as well in Phyllis Gates's 1987 memoir of her marriage to a man whose sexual orientation was clearly obvious to her, despite her protestations to the contrary.[25]

"What's funny about that dialogue," Ellroy continues, "is that Rock had come to Freddie six months earlier about that kid, 'cause he'd brought him back from Italy after doing *A Farewell to Arms.* The kid was making demands and Freddie roughed him up. He had his green card revoked and put him back on the airplane. Those are the kinds of favors Freddie did people in Hollywood. Freddie used to be the security boss at the infamous Hollywood Ranch Market over there on Fountain and Vine, where my father took me in the month preceding my mother's murder to explain to me what homosexuals were. He said any man who wore lacquered sunglasses was a homo, 'cause he could check out your crotch bulge covertly without lowering his eyes. And I believed him for many, many years! My father told me that if anybody grabbed my *schvantz* I was supposed to kick 'em in the nuts and run like hell. Anyway, Freddie busted James Dean for shoplifting at the Hollywood Ranch Market in '54—and James Dean became a snitch for him!

"After Freddie walked from the LAPD after only ten years—he hated the chief, William Parker—he got a private eye's license. Freddie became a guy in charge of verifying stories for *Confidential.* The thing about *Confidential* is, it had the run that it had 'cause everything in *Confidential* was true. I think a lot of these studio people just paid Freddie individually. Freddie left a multi-million-dollar estate. I think somebody slipped Freddie five or ten G's, you know?"

How Otash operated in and around gay Hollywood while spewing his hatred of same-sexuality to anyone who'd listen is an irony

Ellroy finds especially fascinating. "I think a lot of this came down to how Freddie Otash felt on a good day. I went to lunch with Freddie at Jocks restaurant six months before he died—he was having a heart attack and called a cab instead of an ambulance, and that did it for him. Anyway, I'd come into Jocks with my French publisher—a very elegant guy, very well-mannered. When we walked in we notice there's an elderly gay couple sitting nearby. As soon as Freddie walks in, they spot him, and act like they're going to throw up right there. Then Freddie points them out and starts in on his usual bit, real loud: 'Yeah, I busted a fag cathouse over on Havenhurst. I was on a door operation with the Sheriff's back in '51. I popped those two old queens. Rah, rah, rah.' My editor is this very sensitive man, and he's just recoiling from this tidal wave of slime washing over the table from Freddie. So finally one of the gay guys comes over as he and his buddy are walking out and he says, 'Well, Freddie, you're looking *svelte* today.' And Freddie goes, very softly, 'Yeah, yeah.'

"You see, *that's* what's interesting about Freddie," Ellroy says excitedly. "He would talk that 'rah, rah' stuff, but if a homosexual sat down at the table he'd be very respectful. And I think a *lot* of people in Hollywood are that way."[26]

The "scandals" that for a decade were the personal property of *Confidential* and its ilk are part of the "mainstream" landscape today. No one need sneak off to a specialized newsstand when the exploits of a Woody Allen, Marv Albert, Frank Gifford, Charlie Sheen, Christian Slater, Robert Downey Jr., and "Hollywood Madam" Heidi Fleiss are featured items on round-the-clock televised news. In recent years the town's supposed corner on behavioral licentiousness has been put well into the shade by Washington, D.C. Congressman Wilbur Mills's affair with stripper Fanne Foxe and the dalliances of Congressman Richard Jenrette's wife, Rita, which won headlines in the 1970s, seem almost innocent today. Anita Hill's sexual harassment charges against Judge (and now Supreme Court Justice) Clarence Thomas, the tabloid scandal provided by former presidential advisor Dick Morris (who has both a call girl and a common-law wife and offspring to contend with, along with his legal one), and President William Jefferson Clinton himself (a one-man soap opera of charges and countercharges on extramarital affairs, presided over by a "special prosecutor" possessed of blatantly partisan political interests) have turned the nation's capital into a gigantic peep show. Against the backdrop of such heterosexual licentiousness, same-sexuality has taken a back seat. Congressman Barney Frank's involvement with a call boy and Congressman Gerry Studds's affair with a Senate page failed to register in the 1980s as they would have in an earlier time, largely because of the fact that the gay and lesbian civil rights movement had brought same-sex issues onto the public stage as never before. But the lives of public officials are one thing; those of stars and "celebrities" are another. And in the early part of the 1990s "revelations" of gay and lesbian life have found themselves reconfigured as a political weapon of sorts.

Spurred partially out of frustration at garnering support to fight the AIDS epidemic, and partially out of long-standing resentment against the special privileges enjoyed by the gay and lesbian "rich and famous," a series of interviews by novelist Armistead Maupin and columns by journalist and AIDS activist Michelangelo Signorile mushroomed into a wide-ranging debate in both the gay and straight press. At issue was whether the "private lives" of David Geffen, Barry Diller, Jodie Foster, and other Hollywood luminaries should remain veiled by a fourth estate long conditioned to disregard evidence of same-sex orientation even when it was unfolding right before its eyes.[27] The "mainstream" press was, needless to say, "outraged" at the thought of such wholesale candor. And so were any number of gays and lesbians whose lifestyles had nothing rich or famous about them. For many, thinking about the "exposure" of a well-known personality evoked memories of their own fears of being called a "fag" or a "dyke." There was, in short, a sense of solidarity on the part of the gay and lesbian masses with same-sex-oriented stars. The problem was, such feelings went largely unreciprocated.

"Some say 'outing' should be used against the homophobic or hypocritical," gay entertainment journalist Michael Musto noted. "Well, practically everyone who's been outed *is* homophobic or hy-

pocritical. They all seem to have phony hetero relationships or promote an anti-gay product. But even if they didn't, why can't we just
casually say they're gay? Or at least *ask* if they are?"[28]

But as the decade progressed, the real "outing" action wasn't
to be found in the gay press but in the modern tabloids that had not
only replaced the likes of *Confidential* but leaped well beyond them.

The *National Enquirer,* the *Globe,* the *Star,* and their imitators
boast circulation figures far in excess of anything the old scandal mags
ever dreamed of. Moreover, they're not exiled to the upper racks of
selected kiosks but are for sale at the cash registers of every supermarket in the country. There is one major difference with today's tabs.
Unlike *Confidential,* the pieces they publish vary from blatant sen-
sationalism to fawning flattery—often when dealing with the same
subject.

Actress/comedienne/talk-show hostess Rosie O'Donnell is a
particularly interesting figure in regard to current tabloid attitudes.
"Rosie's Secret Marriage," a 1996 *Globe* piece, enthuses that "after
years of torment" O'Donnell has "finally found true love in the arms
of a beautiful Broadway starlet," Michelle Blakely, whom she met
while appearing in the Broadway revival of *Grease.* Illustrated with
candid photographs of Blakely and O'Donnell cleaning up the back-
yard of the latter's home, the article declares O'Donnell's recently
adopted baby will be raised by the couple in their "luxury love nest."[29]
A 1997 *Globe* cover story about "The Real Rosie"[30] downplays lesbianism in the text (which centers on her childhood, her favorite snack
foods, her weight problem, and her incessantly dramatized obsession
with Tom Cruise) but is illustrated with candid telephoto-lens shots
of O'Donnell in her garden embracing a female "mystery pal." By
contrast, "Meet the Ritzie New Rosie," a *National Examiner* story
that appeared the same year, claimed "fear of being linked with gay
'Ellen' prompts desperate makeover."[31] DeGeneres's appearance that
year on O'Donnell's show, where she made coy cracks about her television character revealing herself to be "Lebanese" (as both the character's and the actress's comings out were still in process at the time
the program aired), did manage to produce a far more standoffish
Rosie than usual, but nothing more. A 1998 *National Enquirer* story,

"Rosie's Secret Lover," finds Kelli Carpenter, a television executive with the Nickelodeon cable channel, replacing Blakely in O'Donnell's affections, but on this occasion, only separate, noncandid photos of the women appear.[32] For 1998 has seen Hollywood rise as never before against the "intrusion" of the paparazzi, going so far as to encourage legislation that would curtail telephoto-lens photography as an invasion of privacy. More important, the tabs are still reeling from the uproar over the death of Princess Diana—which was blamed at the time on the paparazzi.

Where the tabloids are planning to go with gay and lesbian material in the future is difficult to gauge. Keyed as they are to a readership in thrall to celebrity, the tabs need to strike the proper balance between shock and acceptance. Being the star of not only the *Dr. Kildare* show but the much-watched and well-remembered miniseries *Shōgun* and *The Thorn Birds*, actor Richard Chamberlain has been both exposed and embraced by the tabs over the years. In neither case has he offered any comment. By contrast, tabloid exposés of such celebrity offspring as Chastity Bono and Jason Gould led to changes in their subjects' lives. Bono became a spokesperson for GLAAD (Gay and Lesbian Alliance Against Defamation), while Gould, already in the process of establishing himself as a performer in his own right, wrote and directed in 1997 an autobiographical short entitled *Inside Out*. Recreating the day he discovered the tabs had run a story about his alleged "marriage" to a male friend, Gould is shown to great comic effect, grabbing copies of the magazine off supermarket racks in a frenzy and piling them into a shopping cart.

Recently several tabs have set their sights at featured performers like Chad Allen of the *Dr. Quinn, Medicine Woman* show, running a clearly uncandid photograph of the actor and another man kissing in a hot tub. "Poor Chad. He's a sweet kid," says publicist Howard Bragman, who's well aware of the difficulties faced by performers unprepared when their "private lives" become press property. "He's going to get on with his life and do his series and ignore the issue."[33] But not entirely, for while Allen has declined to talk about his tabloid "outing," he has continued to support gay and AIDS causes, such as an all-star 1997 benefit reading in Los Angeles of *The Boys in the Band*, featuring "out" performers Bruce Vilanch and Mitchell Anderson.

Still, Allen's "outing" was a mere radar blip compared with what happened on May 2, 1997, when actor Eddie Murphy was stopped by the police on Santa Monica Boulevard in West Hollywood while in the company of one Atisone Seiuli, a "pre-operational trans-sexual" prostitute: a transvestite with breast implants undergoing female-hormone injection treatments, who is still in possession of male genitalia.

As no sexual activity, or monetary transaction, was taking place when the authorities—who were looking for Seiuli in the first place—intervened, Murphy was questioned and released without charge. But the tabloids, which had for over a decade tracked tales alleging the actor's interest in such sexual exotics, went into high gear. The *National Enquirer* and the *Globe* rushed out stories detailing Murphy's "secret life" only days later. But the actor and his lawyers were ready, and on May 13 they launched a lawsuit against both publications.

Murphy's *National Enquirer* lawsuit asked for $5 million in damages plus unspecified compensation for "emotional distress, embarrassment, and humiliation" in an action charging "libel, false light, invasion of privacy, and slander." The suit named the writers of the *Enquirer* piece (Alan Smith, Michael Glynn, Patricia Towle, and John Blosser) as defendants along with transvestites Sylvia Roe and Holly Woodlawn (the latter a "superstar" from the Andy Warhol "factory"), who had claimed in the article to have known Murphy sexually. Seiuli was not targeted by the suit, but the defendants were said to have made "provably false factual statements about Murphy in a sensationalized and malicious effort to profit from the outrageous publication of salacious fabricated stories of and concerning Murphy" with "callous, malicious, and despicable disregard of the truth," having "relied on persons who have demonstrated anger and hostility to plaintiff."[34]

For its part the *Enquirer* released a statement saying it stood by its story and would not "tolerate this legal attack. . . . Mr. Murphy is attempting to rehabilitate himself at our expense. We intend to prove our case in open court." Murphy, in statements made on the night of the incident to the army of reporters that appeared at the police station once word got out, claimed he was "just being a good Samaritan," offering Seiuli a ride home and nothing more.[35]

For appearing on the boulevard, and thereby violating the terms of his probation on a previous prostitution conviction, Seiuli was incarcerated for ninety days. Murphy was left with the much more delicate task of explaining, to a greatly amused press corps, why his "good Samaritan" actions should be unfolding on a thoroughfare known to be trafficked by male prostitutes. "I love my wife and I'm not gay," Murphy told *Entertainment Tonight* on a broadcast the night after the incident. "That's what's weird about this, to have your sexuality questioned and your moral fiber questioned and all that, when all I was trying to do was be nice to someone." But no explanation was needed for the *Enquirer* story's breathtaking opening quote: "Hi, I'm Eddie Murphy. Here's $200. What type of sex do you like? Can I see you in lingerie?"[36]

To no one's surprise, by August of that year Murphy had dropped the *Enquirer* lawsuit. "The actor's spokesman said that Murphy had decided the tabloid didn't act maliciously," the *Los Angeles Times* reported, going on to note that "a separate $5-million suit against *The Globe* over a similar article was settled earlier out of court."[37] If Murphy avoids driving down Santa Monica Boulevard as assiduously as Tab Hunter has turned down "pajama party" invitations, a repetition of these events is unlikely. Moreover, as Seiuli died in an apparently accidental fall from his apartment window in May 1998, no "up close and personal" follow-up to the initial incident should plague Murphy in the future.

But it isn't just the daily press that longs for gay "scandal," *Confidential*-style. Upscale magazines have been on the lookout for it as well, particularly in their coverage of the so-called "Gay Mafia." This sinister-sounding circle (also known as the "Velvet Mafia") has been splayed across the pages of *New York* and *Spy* magazines in stories revealing little more than the fact that media moguls David Geffen, Barry Diller, and Sandy Gallin, designer Calvin Klein, painter Ross Bleckner, and writer Fran Lebowitz are all close friends and spend many hours in one another's company on both coasts. While Geffen, Gallin, and Bleckner have been forthcoming about their sexual orientation, Diller, Klein, and Lebowitz have not—a fact that causes "Mafia" watchers no end of upset.

"Despite being the most-talked-about gay-press-outed man in Hollywood, Diller hasn't 'given permission' for the press to say he's gay," writes Mark Ebner in his *Spy* profile. The problem, however, is that whether "permitted" or not, making something newsworthy out of the sexuality of this merry crew is no simple task. They're rich and they're "powerful." But as this "power" connects with everyday gay and lesbian lives only via the AIDS charities "Mafia" members widely support, there is little for a journalist like Ebner to cluck over. So he goes the *Confidential* route, interviewing unnamed parties who claim to have had carnal knowledge of select "Mafiosi." But the bedroom isn't the best place to learn information, as Ebner discovers after talking to one "actor" whose "experience illustrates another way in which the Gay Mafia can work. On the one hand, he describes how Geffen 'played with me'; on the other, he says there's also a feeling of connectedness that comes with being Geffen's lover. 'He's not exactly my type,' the actor says, 'but to be with someone so powerful was exciting to me.' " In other words, there's no story to his story.

Still, Ebner manages to hit paydirt, albeit secondhand, with his notation of the curious situation that arose when Scott Bankston, "one of Gallin's more serious lovers," left the impresario for Bryan Lourd, a CAA agent who at the time was involved with writer-actress Carrie Fisher, with whom he had fathered a child. "Gallin took it upon himself to 'out' Lourd all over town," claims Ebner of a story no force on earth could have prevented from spreading like wildfire. But such blazes generally run their course within the confines of a group whose members know one another, either personally or professionally. Lourd and Bankston are complete strangers to those outside the industry. And the marketing of the celebrity of industry insiders like Gallin and the other "Mafiosi" is a complex notion. The assumption is that the public is awed by power as a spectacle in itself as, for example, in the picture Ebner paints of the late William Morris agent Stan Kamen.

"A former employee of Kamen's discusses his power. 'He was

the original gay power broker. He was the head of the Motion Picture Department and had every Ovitz client—Barbra Streisand, Steven Spielberg, Robert Redford, Goldie Hawn. He had it all, and the [straight] guys who came off his desk idolized him, and wouldn't mention [his sexuality], or even fuck around about it. It was just not spoken about—ever. It's fear, and a reverence built out of fear. It's not based on intellect, but based on what will happen to you.' [And] what will happen to you is you will get fired, or worse, blacklisted."

In other words, homophobia requires *intellect* in order to operate properly. But Kamen's standing as a "power broker" had nothing to do with gay Hollywood. He was a power broker who simply happened to be gay.

"Does being straight get in the way?" Ebner asks in conclusion. "Is there a heterosexual glass ceiling? Probably not. While entry into the Gay Mafia equals entry into a very exclusive and powerful enclave, one who does not share their similar sexual appetites and tastes wouldn't necessarily be considered an outsider."[38] But the very fact that Ebner feels such a question has legitimacy is indicative of the paranoia that persists around the subject, even in supposedly sophisticated circles—as if a *Protocols of the Elders of Judy Garland* were about to be unearthed at any moment.

The reason for this is the fourth estate's insistence on clinging to the notion that the only gay or lesbian story is that which pivots on a "shocking revelation" of a celebrity's "private life." But this search for "shock" has sometimes resulted in shocks of another sort for the searchers involved. And no better example of this can be pointed to than the October 1997 *Esquire* profile of actor Kevin Spacey.

It begins in an oddly cozy fashion with writer Tom Junod discussing the impending article with his mother. "I told her I was writing a story on Kevin Spacey, and she said 'Well, I hear he's gay.' " How Junod's mother came by such information is never explained. But Spacey's sexuality has been the subject of any number of stories that have circulated through Hollywood over the past few years—few of them flattering in traditional public-relations terms. The most egregious would have it that the actor was discovered *in flagrante* with the lover of a professional colleague. Why Junod would expect that a story this untoward would provide an occasion for the actor to speak about his "private life" as he never has before speaks to a fourth-estate inability to differentiate the "scandal" of same-sexuality from possible scandals of other sorts.

"Spacey is what everyone else has already said," says Junod on meeting the actor during the shooting of *Midnight in the Garden of Good and Evil,* "which is that he is supposed to be very smart, that he is supposed to be very private, that he is supposed to be extraordinarily committed to the protection and development of his extraordinary gifts as an actor, and that he is supposed to be gay." Thinking that the fact Spacey plays a gay man in *Midnight* will provide him with an opening, Junod approaches his quarry stealthily—not realizing that playing a gay character has become in recent years less an invitation for personal inquiries than a shot at getting an Academy Award nomination.

"In my research," Spacey tells Junod, "I found a very different Jim Williams. He was a southern gentleman. He was very at ease with his sexuality. He was *not* hidden and I do not play him that way." But rather than explore this rather questionable reading of the central figure of the Clint Eastwood film based on John Berendt's nonfiction bestseller, Junod gets achingly coy.

"The thing is, it's always right there. The secret, I mean— Kevin's secret: It's always right there, in front of you. You have to look, of course—you have to open your *eyes*—but you don't have to look very far. . . ." But Junod isn't talking about Spacey's sexuality at all, it emerges, as Junod declares: "And that's it. That's the truth. And that's Kevin's secret, the one that's always there for the taking. He's a movie star. He *wants* to be a movie star."

One would have to go back to Adela Rogers St. John's 1944 *Photoplay* examination of the "secret" of Irene Dunne—which after no small amount of soul-searching reveals that "Irene Dunne makes being good more fun, more dramatic, more beautiful"—to find an equivalent to Junod's prolixity. It comes as something of a shock when he finally pops to Spacey the $64,000 Question.

"Look," says Spacey, "I don't see anything wrong with sexuality. And so I'll put it to you this way. I live in a world in which I work with many different people all day long. They're my friends and I *love* them. And many of these people *are* gay or homosexual. And I can't imagine feeling the need to jump up and say 'I'm not one of them.' If anyone wants to think that, they're absolutely free to think that. I have no interest in confirming or denying that *at all*. It's just of no interest to me. So *what*? So . . . what."[39]

The reaction to Junod's piece was swift and severe. *Time* magazine reported that "Spacey's agent, Brian Gersh, went so far as to suggest that he would discourage anyone William Morris represents from working with *Esquire*, a statement others at the agency—which has 3,000 clients, including Clint Eastwood and Bill Cosby—later backed away from."[40]

"I did not expect to 'out' Kevin," a contrite Junod informed the *Advocate*, "because I thought he *was* 'out.' I had heard so many people say, 'You know he's gay'—as the first or second thing that they said. Then I go out there, and suddenly it's a completely different thing."[41]

But the real "difference" has nothing to do with either Spacey or Junod, but with the press. "Junod's decision to structure the story on the rumor that Spacey might be gay—a potentially career-altering designation made not by reputable sources, but by Junod's 80-year-old mother—left other magazine editors drop-jawed and publicists looking to hide women, children and clients from the newly revamped *Esquire*," wrote *Daily Variety*'s Michael Fleming, going on to note that the story "also left many feeling that a spate of celebrity-scorching features indicates that the leverage once held by publicists is switching back to magazines and their star byliners."

Fleming went on to detail that Spacey's managers felt "duped" by Junod; they reportedly had been told the profile would be about his acting, not his sexuality. In a statement, Wolfe Newman said, "*Esquire* has made it abundantly clear that they have now joined the ranks of distasteful journalism, and this mean-spirited, homophobic, abusive article proves that the legacy of Joseph McCarthy is alive and well."[42]

In a way, it's appropriate that Fleming cited the McCarthy era, in that so many of its key figures (Roy Cohn, Whittaker Chambers,

J. Edgar Hoover, and McCarthy himself) were closeted homosexuals whose anti-Communist zeal was spurred by fear of being found out. But that was close to fifty years ago. And Kevin Spacey isn't a Communist.

Feeling the heat as never before, *Esquire* declined to comment any further on the story, in the clear hope that it would all go away of its own accord. But the most interesting insight of the Spacey/Junod contretemps can be found in the remarks of *Variety's* Fleming when questioned about his criticism of the story.

"It's like you're playing around with a lighted stick of dynamite with that *Esquire* piece," says Fleming, anxiously. "The bottom line is, who gives a rat's ass about Kevin Spacey's sexuality? He's not some gorgeous leading man who women just fawn over. This guy has become a star based on his ability to act pretty much better than anyone else out there. I just think that revelation—aside from being an invasion of someone's private life—is just a complete nonstory. Who cares? Why would anybody give a *crap* about someone's sexuality?" Fleming has a point in that Spacey's name doesn't arise when Tom Cruise or Brad Pitt or Leonardo DiCaprio proves unavailable.

But Fleming has put Spacey aside by now, turning his attention to Ellen DeGeneres and Anne Heche, whose love affair has become one of the biggest entertainment news stories of the last decade.

"You want to know the truth about that?" Fleming asks unbidden. "If you talk to her manager he will tell you point blank that they basically came out and declared themselves a couple because they just had no peace. They were a target, and they had to worry about someone trying to photograph them in the clinches every single time they were together. I don't believe they came out because they wanted to. I think they came out because they wanted to be accepted and live their life in peace. I don't applaud someone being pressured into making that decision, based on those parameters."

Such a notion is in striking contrast with everything DeGeneres and Heche have ever said to the press about their relationship and their careers. But it should be noted that neither DeGeneres's manager, Arthur Imperato, nor her publicist, the ubiquitous Pat Kingsley, had, when questioned, anything to say about Fleming's outburst.

"My feeling is just simply *so what?*" screams Fleming in conclusion. "*I don't care!* I don't care if someone goes to leather bars. *I don't care!* For me it's *just not a concern!*"[43]

Kevin Spacey himself couldn't have put it more dramatically.

FIVE

CLOSET PRIVILEGES

—

ARE YOU A HOMOSEXUAL?"

"No, sir," replied Liberace.

"Have you ever indulged in homosexual practices?"

"No, sir, never in my life."

"What are your feelings about it?"

"My feelings are the same as anyone else's. I am
against the practice because it offends convention and
offends society."[1]

Liberace was, of course, *lying*.

The popular pianist had for many years "indulged in homosexual practices" when he told a British courtroom otherwise in 1959, and he would continue to do so for the rest of his life. To state that his "feelings about it" were "the same as anyone else's" in that it "offends convention and offends society" doesn't elide the truth of his lie. It merely denotes Liberace's willingness to conform to standards long established by the ruling heterosexual middle classes as a "norm."

If "asked," he would "tell" . . . a lie.

It goes without saying that Liberace's lie must be seen in its proper context. "To call homosexuals liars," claims Michel Foucault, "is equivalent to calling the resistors under a military occupation liars. It's like calling Jews 'money lenders,' when it was the only profession they were allowed to practice."[2] But there is an enormous difference between a person of average ways and means lying about his or her same-sex affinity in order to keep a job, a residence, or family peace, and the lie of a highly paid and well-connected show-business figure who had successfully promoted modest pianistic ability into a career in nightclubs, concert halls, film, and television. Moreover, an overt appeal to the sexual sensibilities of his audience was very much a part of Liberace's act.

"I spoke to sad but kindly men on this newspaper who have met every celebrity arriving from the United States for the last 30 years," said "Cassandra" (the pen name used by London *Daily Mirror* columnist William Conner) in the 1956 article that prompted Liberace to press libel charges. "They all say that this deadly, winking, sniggering, snuggling, chromium-plated, scent-impregnated, luminous, quivering, giggling, fruit-flavored, mincing, ice-cream-covered heap of mother love has had the biggest reception and impact on London since Charlie Chaplin arrived at the same station, Waterloo, on Sept. 13, 1921. He reeks with emetic language that can only make grown men long for a quiet corner, an aspidistra, a handkerchief, and the old heave-ho. Without doubt he is the biggest sentimental vomit of all time."[3]

To anyone familiar with Liberace, "Cassandra"'s remarks

would appear to be perfectly fair comment. Turning performances of classical music into a form of parlor trick, Liberace adapted fragments of Chopin, Tchaikovsky, and other great composers into "tunes" displayed with ostentatious flourishes of the arms and wrists, vigorous shakes of his curl-encrusted head, and an implacable, face-wide smile. Long before a series of increasingly bizarre costumes (jeweled capes, sequined shorts) and props (a harness rigged to make him fly across the stage, a fake-jewel-covered limousine) that dominated his later years, Liberace's act centered on a display of blatantly "effeminate" mannerisms that stood in polar opposition to the (equally ostentatious) "masculinity" of a John Wayne. Liberace knew exactly what he was doing: just how far to go "too far." His every word and gesture was crafted to raise the question of his sexual identity in the minds of his adoring fans, only to stave off their actually bringing it up in earnest at the last minute. Constant flattery ("Oh, you're so wonderful to me, ladies and gentlemen!") was Liberace's primary method of stopping his worshipers in mid-thought. His feelings about homosexuality *were* "the same as anyone else's"—in public relations terms. He didn't seek to challenge "convention" or "society"; therefore, he would never acknowledge the truth. His only "offense" would pertain to taste—which was in fact the heart of the "Cassandra" broadside. What the case provided for Liberace was a publicity bonanza. He would take on "Cassandra," and by doing so silence the snickers of his legions of detractors. He would "prove" he wasn't homosexual—even though he was.

"Liberace complained that the word 'fruit' is a widely known euphemism for a homosexual and that its use by Conner implied the pianist was one," the *Los Angeles Examiner* reported. "The jury deliberated three hours and 24 minutes in concluding that William (Cassandra) Conner had implied that Liberace was a homosexual when he wrote in the *Daily Mirror* that the forty-year-old piano player was 'the summit of sex—the pinnacle of masculine, feminine and neuter; everything that he, she or it can ever want,' " the *Los Angeles Times* explained. And so, because "Cassandra" had, in effect, called him a "fag" and thereby (presumably) undermined his reputation, Liberace was awarded $22,400 in damages.[4]

What Liberace and his lawyers clearly understood was that with the libel issue posed on this narrow "damage" question alone, the pianist would win. To imply that Liberace might be anything other than heterosexual, it was argued, was damaging on its face—notwithstanding the fact that Liberace's entire performing persona ceaselessly exploited the notion that he might be other than heterosexual. For their part, "Cassandra" and his lawyers were stymied from the start, as they apparently had neither the means nor the inclination to testify that Liberace was indeed same-sex-oriented. And in an England still reeling from the impact of the Oscar Wilde trials, such timidity is no surprise.

When, in 1895, the Marquess of Queensberry, the father of Wilde's lover, Lord Alfred Douglas, sent a card to the writer reading "To Oscar Wilde posing Somdomite" (a misspelling whose meaning was nonetheless clear), Wilde instituted a libel action against the Marquess, much along the lines of the one Liberace brought against "Cassandra." His mistake came from his belief that the Marquess wouldn't risk a breach in social decorum by upsetting the virtual "don't ask, don't tell" policy under which Victorian society had lived, and Wilde had prospered. But Wilde lost his suit against Queensberry, and as a result found himself facing the state on charges of "gross indecency" and "immoral" behavior. Completing the process the Marquess had started, Her Majesty's government produced a parade of lower-class men whom Wilde had paid for sex into court to testify against him. "Cassandra," however, was no Marquess of Queensberry, and so, half a century later, Wilde's loss became Liberace's gain.

Liberace's win against "Cassandra" strengthened the public-relations hand that he had played two years before with *Confidential*. His not being in the city in which the magazine claimed certain same-sex assignations took place didn't alter the truth of his sexual identity, but it kept that truth from being unambiguously stated in a public forum. Likewise, the perceived damage of "Cassandra" 's snideness was a separate issue from Liberace's sexuality. But in the court of public opinion it was a slam dunk. As Liberace had twice sued and won against those who had (albeit virtually rather than literally) called him a homosexual, it therefore followed that Liberace was *not* a homosexual. Truth be damned.

Liberace's legal victories, absurd as they were, managed to hold his carefully constructed public image in place until 1982, when Scott Thorson, an ex-lover who had worked as the pianist's chauffeur and appeared as a performer in his act (driving the fake-jeweled limo), sued the entertainer for $113 million in "palimony." The action was spurred by Thorson's claims that four men working for Liberace had thrown him out of the pianist's Los Angeles apartment.[5] In May of 1983 Thorson filed a separate $6 million lawsuit against the *Globe* for publishing a story Liberace reportedly gave them attacking Thorson.[6] In December 1986 Liberace settled with Thorson for $95,000.[7] And two years later, living up to the bad light the *Globe* had cast upon him, Thorson was sentenced to three years' imprisonment for armed robbery. All of this, of course, was made moot in 1987 when Liberace's death opened a floodgate of stories about his sexuality the press was loath to publish while he was alive.

Still, in the period just before his death Liberace himself had begun to loosen up a bit. "Despite everything, it is difficult not to like Liberace," claims interviewer James R. Gaines in a 1982 *People* profile.

> He has become a more interesting man with age, and far more open about himself. . . . Now he frankly admits the gay drift of his show and speaks sympathetically of all sexual preferences. "My act is just *that far away* from being drag," he says "but I would never come on stage like, say, Danny La Rue [the British female impersonator and music-hall star], who is a very dear friend of mine. I have a general family audience appeal, and I don't want to develop only a gay following. It's going to take many, many years for this kind of an audience to accept people who are totally gay or come out on Johnny Carson. I've seen careers hurt by that kind of thing—look at Billie

Jean King. But with a name like Liberace, which stands
for freedom, anything that has the letters L-I-B in it I'm
for, and that includes gay lib."[8]

"Liberace was tougher than people imagined," John Rechy recalls. "I saw how he worked. It was really extraordinary. I saw the
bodyguards he had to protect him. But he did take care of people who
stopped being his main boyfriend. He would hire them to work for
him. I knew two of them. We were at a dinner party, and I didn't
realize that I was being offered to him by my hosts. He put his hand
on my crotch right under the table. This was rude. You don't want to
say anything, because it's a dinner. So when he left, he wanted me to
go with him, and there was this big fuss because his bodyguard was
with him and saw what was going on. Later he called back. He was
crying: 'Please come, I'm so lonesome. Please, please come!' I
was truly moved. So I said I'd come over. I really thought I was being
humane. But I was naive too. So I went into that incredible black-
and-white house he had in Los Angeles. He had these poodles that
were black and white. They were running all over, and suddenly *I*
was running all over because he was actually quite aggressive. He
was an incredibly, incredibly aggressive man. He was just *determined*
to get sex. He offered to show me the house, and every time we turned
around it was another bedroom. Finally there was his big one. I had
to run out. I certainly wasn't innocent, but . . ."

Rechy pauses for a moment to reflect, and then remarks, very
simply: "He was a *nice* man.

"I think it was very obvious," the novelist continues, after another pause, "that his appeal was to women who wanted a gay son, or
had a gay son. More than anything else, it was women who saw him
as the ideal son who loved Liberace. He would be kind to them. He
would perform for them. And he would *always* return to Mom. He
would never marry. He would never leave them. I think that was the
basis for his popularity."[9]

And so it would follow that any indication that Liberace was
straight was just as threatening to his performing persona as any con-
firmation of the fact that he was gay. That situation arose in 1954

when stories began to appear in the press that Joanne Rio, a dancer Liberace had been publicly dating, was engaged to marry him.

"There isn't a word of truth that I am engaged to marry. I was misquoted and I am very embarrassed for Joanne," Liberace told Louella Parsons.[10] Whether Liberace or Rio was responsible for suggesting that an engagement was imminent will never be known. But it's clear from such stories as "Girl Friend Tells: My Dates with Liberace"—with a photo of Rio, captioned with inadvertent irony, "The tomboy developed an early crush on the gay pianist"—that the dancer was making the most of her association with him.[11]

In 1974, Rio reappeared in Liberace's life to complain of an autobiography he had written and a piece about it published in the *National Enquirer*. Suing both Liberace's publisher, G. P. Putnam and Sons, and the *Enquirer*, Rio contended that she never profited from articles written about her dates with the pianist, as she claimed he had implied. Moreover, her suit contended Liberace used " 'innuendo' to indicate she was intimate with the pianist, which further destroys her reputation, by making her appear unchaste."[12]

Like most celebrity-related lawsuits Rio's evaporated over time. Still, her legal efforts were no less curious than the one launched years later by Joel Strote, the executor of Liberace's estate, against the performer's manager, Seymour Heller, in order to "prevent him from disclosing confidential facts in a television movie about the pianist's life."[13] It would be hard to imagine what was left to be disclosed about Liberace at the time of his death. He was gay. He was sued for palimony by an ex-lover and settled out of court. He died of AIDS, a disease whose contraction he had denied as vociferously as he had his sexual orientation. But as anyone connected with all things Liberace is well aware, simple truths are out of the question. Even in death the lie must remain in place. In fact Heller, the defendant in the abovementioned action, had launched a suit of his own against the *Las Vegas Sun* for reporting that Liberace had died of AIDS.[14] Needless to say, none of this could hold for long, as the Riverside County coroner came forward to accuse Liberace's doctors of trying to hide the cause of his death.

"Somebody along the line wanted to pull a fast one on us," the

coroner, Raymond Carrillio, announced at a news conference shortly
after Liberace's passing. "Microscopic tissue analysis showed that
Liberace died because of cytomegalovirus pneumonia due to human
immunodeficiency virus disease," *The New York Times* reported. "Dr.
Ronald Daniels, a physician who treated Liberace, said last week that
the entertainer died of cardiac arrest due to heart failure brought on
by subacute encephalopathy, a brain inflammation. The Coroner said
that Dr. Daniels' failure to report the correct cause of death would be
reported to California's Board of Medical Quality Assurance."[15]

And so even in death, the "truth" about Liberace had all the
stability of an ace in a three-card monte game. To admit he died of
AIDS would be tantamount to admitting that he was gay. And even
though the world had known that simple fact for years, public-
relations tradition demanded that it never be broached under any
circumstances.

Hollywood lies about homosexuality. But it would be wrong to
regard this lie as any sort of exception to the rule. Hollywood
lies about almost everything—be it overwhelmingly important or utterly trivial. Clark Gable wasn't the rugged outdoorsman MGM publicists led the world to believe. His hunting trips were a show as
carefully contrived as any Rock Hudson date. Likewise, Bing Crosby
and Bob Hope weren't the bosom pals offscreen their onscreen interplay would lead one to believe. They were simply professional col-
leagues. And in the immortal words of Carrie Fisher, issue of the
ceaselessly publicized pairing of Eddie Fisher and Debbie Reynolds,
"My parents' whole relationship was basically a press release."[16]

"For a long time American society was a great deal more innocent than it is today," journalist Kevin Thomas explains philosophically. "I'm old enough to remember that Howard Strickling at
MGM did, innately, understand the power of *noblesse oblige*—a term
he may never have heard of, or could pronounce. But he did manage
to pull off that fabulous image-building thing with performers when
he was head of publicity there. He taught the stars how to deal with

the press. Today, television takes you right into people's living rooms, and people see things they never saw before. But I have met stars of the 'golden age,' and there is this *aura* about them. They glitter like mad, and you know that the person isn't really like that—but you're still taken in. It's often said some of our greatest actresses gave their greatest performances in the interview. I somehow go along with that, because they do it so well, and work so hard at it."[17]

But even in optimum circumstances, with star, press agent, and journalist working in concert, like a well-oiled machine whose sole goal is to cast an actor in the best possible light, same-sexuality can come to haunt circumstances where its presence would never be acknowledged.

"How are the fan magazines to keep presenting these profiles to their swooning girlish readers as ardent, romantic personalities, and how are they to explain the fact that these movie idols seem to be so oblivious of the opposite sex?" veteran journalist Ezra Goodman muses, with no small amount of amusement. "The fan magazines turn themselves inside out trying to drum up romances for these unsusceptible swains, and they trot out such tricky and evasive verbiage as 'Trying to escape from any romantic involvement'; 'He wants a free life'; and 'Few women have been able to really get close to him.' "[18]

And this rhetorical evasiveness persists today in a world where questions about sexual orientation are being raised in ways that would have been considered unthinkable in the past. A perfect example of this careful sidestepping is *The Gossip Show* on cable television's E! channel. Featuring a crew of columnists that ranges from gay *Village Voice* scribe Michael Musto to *New York Post* doyenne Cindy Adams to Janet Charlton of the *Star*, it displays them at their office desks, or seated at restaurant tables, or lounging on cushion-covered sofas in swank hotel lobbies, briskly dispensing sound bites, with no pretense of depth or insight whatsoever. The 1997 "coming out" of Ellen DeGeneres and Anne Heche might have provided these "gossips" with a prime opportunity talk about gay Hollywood in general. But it wasn't taken. "Dish" about Ellen and Anne was supplied at length,

but as far as any other gay or lesbian performers or industry luminaries were concerned, the silence from *The Gossip Show* was deaf-
ening.

"There are certain unspoken rules in the fun and frivolous
world of gossip," notes the show's producer, Gary Socol, in an article
written for the gay magazine *Genre*. "Never report the drug habits of
a celebrity—unless he or she has officially entered the Betty Ford
Center. Never divulge the details of a diva's plastic surgery—unless
it's Joan Rivers, who boasts about it. And never, ever discuss the love
life of a gay celebrity—unless he or she is out of the closet." Socol,
who is himself gay, freely admits such strictures are necessary to keep
a show of this kind on the air. But the fear of lawsuits doesn't play
any real part in this "don't even think about asking, much less telling"
policy. *The Gossip Show* is a lightweight affair, the bulk of whose items
are supplied by celebrity publicists. Were the show to seriously investigate the offscreen lives of the stars it covers, be they gay or
straight, access to such "softball" items would be withdrawn in an
instant. Socol claims "blind items" are a possibility for use on the
show, noting, "Right now, I see a male TV star asking his lover to
leave the house when a *People* magazine reporter is due, and a movie
hunk who denies he's gay (or even bisexual), despite the fact that he
has a propensity for picking up guys at the mall (and refusing to
shower)." But such teasing tidbits rarely make their way before the
cameras, for much the same reason the franker items fail the test;
publicists wouldn't like it.[19]

For all that's happened to alter gay and lesbian life across
America over the past two decades, same-sexuality is still regarded
as an acceptable "secret" in Hollywood. And it is *secrecy*, rather than
"privacy," that is at issue. For stars are in the business of selling their
"private lives" to the media on a daily basis. Open any magazine or
watch any entertainment news program, and chances are you'll be
able to find out far more than you ever wanted to know about superstar
Sadie Glutz's new boyfriend or new husband or new baby or new
breast-augmentation surgery. In fact, these "bites" of audiovisual "in-
fotainment" often as not put Sadie's new movie or television series or
ghostwritten "tell-all" autobiography in the shade. And that's as it

should be. Movies, books, and television shows come and go, but Sadie must remain in public view as much as possible in order for her career to survive. And to that end information once considered untoward is now regarded as a perfectly viable means of keeping Sadie in the spotlight.

Sadie's addiction to controlled substances may be a career embarrassment, but her struggle to overcome it can serve to stir the sympathies of her old fans and attract new ones. Likewise, the dissolution of her marriage may have been bitter, but a sympathetic *People* cover story, or Oprah Winfrey or Barbara Walters interview, can place it in a light divorced women everywhere can appreciate and empathize with. However, the fact that Sadie, just prior to the debut of her new talk show, approached a noted film marketer at an industry party, complained about said marketer's handling of a recent low-budget sapphic item, and loudly declared, "I'm a lesbian woman and I want to see more lesbian films!" isn't to be broached in print or broadcast under any circumstances, for to do so would be to break with standards of heterosexual middle-class decorum to which all stars and celebrities, no matter how singular their lives may be, continually pay homage.

"I would bet every penny I have that their marriage is totally legitimate, that they're in love and that it's the best thing that's ever happened to him," gay media mogul Sandy Gallin declared in a 1994 *Out* magazine interview on the occasion of the nuptials of self-styled "King of Pop" Michael Jackson and Lisa Marie Presley. "He is happy and together and it is without a doubt a real marriage."[20] Needless to say, this marriage, which barely lasted the span of a few months, was as "real" as anything else surrounding this former child star who has spent the better part of his adult years altering his facial features and lightening the complexion of his skin. The marriage came in the wake of a child-molestation scandal that kept Jackson in the international media spotlight throughout 1993—and which the performer paid a reported $40 million to settle out of court. The marriage's end was quickly followed by the announcement that Debbie Roe, office assistant to Jackson's plastic surgeon, Dr. Steven Hoefflin, was carrying a child the singer had fathered. Following the birth of this offspring,

Roe and Jackson were married. But, unlike the overwhelming majority of newlyweds, they elected not to live together. Jackson took charge of the upbringing of the child (whose physical resemblance to the singer can at best be called slight), while continuing to "date" Presley periodically and, as has been his custom, travel about with an entourage of underage boys. Consequently, while his musical career is in limbo, Michael Jackson's profile as a tabloid-newspaper sensation is as high as ever. With Roe giving birth to a second Jackson-sired offspring in 1998, even while continuing to maintain physical distance from her husband, any sense of this second marriage creating a "normalizing" effect on Jackson's public image would appear to be beside the point. It's as bizarre as anything else about him.

A be, it's absolutely true. I asked Nancy to marry me," producer Ross Hunter tells columnist Abe Greenberg in 1967, announcing his intended betrothal to the ex-wife of singer Frank Sinatra. "You know how wonderful a person she is, and we've been seeing a lot of each other now for quite a while and we're good for each other."

Why was the fifty-one-year-old producer, famed for his glossy melodramas (*Imitation of Life*) and frothy comedies (*Pillow Talk*) contemplating marriage for the first time in his life? The uncharitable might suggest that the release of his latest film, the Julie Andrews–starred musical *Thoroughly Modern Millie,* might have had something to do with it. Whatever the cause, such plans were tentative at best, as Hunter himself freely admitted. "Nancy hasn't accepted, nor has she turned me down completely. She's put me off, at least until such time as she can get her own personal problems resolved. And there it is in a nutshell. We'll keep seeing each other, and I'll keep wooing her."[21] Three years later, Hunter is still in that nutshell, telling a *Los Angeles Herald-Examiner* reporter that until a marriage commitment finalizes, "we plan to see each other as often as possible."[22] At that time, Hunter was basking in the glow of *Airport*—his biggest hit to date. And in the mountain of coverage that blockbuster inspired, a story that appeared in *Los Angeles* magazine (appropriately entitled

"On the Crying Need for a Ross Hunter Film Festival"), is especially interesting:

> It was Hunter's birthday and a lady rushed over to Executive Producer Jacques Mapes, who was also standing around and observing, and screamed, "Happy Birthday, darling!"
>
> Somewhat annoyed, Mapes said, "It's not my birthday. It's Ross's."
>
> "So what," said the lady, kissing him. "Happy birthday anyway. I'll send you both a gift."[23]

Hunter is a singular figure in his insistence on publicizing an intention that never reached fruition. He died in 1996 without ever having married Nancy Sinatra Sr. For at the same time, other Hollywood figures of his generation found nonmarital alliances were perfectly viable. Merv Griffin's relationship with actress Eva Gabor was established well in advance of the "palimony" suit launched by an ex-employee in 1991.[24] It cushioned the blow of many a tabloid tale. On the other hand, Malcolm Forbes's elaborately publicized "dates" with Elizabeth Taylor made postmortem revelations of his same-sex liaisons seem even more bizarre than they would have outside that context.[25] But whether "believed" or not, heterosexuality need only be *mimed* to accomplish its purpose: the pairing of male and female in the public's mind. The only problem comes when an effort is made to ignore the necessity of such a pairing.

D o you have a boyfriend?" Ellen DeGeneres asks herself in a "self-interview" published in *US* magazine in 1994. "That's personal. I don't talk about my private life," she replies, as countless others had done before her when pressed by the press.

"But people want to know," interviewer DeGeneres insists. "Why?" actress DeGeneres answers. "Let's say I do. OK, great. 'She has a boyfriend.' What's next? What's his name? What does he do?

Are we happy? It's hard enough to have a healthy relationship without all the pressure of people watching you, scrutinizing everything. Now, let's say I don't have a boyfriend. What's the next question? Why not? What's wrong with me? My private life is just an area I choose to keep private. Hence the name *private life*. Maybe some day I'll change my mind, but not yet."[26]

Clearly, Ellen DeGeneres knew the rules of the game she was ever-so-coyly playing. Being a star means talking about yourself. And if you're gay, that "self" is problematic. Moreover, as everyone in Hollywood knew the answer to the question the entire press corps longed so desperately to ask, it was no wonder DeGeneres had elected to become her own ventriloquist's dummy.

"She is mum about her personal life now," claims *TV Guide* in a profile that appears the same year as the self-interview. " 'I mean, I'm in a relationship and I'm happy and I'm not hiding some secret—like I'm really an Hispanic male.' "[27] But as time wears on, a sense of editorial desperation begins to overtake *Ellen* (and Ellen) press coverage. "She also is challenging Hollywood's fixation on things like romance and dating and girl's-gotta-want-a-guy," claims an only-tryin'-to-be-helpful Tabitha Soren in a 1995 *USA Weekend* piece. "DeGeneres says there's more to life. As for her own love life? Private. 'What's the issue?' she has said. 'If it's important to someone what my sexuality is, then I'm sorry.' "[28]

Still, as DeGeneres and her representatives had come to realize, it *was* important. She had no "self" to sell the media whose attention she required to keep her career afloat.

"The show also features a new color palette of warmer tones for a warmer look and a number of other details to support the show's characters," writes Debra Kaufman, desperate to find a "hook" for her DeGeneres cover story published in the February 1996 issue of *Producer* magazine. "In Ellen's apartment, for example, look for some new whimsical items strewn about that will reflect the comedienne's own offbeat personality."[29] That same month, on the verge of uttering the "yep" heard round the world, Ellen went one more round with *TV Guide*, claiming, "It's an amazing thing to me that everyone thinks I have a responsibility to divulge my personal life. The more people know about me, the harder it becomes for them to accept me in different roles."[30]

But there was no sense anywhere in Hollywood that DeGeneres would be considered "acceptable" in "different"—which is to say conventional—roles. Her big-screen comedy, *Mr. Wrong*, had by then debuted to press and public indifference. In both manner and appearance, DeGeneres had made no effort to appeal to accepted notions of the feminine. At the same time, she was far from confrontational or "in your face" about anything—sexuality least of all. Her professional "image" was floating in an iconographic limbo. She wasn't Lucille Ball, but she wasn't Rita Mae Brown, either.

"It's a tremendous amount of pressure, and I'm getting better and better at handling it, and I'm feeling more and more confident of who I am," DeGeneres told an audience at a Museum of Television event celebrating the *Ellen* show. "I'm really proud of who I am. And I think the character is someone who is very likeable. . . . So I think it would be great to be able to do great things for a lot of people with this character."[31]

But by the time DeGeneres made these remarks, likability had nothing to do with it. The word was out in Hollywood that Ellen Morgan of the *Ellen* show would be coming out that season as a lesbian. And that in turn meant that Ellen DeGeneres, the actress/comedienne who played her, would *also* be coming out as a lesbian. On one level, there was nothing "shocking" about this. DeGeneres had never hidden her sexuality from view, having appeared in public places on any number of occasions with women who were clearly more than friends. The press was well aware of this but would not report it. That they might be forced to do so was what they truly found "shocking." For when Ellen came out her sexuality was no longer a dirty little secret the fourth estate could snort over in private. They would have to mention it, if only as a simple matter of fact. And that is something for which they had neither the training nor the preparation to accomplish.

The same not-having-to-ask-but-never-dreaming-of-telling syndrome that haunted press coverage of Ellen DeGeneres prior to her coming out has existed for many years with Jodie Foster. But unlike Ellen, Jodie has never posed a problem to the press. Prior to the regrooming of her image that came in the wake of her winning the 1988 Best Actress Oscar for *The Accused*, it was quite common to see the actress (resplendent in the "grunge" attire she affected at that time) going around town accompanied by young women whose relationship to her might be described as "ambiguous." One evening in 1987, at an "all media" press screening at the Academy of Motion Picture Arts and Sciences' Samuel Goldwyn Auditorium, Foster appeared with another woman toward whom she extended no small degree of attention. The next day, at the offices of the *Los Angeles Herald-Examiner*, where I was employed as a film critic and entertainment feature writer, I inquired of others if this was an unusual event and was informed that it was not. Could there be an announcement of some sort in the offing from Foster? Should her date with this "gal pal" (the preferred tabloid term) be noted on "Page 2," where opposite-sex dates of all sorts were tallied on a daily basis? Jeff Silverman, "Page 2"'s editor, was fascinated by this prospect. Had we entered an era where a female couple could be casually noted in passing, as male-female ones commonly were? Was there a story here worth exploring? He decided to check with the newspaper's editors about it before acting one way or another, and was told no, in no uncertain terms, and without any explanation as to why.

It goes without saying that had any attempt been made to discover who Foster had attended the screening with that evening, and what her relationship to the actress might have been, it would have met with the resistance of her managers and press representatives. Yet such is the state of affairs in Hollywood regarding same-sex relations that no assumption drawn from casual observance (as would be the case in an opposite-sex pairing) can be permitted. Admittedly, any coverage of Foster was rendered problematic by the 1981 assassination attempt on then-President Ronald Reagan by John Hinckley, a disturbed youth who claimed his actions were undertaken specifically in order to impress the actress. This unfortunate circumstance didn't appear to impede her social life in any way, yet it put a considerable damper on press coverage in general. Questions of any sort had to be asked *carefully*.

"A certain steeliness comes into her voice and manner," reporter Francesca Stanfill notes in a 1987 interview when she mentions Hinckley to Foster in passing. " 'I never talk about that,' she says firmly. It's the same voice she uses to respond to queries about her personal life. 'I'm not involved with anyone now—and if I were, I wouldn't tell you.' "[32] To a community torn with doubts about the value of "coming out" in face of the personal and professional risks involved, Foster's desire to keep even the most mundane mention of her "private life" off-limits was embraced by some. But others in Hollywood's gay and lesbian community felt frustrated, particularly in light of *The Silence of the Lambs.*

While the actress received no end of praise for her performance as a dedicated FBI agent tracking down a serial killer, the film itself was criticized by many in the gay and lesbian community for its portrayal of that killer as a gay transvestite consumed by hatred of women. Coming at the end of a long line of increasingly egregious gay-unfriendly Hollywood releases, *Silence* inspired considerable debate. By the time the 1991 Oscar ceremonies rolled around (in March of 1992), protests were planned. The "mainstream" press went into high gear, as stories that gay and lesbian activists would disrupt the ceremonies and "out" stars during the broadcast began to spread like wildfire.[33] The gay and lesbian biweekly the *Advocate* faced a steady stream of "mainstream" inquiries regarding whether a Foster "outing" was in the offing. The *Advocate* knew no more, and no less, than anyone else. But both the industry and the general public seemed poised for an onslaught of some sort.

Meanwhile, as the pros and cons of protest were being debated, the *Village Voice*'s Michael Musto noted, "There's been a wave of pre-Oscar press lately heterosexualizing Jodie Foster. The *Enquirer* wrote up her alleged live-in male lover, and in *Ladies' Home Journal* Foster breaks her own rule of not discussing her personal life to wax romantic about her first boyfriend! I liked it better when she kept quiet."[34] But in the end it wasn't Foster's "quiet" that was at issue. For in spite of an avalanche of hype, there were no gay/lesbian activist disruptions at the 1991 Academy Award ceremonies. Jodie Foster won her second Best Actress Oscar for *The Silence of the Lambs* (which also won Best

Picture, Actor, Director, and Screenplay), and in her acceptance speech she thanked "the people in the industry who have respected my choices and who have not been afraid of the power and dignity that entitles me to." It would seem that any questions about her "personal life" were now off the table for good.

"The usually animated Foster, who will affectionately grab one's arm to stress a point, goes suddenly very still, her face a mask of contempt. 'Even to respond to that kind of journalism would be wrong,'" she tells a British journalist in the wake of her Oscar win when questioned about the *Silence* controversy.[35] Three years later, in a *Vanity Fair* profile, writer Michael Shnayerson tries to walk her through things *very* carefully—to no effect:

> Foster is famously guarded about her personal life, and rather than risk being bonked by a hand weight, I circle the subject as we circle the lake. *Are you happy being alone?* "Yeah, I like it." *Can you be alone for a whole weekend and not get depressed?* "I always need one person. I just need someone to be in the room, but I don't need them to talk to me." *Is there anything, Miss Foster, you wish to say on the subject of relationships at this time?* "Nope." She pauses. "If you've been in the public eye as long as I have, your life is more important than the trivialization of your life to feed some sort of curiosity machine."[36]

The "curiosity machine" has been fairly quiet in recent years. An unauthorized 1997 biography of the actress, written by her brother Buddy Foster, made mention of an older woman she lived with in Paris during the shooting of *The Blood of Others*.[37] But this barely registered with the media. Yet in 1998, Foster herself vouchsafed to columnist Liz Smith that she had become pregnant, and she cooperated with a *People* magazine cover story about the pregnancy. "Close friends" were quoted in lieu of a statement from Foster herself, and no information was offered as to "the man or the method" of conception.[38] Apparently, childbirth is less "personal" than dating.

*   *   *

In many ways, the ambivalence of today's press when dealing with same-sexuality echoes the politesse of a previous generation of Hollywood denizens, both gay and straight. In a 1958 diary entry concerning Anthony Perkins, Christopher Isherwood notes the actor's frequent trips to his analyst "apparently to get over the effects of splitting up with a roommate. He didn't say who. And we couldn't *quite* ask him." Yet a few years later, the writer mentions his delight at Laurence Harvey's ability to offer a casual embrace at a party at Chasen's restaurant. "That's the kind of thing which sets him apart from most actors. Olivier would do it. Almost no American."[39]

"I remember the fear that used to grip us when we walked into a bar in the sixties and saw someone from the industry," publicist Harry Clein recalls. "Obviously we were there because we were gay, but we didn't want to talk about it with each other. I remember going to the baths once in San Francisco and running into someone I knew, and it was 'Ah ha!'—just for knowing I had other passions besides literature and music and film. But this is how twisted we all were then. There was almost as much hiding from each other and ourselves as from the world."[40]

And it's in *this* context of hiding—from himself, far more than the world—that Rock Hudson must be understood.

"Rock was about as one-hundred-percent masculine a man as you could ever meet in your life," says Kevin Thomas. "He was *profoundly* masculine. When I met him, it really shook up the stereotypes one internalizes, especially when one is a little *obvious*, shall we say. I have since met men like him. But he was a world-famous movie star. This great deep voice. This spectacular-looking giant of a man. It was difficult to get to know him really well. He was a little wary at first. Later on he was very gracious. I *did* know, much better than I knew Rock, Tom Clark. He worked at Metro for many years. Tom was a great big man like Rock. He was not handsome, however. He was a sweet guy, and an outstanding publicist. He was totally devoted to Rock. Rock was very lucky to have him in his life."[41]

Because of that, one would have hoped Clark's memoir, *Rock*

Hudson—Friend of Mine, would offer the sort of insight the numerous books and articles that appeared in the wake of the actor's death did not. But Clark's attempt to "set the record straight" on Hudson does just that. Once again agent Henry Willson is castigated as a "diabolical" creature who "went to his well-deserved grave." Willson is certainly a fascinating figure in Hollywood history, moving from a talent scout for David O. Selznick to a force all his own, capable of creating careers for incredibly good-looking (if on the whole minimally talented) young men, and pinning curious first names on them. But if Rock Hudson, like Guy Madison, Tab Hunter, Troy Donahue, Clint Walker, and Ty Hardin, may have been given his "break" by Wilson, it was up to studio management to truly shape his career.

Living as he did with Hudson for so many years, Clark could claim authoritative knowledge as to his lover's personality. But their affair isn't discussed. Neither are any of Hudson's other romantic alliances with younger men, save for Marc Christian—about whom Clark is angry chiefly for not returning some record albums he had borrowed. Outside of Hudson remarking, "I want to have a lot of men in white coats on the yacht to serve drinks and empty ashtrays," his life with Clark would appear to consist solely of bridge games.[42]

That Clark went to his death without making any additions to this "official" record doesn't surprise writer Armistead Maupin, who came to know them both in 1976. "It was one of those roundabout gay ways that you meet somebody," the *Tales of the City* author recalls. "A guy that I'd picked up at a bar—the Lion Pub in San Francisco—invited me to a gallery opening in Palm Springs where Rock Hudson was expected to be present. We went to Palm Springs and met a whole lot of young men who knew Rock Hudson in one way or another. We never met Rock but during that weekend I fell into bed with one of those guys, Jack Coates. He turned out to be an ex-lover of Rock's. Some weeks later Jack took me to San Bernadino to see Rock onstage in *John Brown's Body*. Afterwards we went backstage to say hello. At the very moment I extended my hand to shake hands with him, there was a blackout in the theater and the place went pitch dark. So I'm standing there in the dark holding on to Rock Hudson's hand, and I made a very feeble joke about 'This is the moment I've waited for all my life!'

"That was our initial meeting. A couple of weeks later he came to San Francisco with *John Brown's Body* and assembled a group of us for dinner at Mama's restaurant on Nob Hill. We hit it off right away. That evening just happened to be the night before *Tales of the City* first appeared in the *San Francisco Chronicle*. After dinner Rock invited a number of us up to his suite at the Fairmont. Unbeknownst to me he had bought the 'bulldog' edition of the *Chronicle*—the one that comes out the night before. When he had everyone assembled in the room, he stood up and did this sort of drunken reading of the first chapter of *Tales of the City*, playing the roles of both Mary Ann and her mother. And the irony was, in that chapter Mary Ann's mother actually makes reference to *McMillan and Wife*, when she's warning her daughter to watch out for what goes on in San Francisco! I was very touched by it, because here was this icon of my youth reading my words in an affectionate way. So Rock and his lover, Tom Clark, invited me to dinner the following night. We went to a restaurant down in the Tenderloin district at the end of an alleyway. They got very polluted, as was their custom, and I suppose I got a little drunk myself, keeping up with them.

"What happened at dinner that night was interesting," Maupin continues. "Here I was, newly out of the closet and completely high on the exhilaration of that experience. I had a career starting, finally, at the age of thirty-two, and I was a happy gay man living in San Francisco. Rock Hudson was a mythic figure at that point who had been privately celebrated as gay for as long as I can remember. I remember thinking, I'd better meet him soon, cause I'm beginning to feel that I'm the only gay man in California who hasn't! For many of us he was the first gay person we ever heard about. There was some strength in knowing that he was this studly guy who made hearts beat faster. So when I had a moment at dinner with him and his lover, I approached him with an almost evangelical fervor about coming out— scaring the holy fuck out of him. I told him, 'You really should write a book and tell it all before somebody else tells it. You can be dignified about it. You can make a difference in the lives of so many young people.' I made the whole pitch. And his lover looked at me very sternly, took me aside afterward and said, 'Not until my mother dies!' Now this guy was in his fifties at that point, and the notion that some seventy-five-year-old bat was going to be horrified to find out that her son was sleeping with the heartthrob of the Western world struck me as patently absurd.

"Rock, who had an engaging way of trying to accommodate everybody, listened to me very carefully, and in fact for years afterward talked about something he referred to as 'the book.' It was this mythical tome that was going to contain the truth of his life and was going to be published 'one of these days.' When anything funny or off-the-wall would happen, he'd say, 'That'll go into the book.' It was his way of coping with the growing enormity of the lie he was having to live with. So on my first meeting with him I made that attempt, and it sort of defined me for him. Whenever we would get together subsequently, he would make some pathetic effort at sounding like a gay libber.

"A few years ago, *Tales of the City* was honored by the Museum of Radio and Television. Marc Christian was waiting in line for my autograph after the program. He was very polite. He said, 'We met at Gore Vidal's house, back when Gore was running for the Senate. And I was Rock Hudson's last boyfriend.' I immediately knew who that was, and I said, 'Marc—I was wondering when our paths would finally cross.' He told me that Rock used to say to him that I came closer than anyone to getting him out of the closet—which I was very moved to hear. Because I wasn't sure if he ever listened to me at all. But he said Rock used to say to him, 'He almost got me out. He almost got me out.'

"Rock buried a lot of his feelings under booze and anger. He was a very sweet man, but he could get quite nasty drunk. And when that happened he was completely out of touch with everything and everybody. He had a groove in his thumbnail—a very serious deformity that ran down the middle of it. I asked him one time what it was. He said it was a 'war wound'—an entirely facetious remark, but I believed it. Later, when I made reference to it to Mark Miller, his personal assistant, he laughed and said, 'That's no war wound, that's just Rock.' I observed him after that and I realized what Mark meant. Rock had a way of taking his forefinger and rubbing it continuously against his thumbnail. He'd done this for so many years he'd actually deformed his thumb in the process. It was a low-key form of self-mutilation. If that doesn't define the burden of the closet, nothing does."[43]

Actress Piper Laurie's memories of Hudson are no less warm, though at some remove from the sociopolitical arena Maupin traverses. "Rock Hudson was a great pal of mine," says the co-star of *The Golden Blade* and *Has Anybody Seen My Gal?* who emerged from the Universal contract-player stable to become a well-regarded serious actress in such films as *The Hustler, Carrie*, and *The Grass Harp*. "We met when I was seventeen. We did our screen test together. He took me to my first circus. He used to come to the house a lot. My mother loved to cook for him. He was a great eater. After a while I used to wonder why he never made a pass at me. I don't know; it was never like an epiphany or anything that I discovered that people were homosexual—I just suddenly *knew*. And I never really thought about it. I remember watching him doing a love scene in class with one of the actresses and I thought, God he's so passionate, so physical. Later I wondered if that had something to do with it. But we continued to be friends all through that time. Just recently I saw *The Golden Blade*. It wasn't as bad as I thought it was. And I actually seemed to be having fun, which I never did. And the reason I seemed to be having fun was because I was working with Rock.

"I saw him about a year before he died. He was very thin. He had some sort of reason for why he was so thin. But he was the same old fun person. Oh, and I remember another time, several years before that. I was walking on upper Broadway in New York with Maureen Stapleton. To her Marlon Brando was just this kid she knew and worked with. He was nothing special. But to Maureen a movie star was Rock Hudson. We had been playing in a production of *The Glass Menagerie* for a long run, so we had a lot of time to talk about that. Rock Hudson was her idol. And we spotted him, just right around the corner from where she lived. We hollered at him. I hadn't seen him in ten years, fifteen years. He didn't turn around, 'cause he thought it was just fans. But we started running after him. The faster we ran, the faster he ran. It was awful. Finally there was a red light and we managed to get close to him. He turned around and said, 'Piper!' He grabbed me and lifted me into the air. I love that picture of Maureen and me running down the street—both of us overweight, and acting like teenagers."[44]

There's no reason for Laurie or Stapleton to have behaved otherwise. Rock Hudson was a fantasy figure to be enjoyed by all and sundry. The "truth" of his sexuality had no real bearing on his appeal. But the "unmasking" of that truth is another matter, not just in Hudson's time but right now.

"I think the closet is still an extremely viable institution in Hollywood," Armistead Maupin declares. "Closeted people have just gotten more sophisticated in dealing with it. The current politically acceptable line is 'I'm not gay, but I take it as a compliment that people think that I am.' You utter those words and no one is offended. That still allows the privilege of lying. We still haven't reached the stage where being gay is just a fact. We're closer to that point, but we still haven't reached that stage, because there are no major male movie stars who are out of the closet.

"My observation is that agents and managers are the keepers of the closet keys," Maupin continues. "They are the ones who are continuing to promulgate the myth that stars should not come out under any circumstances. Therefore it's a little annoying to me to see these people showing up at GLAAD functions acting as if they're doing all they can to eliminate homophobia in Hollywood, because they *aren't*. They're still hanging on to the single belief that keeps the prejudice going: that it's okay to be in the closet

"They all say, 'Why should I when everybody knows?' That's never been the point. The point is whether or not we have the dignity and the pride to state it matter-of-factly in a public way. That's what it's all about. And it's always the people who work so hard to keep it from being official that claim that everybody knows. We *know* that everybody knows. It's the fact that everybody knows, and can do nothing about it, that suggests that there's something wrong with it."[45]

Writer-director Bill Condon agrees with Maupin and cites an incident to illustrate. "There's one really good story I've got to tell you about attitudes toward gays in Hollywood. I went to see the Matthew Bourne *Swan Lake* with Curtis Harrington, who was actually—weirdly enough—slightly the inspiration for the Edmund Kay character, the gay horror-movie buff in *Gods and Monsters*. Roddy McDowall was at *Swan Lake*. I'd never met him, but he knows everyone involved in this project—Clive Barker, Ian Mc-Kellen. He knows *everybody*. So Curtis told him I was doing the ad aptation of this novel and Roddy scowled. He talked about what a close friend he was of George Cukor's; then he turned to Curtis and said—very pointedly—'I've never met *anyone* who had a good thing to say about James Whale.' It was so interesting to see, some forty years later, that divide between people who were just a *little* more open about things and everyone else. We thought that dynamic had totally disappeared from Hollywood, but it's still there. There's still a vestige of it in Roddy McDowall."[46]

I f you understand how casting agents work, you know they're looking for reasons to red-light you," notes publicist Howard Bragman. " 'Nobody will buy him as a lead—he's a fag!' is an excuse for not hiring. Many straight men have been awarded for playing gay guys. Many gay people play straight their whole lives. It's not the hardest job in the world to do. You just make yourself a little less interesting, don't dress quite as well as you usually do, watch your movements— no living large with the gestures—and people think you're straight.

"But I look at the sadness of somebody like Tony Hamilton," says Bragman regretfully of the star of the *Cover Up* spy adventure series and the *Samson and Delilah* made-for-television spectacular of 1984, who expired from AIDS in 1990. "He was unable to make the difference that someone like him could have made if he'd come out. It's really sad.

"Look, I'll even say this on the record and have her come after me," says Bragman sharply. "Lily Tomlin has never officially come out and said 'I'm a lesbian.' Now I think there's a huge irony here.

All the decision makers in town know that Lily Tomlin's a lesbian. She's well established in the gay and lesbian community, yet she won't go out on a stage or before a camera and say four simple words: 'I am a lesbian.' And you know what? I don't mean we have to label ourselves, but as long as teenage kids are committing suicide, and as long as they're trying to deny us our rights, I think we have a certain obligation to use what we have to change things. I think it's silly that at the Gay and Lesbian Community Center's twenty-year anniversary she said, 'We've been gay and lesbian twenty years,' and then the next week we hear her publicist backtracking: ' "*We*" meaning the crowd there—she didn't necessarily mean herself.' I just think you lose a measure of respect.

"Look, I don't mean to pick on her," Bragman continues. "Lily has done more for the gay and lesbian community than 99 percent of the actors in this town. But you know what? I was with Marta Kaufman and David Crane, the writer-producers of *Friends,* the other day, and we were talking about the airing of an episode of *Dream On* that had a gay character in it. They said, 'Isn't this great?' and I said, 'It's great, but what you need is a regular recurring gay character.' They said, 'How much do we have to do?' and I said, 'Those of us who have the courage have to do more for those who will never do it.' So Lily, if you're reading this, you've done more than enough—but *not enough.* She's a handy example of someone whose career is not going to be hurt by her saying that she's a lesbian. I don't see huge commercial endorsements out there that would be coming her way for not saying so.

"I'm forty-one, and I look at my friends who are a generation older than me. They say, 'It's nobody's business. We don't have to talk about it.' That was sort of the liberal accepted thing of the past. It's not the same anymore. I look at the kids coming up—eighteen- and sixteen-year-old kids—saying, 'I'm gay and I'm starting a club at my high school, and I'm not going to stay in the closet.' There are people who are saying, 'I don't care if I'm a hundred-million-dollar star, I'd rather be a fifty-dollar star and have my dignity.' That's the point where we're getting. So many people have chipped away this thing: Elton John and Melissa Etheridge, and Martina Navratilova in the sports world. So we're getting a TV lead with Ellen. Now we need a big movie star—male or female. And you know what? People's movies are going to open regardless of their sexuality.

"What's happening now with gays and lesbians is the same thing that used to happen with blacks," Bragman continues. "If it was twenty-five years ago and someone wanted to cast Whoopi Goldberg in *Ghost,* it would be, 'We don't want a colored person in that movie.' Now she was cast—and it worked. So you change your thinking. And with the liberal hierarchy hopefully in place, I would pray there wouldn't be a casting agency where they would say, 'We're not going to put that fag in—nobody will believe him.' They might come up with other excuses, but they wouldn't say that out loud, because they don't know who they're saying it to anymore. Homophobia in Hollywood is taboo. And it's one of the first industries where it is taboo.

"The elders of the community used to say to me, 'You don't need to be so in people's faces, Howard.' And my answer was, 'Yes I do.' I was a suicidal teenager. For the grace of God I'm here and have some opportunities other people didn't get. And I do need to be in their face. I'm sorry. I don't see anybody hiding their religion in this town. I don't see people hiding their weddings in this town. And I'll be goddamned if I'm going to be a partner to people hiding their sex life in this town. It's not that big a deal, and the bigger deal everybody makes about it makes it a dirty little secret."[47]

It's no secret of any sort for Ian McKellen, who credits his mid-career "coming out" with aiding him both personally and professionally. But at the same time he's aware that the pressures on performers haven't lessened.

"I know actors who are Brendan Fraser's age who are gay. Looking at what happens, I suppose I would stay closeted if I were in their position. There are very few young actors who are out in movies. For that reason, I think Anne Heche's coming out is more significant than Ellen's. Ellen can always go to clubs or out on the concert stage on her own and earn a living, but Anne Heche always has to be employed in film. I remember when Anthony Sher came out. He was asked by the *Times* of London, What about a film career?—which he was just beginning to have. He said, 'Look, if people don't want to work with

me because I'm gay, I certainly don't want to work with them.' And
that's what I feel. I don't want to work with second-rate people. In the
hope of becoming very rich, I don't want to have to lie. I know English
actors like Miriam Margolyes who are out at home, in London. She
said to me, 'You understand that in Hollywood I'm not a dyke.' So
what does her girlfriend think about that?"

McKellen is greatly amused by Hollywood's reaction to the El-
len/*Ellen* story, finding DeGeneres's appearance on *The Rosie
O'Donnell Show* to be particularly interesting. "All she said to Ellen
was 'I like the show.' Of course she *hated* the show. It brings her one
step closer to the day when she'll have to deal with her own problems.

"People have odd ideas about what being out is," McKellen
continues. "I think Lily Tomlin would probably say that she's out, but
she's not out. And goes to great, considerable lengths to avoid being
out. When she read the narration for *The Celluloid Closet*—which
Vito [Russo] asked me to do, but the producers wanted her—she
helped get it made. She helped with the financing. Armistead [Mau-
pin] asked, 'Who's going to read the narration?' And they said, 'Lily
Tomlin.' He said, 'No, I'm not going to write for a closeted dyke!' They
said, 'No, it's fine. She's going to use this opportunity to come out and
be honest.' So Armistead wrote her coming-out speech. And she *cut*
it.

"Do you know," says McKellen with no small degree of amusement, "that you can buy bits of her hair in the classified ads in the
Advocate? I don't know where the hair comes from."[48]

The classified ads in the *Advocate*, as well as many other gay
publications, feature personal ads for "escort" services. Many of
them proudly offer the services of gay porno stars. And that in turn
opens the door to the very contemporary phenomenon of "porno culture."

"It's become really chic in Hollywood over the past few years
to be into dating porno stars," says journalist/filmmaker Richard Natale with a mixture of amazement and amusement. "For some people
it's a badge of honor to be dating somebody who's a porno star/hustler.

It makes sense in a way, because they're the most desirable people. They're very attractive. They're stars in their own right. And it means *you* must be very attractive, because it means they want to sleep with you—not to mention anyone else who pays them. That's the new aesthetic. People who want to date porno stars or look like them—that sort of white, suburban, hairless, buff body. That's what people want."[49]

Of course, dalliances with same-sex professionals are no new thing in Hollywood. But the atmosphere has shifted sharply over the past two decades, as those who have "kissed" have been increasingly willing to tell. In 1993 a crisis of sorts arose when Gavin Dillard, star of *Track Meat* and other gay erotic features, attempted to publish his memoirs, *In the Flesh: Undressing for Success*, through Harper*Collins*. When David Geffen and Barry Diller learned that the book contained detailed allegations of their relationships with Dillard, libel action was threatened. Five years later the memoir found a home at Barricade Books—with the moguls' real names replaced by pseudonyms.[50] A lot had happened in the intervening years, with Geffen coming out and using his clout to help gay and AIDS causes in numerous ways, and Diller likewise pitching in—while insisting a veil be maintained over his "private life." Yet for all the loosening of the atmosphere surrounding same-sex relations in Hollywood, sex-for-hire remains a bit of unsettled social business—for all the "chicness" it may evoke for some.

"People should have more respect for whores. They never know who they're dealing with in the long run," says Steven Dornbusch, a key grip with a worldly-wise attitude toward gays in the industry—himself included. "Some really fascinating people are prostitutes. They know who they are. It's a personal choice. What people experience as prostitutes is a fascinating view of the world. Looking up from the bottom at everything rather than down from the top. There's no smoke and mirrors. I'm not talking about street people versus being kept. It's all the same. It's a business. There are people who are prostitutes when they're younger. Male and female. And I think part of the reason they became prostitutes is because they're adventurous. With some people you don't even necessarily have to have sex. A lot of people are dysfunctional and just want people to *think* they have sex. They want to be listened to. They can treat you like a bartender— a person who's paid to listen. The other thing is that prostitution can expose you to things in a different way that you might not have seen. Usually it's secret, sometimes it's not. But rarely do they make a point of it like Rechy or Genet.

"I'm not into reforming people," Dornbusch continues philosophically. "I'm not prudish; I simply don't like people like that. To put it real simple, I don't like johns of all types. I don't like the johns driving around in station wagons looking to get a blow job. I'm suspect of any male who says he's bisexual. I don't trust them. Scientifically there's no one who isn't bisexual. It's just that socially, women get points for pretending that they're homosexual, men get points for pretending that they're heterosexual. There are a lot of people who don't want to be called 'homosexual' or 'heterosexual.' If—eventually— there's a more just and healthier world, these categories will fall apart, disappear, and be integrated into the culture."[51]

To Dornbusch, hiring a prostitute is less about sex than it is about control. And in Hollywood control—over profits, people, and social situations—is the most desirable of all commodities. It's no wonder then that in recent years Scientology, a self-help technique that has evolved into what its followers claim to be a religious practice, has become so attractive in Hollywood. Religious and "personal growth" fads blossom and wither in the California sun on a regular basis. But this particular one, founded by the late science-fiction writer L. Ron Hubbard, has been able to boast of the likes of Tom Cruise, Nicole Kidman, Mimi Rogers, John Travolta, Kirstie Alley, and Jenna Elfman among its members. As Hubbard's writings evidence an apparent antipathy to same-sexuality, it has been suspected by many that the "church" has provided a "closet" for select celebrity members. Publicist Doug Lindeman, a former church member, who broke with it several years ago in the wake of coming out, has decidedly mixed feelings about the situation. While no longer part of the church, he still stands by many of its tenets. But when it comes to sexuality he remains much as he did five years ago when he first broached the subject to Michelangelo Signorile.[52]

"I got a call from someone in the church who was mortified to read about it and wanted to know if they could help me with any legal action," Lindeman recalls with some amusement. "I said no. I said, 'I did that interview and I hold by it. This is true. You're homophobic. You view homosexuality as antisocial behavior, and that's your problem, not mine.' I respect Scientology, but, hell—I'm sure the Orthodox Jews are homophobic, I'm sure the Buddhists are homophobic, I'm sure the Mormons are homophobic. Most religions come from heterosexual society, so give me a break. Every religion says they're right. The problem with being right is everybody else is supposed to be wrong—except for those who agree with you.

"Scientology also has, in my understanding of it," Lindeman continues, "the disadvantage of Hubbard's son, Quentin, who killed himself. The assumption was Quentin was gay and was quite tormented, being deeply steeped inside the paradigm of Scientology, and not being able to manifest this and not being able to have the recourse of counseling to help himself get over his sexuality. Most heterosexuals are not out to 'promote' heterosexuality. As a homosexual man, I'm not out to 'promote' homosexuality—just peace on earth. But some in Scientology are kind of trapped because Hubbard had his understanding of homosexuality from a heterosexual viewpoint in a very homophobic society. And his own experiences with homosexuals were probably not positive ones. John McMasters, the first 'clear' [the church's term for the most enlightened] in Scientology, I'd heard, was a homosexual also, and left the church. I'm sure there were a lot of others because 'clears' didn't have their act together back in 1950 when Hubbard was organizing Scientology.

"Scientology is very nuts-and-bolts," Lindeman claims. "It's a workable technology. You can get observable, verifiable results. You can see conditions in your life change. But they happen to have some false information about homosexuality. I expect that over the years it will evolve and they'll lighten up this homophobia. It's going to be like the last horse in the caravan if it doesn't.

"I've heard all the rumors," says Lindeman of Scientology's biggest stars. "I've never slept with Travolta. I've never slept with Tom Cruise. I don't know whether this is true or false. They're human beings transmogrified into gods to serve the culture and the mass media and everything else. If these people are using Scientology or anything else to try to rectify their life, that's fine. It's pretty small to talk about Scientology without being inside it. You can't talk about what the Sikhs are up to. We like to talk about the Scientologists because it's been turned into tabloid fodder.

"This whole thing has always been the heterosexual community's problem, not ours," Lindeman continues. "We're rather blessed by being queer, because we're *not* saddled with role models, we're *not* saddled with societal expectations. We're unencumbered. People who want us to lie about our sexuality are saddled with old, unexamined societal rigor mortis. They're in no position to examine what is true and what is honest. If someone has a problem with my being gay, they should get help. Go seek professional counseling. That's what we have to learn as queers. It's *their* problem, not ours.

"Being an actor is kind of like being queer in society. The actor that people are adoring on the screen is an illusion. This is a person who has taken on a role, is speaking somebody else's lines, doing what somebody else says. Everybody has taken this blank piece of paper and created something out of it. An audience member falls in love with this person and knows that they know nothing about the person they've fallen in love with. It's loving an illusion. You want to substantiate it with some real information. You know when you see an actor in public, how unnerving it is? You recognize them, but you know they've never met you. What's that all about?

"I happen to live next door to Sandra Bullock. I knew her before all this success happened to her. She was just an actress working in Hollywood—and then *Speed* hit. She said it was a wave, she was riding it, and she's hoping that people still want her to work five years from now. It's been like watching lottery tickets land in her backyard! So I'm seeing her picture on magazine covers and think, 'Sandy would never dress like that, or walk around and pose like that.' But there it is on the cover of a magazine, being used to get your attention.

"Celebrities are more astute about keeping their private lives out of the public eye than ever before," Lindeman continues. "I think there's much more of a professional respect between the community of celebrities and publicists and the editors. I think they realize they're in it for the long haul, and it's not in the best interest to cover every aspect of everybody's private life. They have to keep their icons intact, because if they pull the icons off the wall they're not going to have them to put on the front cover."[53]

Mark Miller, an editor at *Newsweek*, is keenly aware of "front cover" pressures and the media's curious role in detailing gay and lesbian issues and celebrity lives in recent years.

"There's this collusion between source and press to keep what is known to all of us, and known to large numbers of people, a secret simply because of our own squeamishness," Miller declares. "The only way to effectively overcome this is for people to come out. Now if Jodie Foster were living a completely closeted life, that might be one thing, but there's no reason not to report things that are happening in front of you. We had this interesting thing at *Newsweek* where Nathan Lane thought we had outed him. Jack Kroll, the theater critic, did the piece. *Birdcage* had come out and Lane was about to open in the revival of *A Funny Thing Happened on the Way to the Forum* on Broadway."[54]

Kroll's offense? A passage in the piece where he quoted Lane:

> "A lot of actors didn't want to play that role because it was so flamboyant. But I just instantly knew who the man was." Well, sure as a gay man, he would know, right? Lane, who could play dueling face muscles with Jim Carrey, hoists his eloquent eyebrows, flares his nostrils and corkscrews his mouth, composing a perfect line drawing that says "None-of-yer-bizness." He's right. And he's not worried about being typed as the gay guy of choice.[55]

"Jack thought it was perfectly fair that he didn't want to talk about his private life, and he moved onto the next part of the interview," says Miller. "But when the piece came out, Nathan Lane was apoplectic and accused us of outing him. Jack and I had this conversation about this. He was horrified he had done something like that because he really didn't think of it that way. And *I* didn't think of it that way. 'Cause here is someone who goes to the bars, goes out, and is known, and has chosen these roles—and he did raise the subject *himself*. But he expected us to participate in the secrecy. He just assumed that that part of the conversation would never be reported."[56]

Lane's ambivalence was apparent from another profile that came out that same year, in *Esquire*. "Someone asks me a question and I just answer it. I don't see any point in not being honest," Lane first tells interviewer David Blum—only to inform him several paragraphs later, "I just sort of take the unpopular stance that my personal life is my own and nobody's business."[57]

Like Lily Tomlin, Lane has shown no shyness about appearing at gay-supportive events, such as the annual "Broadway Bares" AIDS benefit at which, as columnist Michael Musto succinctly puts it, "the usual procession of half-naked gypsies [display] their metaphorical Tony Awards. After the show, host Nathan Lane told the crowd, 'For those of you out there who like to mentally undress people, I guess this evening has been a real disappointment.' As the audience got more and more heated, Lane decreed, 'Get out the poppers, we'll sing all night.' We didn't, but Lane did give his take on the production number that had a guy with a giant net rounding up a gaggle of boys dressed like fishies: 'Very Ernest Hemingway.' "[58]

And yet, according to *New York* magazine, "Lane has remained tight-lipped about his sexual orientation, and had reportedly turned down the chance to reprise Buzz [the role written especially for him in the play *Love! Valour! Compassion!*] on film in order to distance himself from gay roles."[59] Meanwhile, Michael Musto noted that "the fabulous Nathan Lane was recently spotted at the gay cruise bar Splash, and told a fan who went up to him that he was taking a big risk being there alone. A shock wave went through the room as everyone realized Nathan thinks he's not 'out'—and what's more, that indeed he isn't. But my spies say that all was forgotten as, moments later, the comic actor busied himself with a slender stud and the birdcage door flung wide open."[60]

By 1997, things had calmed down somewhat. "He had a highly

publicized spat with [playwright Terrence] McNally when he wouldn't appear in the movie version of *Love! Valour! Compassion!*," a *Los Angeles Times* profile noted. "Accusations flew that Lane didn't want another gay role, although he maintains that he bowed out because of scheduling conflicts. At any rate, he says, it was blown out of proportion by the press."

Still, in the same article, Lane continues to express the feeling that his sexuality, onscreen and off, was having an effect on his career. "I had a meeting with a studio executive who said, 'Gee, we're not doing any broad comedies, or anything with gay characters in them.' And I thought 'Is that all you think I can do?' Whether you like it or not, you can get stuck. It'll be interesting to see what will happen with Rupert Everett. You try to keep them guessing."[61] But there was nothing to guess—as Lane finally admitted ("You do the math!") a year later in an *US* profile.[62]

Like many gay and lesbian performers, Nathan Lane has been trying to navigate his way through uncharted waters in uncertain times. His skill at flamboyance has won him accolades. But can that very winning factor pigeonhole him into certain roles? Hardly. His abilities are such to inspire the now legendary statement (attributed to Neil Simon) "If Nathan Lane can't make it funny, it's not funny." Consequently, the presence of Nathan Lane in any given role doesn't portend "gayness" but, rather, guarantees laughter—of every sort imaginable. Part of the problem has to do with the context in which celebrity gayness has come to reside. Merely acknowledging one's sexuality shouldn't be regarded as a political act. Moreover, "coming out" can be awkward for those who, in all honesty, have nothing to say about their sexuality. Producer Scott Rudin is "out," but he's had nothing particular to add about it. He'd rather just make movies. But producers aren't presented to the public the way performers are. Nathan Lane is a supremely skillful interpreter of other people's words. He is capable of playing any sort of part that's offered to him. That should be enough. But of course, it isn't.

"Right after Ellen came out, Liz Smith had this column saying that a major television icon would come out too," says Mark Miller. "Whoever it was supposed to be, it didn't happen. But then there were stories about Anne and Ellen breaking up. I had a discussion with a reporter about making some calls to see if they had broken up or not. It's a straight reporter and he's saying, 'Oh, it's so personal. I don't know if I could do that.' And I was saying, 'Look, they went to the White House together and were photographed, they've gone on *Oprah* together, they've made their relationship a public issue—if they break up, it may not be earth-shattering news, but it's news.' He didn't want to go near it. The whole subject is still a problem for many, many people. It's different for men than with women. There's more squeamishness about, even more reluctance to do something about male homosexuality in *Newsweek* than female. It's like Bertolucci said about showing the penis in one of his movies: 'It's more personal than the breast.' I think that's the way a lot of media has been. It's run by men, and they're so scared of the idea of male homosexuality."[63]

Jenny Pizer of the Lambda Legal Defense and Education Fund has dealt with any number of issues related to gay and lesbian civil rights nationwide, from job and housing discrimination to the ever-headline-grabbing gays-in-the-military controversy. She also follows Hollywood affairs closely, as she feels they're often a harbinger of things to come in other areas of the culture.

"We in the advocacy organizations are trying to change public understanding so it will not be considered a bad thing to be gay," says Pizer, seated amidst piles of documents in the organization's Los Angeles office. "It shouldn't still be existing in the law that being gay is so horrible that when someone is falsely accused of it they don't have to prove that it's damaging—that the accusation is seen as damaging on its face. People should have to *prove* that it's bad."

"It seems to me you have two different relevant doctrines that are involved making someone's sexual orientation known," says Pizer of the "outing" controversy. "There's the defamation doctrine, and then there's invasion of privacy: public disclosure of private facts, information somehow gotten improperly, and so forth. If a person is in a public place displaying same-sex affection, they can't claim invasion of privacy. That's one thing people get in trouble for. If they're

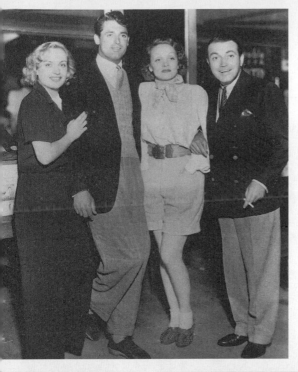

A NIGHT out in the 1930s: Carole Lombard, Cary Grant, Marlene Dietrich, and Richard Barthelmess. (PARAMOUNT PICTURES)

H IDING in plain sight: Cary Grant and Randolph Scott sur la plage, Santa Monica, circa 1932. (BABY JANE OF HOLLYWOOD)

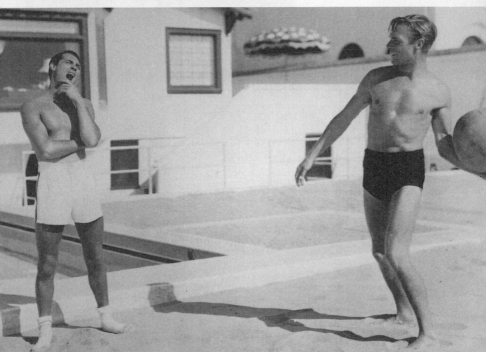

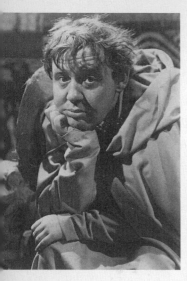

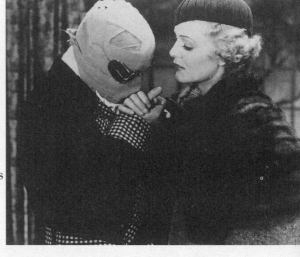

It was so safe": Charles Laughton in *I Claudius* (1937). (JOSEF VON STERNBERG)

Too visible?: Claude Rains and Gloria Stuart in James Whale's *The Invisible Man* (1933). (UNIVERSAL PICTURES)

Gay killers confront their straight mentor: James Stewart, John Dall, and Farley Granger in *Rope* (1948). (UNIVERSAL PICTURES)

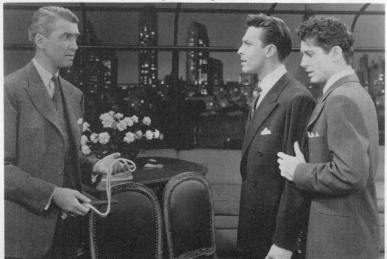

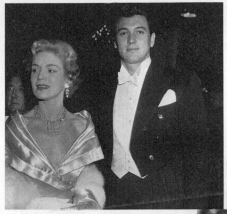

IT'S a date: Rock Hudson and Veronica Hurst attend the Royal Command film performance of *Because You're Mine* at the Empire Theatre, London, 1952. (HOLLYWOOD BOOK AND POSTER)

GAY: James Dean in *East of Eden* (1955). (WARNER BROTHERS)

CLEANING his room: Tab Hunter circa *Battle Cry* (1955). (WARNER BROTHERS)

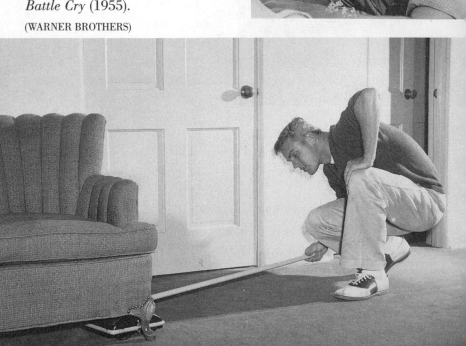

SECRET identities:
Anthony Perkins and Janet
Leigh in *Psycho* (1960).
(UNIVERSAL PICTURES)

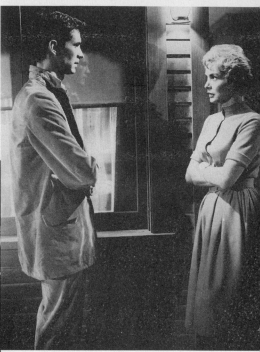

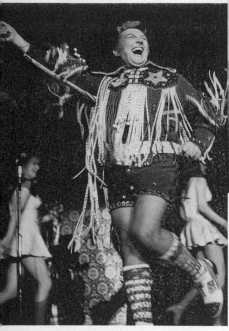

FAMILY entertainment:
Liberace onstage, circa mid-1970s.
(HOLLYWOOD BOOK AND POSTER)

UNFINISHED business:
Randy Shilts at town meeting,
San Francisco, May 29, 1992.
(DAVID EHRENSTEIN)

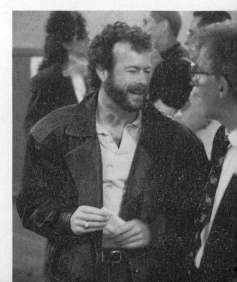

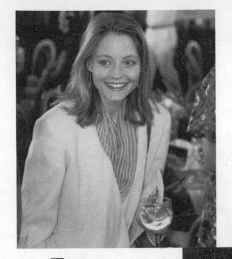

JODIE Foster at the Independent Feature Project Awards, Los Angeles, 1992. (DAVID EHRENSTEIN)

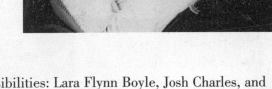

FROM avant-garde to "mainstream" in only five years: Gus Van Sant at the Chateau Marmont, June 1992. (DAVID EHRENSTEIN)

CONSIDER the possibilities: Lara Flynn Boyle, Josh Charles, and Stephen Baldwin in *Threesome* (1994). (TRI-STAR PICTURES)

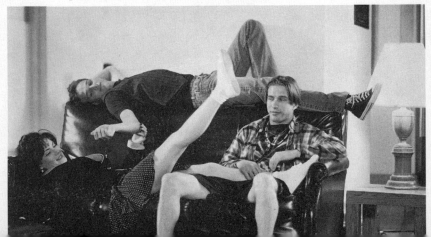

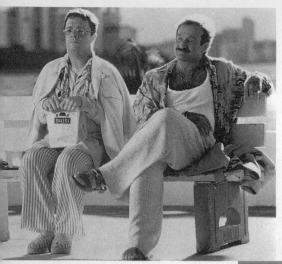

"OVER the top" with "mass appeal": Nathan Lane and Robin Williams in *The Birdcage* (1996). (UNITED ARTISTS)

THREE little words: Jeffrey Friedman, Rob Epstein, and Lily Tomlin (1996). (TELLING PICTURES)

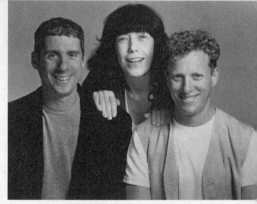

THE gays next door: Jack Nicholson, Cuba Gooding, Jr., and Greg Kinnear in *As Good As It Gets* (1997). (TRI-STAR PICTURES)

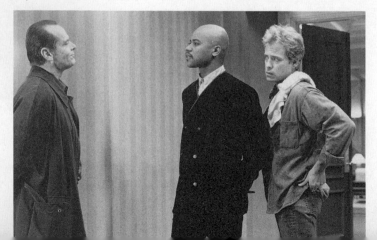

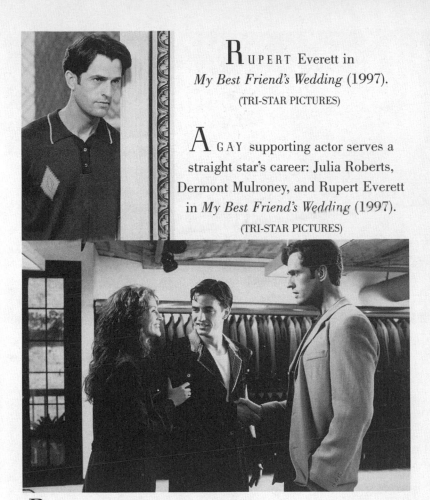

R UPERT Everett in *My Best Friend's Wedding* (1997). (TRI-STAR PICTURES)

A GAY supporting actor serves a straight star's career: Julia Roberts, Dermont Mulroney, and Rupert Everett in *My Best Friend's Wedding* (1997). (TRI-STAR PICTURES)

P LAYING gay: Kevin Spacey and Jude Law in *Midnight in the Garden of Good and Evil* (1997). (WARNER BROTHERS)

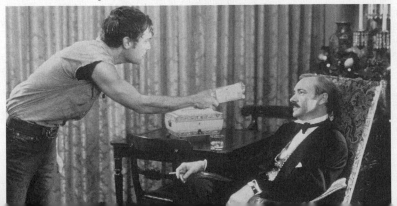

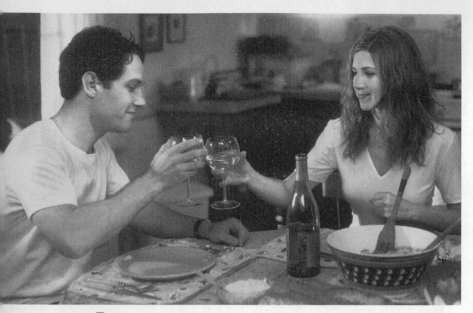

A NORMAL life: Paul Rudd and Jennifer Aniston in
The Object of My Affection (1998). (TWENTIETH CENTURY-FOX)

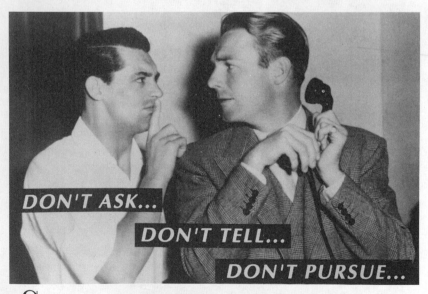

C ARY Grant and Randolph Scott in Mark Rappaport's *The Silver
Screen—Color Me Lavender* (1998). (PLANET PICTURES)

outed that way, privacy wouldn't apply. As for defamation, truth is an absolute defense.

"Under California law," Pizer continues, "there are certain categories of statements about a person that are presumptively harmful to a person's character. For example, if someone's a surgeon and you say of them, 'The guy has such shaky hands he can't hold a cup of coffee,' that's presumptively harmful to his business. If it's true, you can say it, because truth is a complete defense. If it's a false thing being said, he doesn't have to come forward and say why he's damaged—we presume that harm.

"Now what is totally fascinating to me is the way sexual orientation is now in flux. If it isn't something we presume is harmful, we take it to a jury. Is the nature of the statement such that a reasonable person hearing it would think badly about the person of whom it is being said? Sometimes it's a matter of knowing extra facts. If something were said about Jodie Foster, and she brought an action against them, would a reasonable person—this is the standard in tort law—think badly of her? For example, what if a person in their business is an interior designer? Maybe people don't think well of gay men, but when it comes to interior designers, many people in the business world would think, Oh, he's probably a better designer if he's a gay man. If he comes forward claiming damage, a jury could very well say that given his line of work, we don't think he's damaged or could be damaged by such a remark.

"There's a case where a man in the workplace was sexually harassing a woman who rebuffed his advances. To get back at her, he said to other people—falsely—that he had seen her in bed with another woman. Now the standard under California law has been that you are presumed to be harmed if someone imputes impotence to a man or 'unchastity' to a woman. So this actually was imputing unchastity to her, but the case has been misconstrued as implying homosexuality. We have this situation in California where the person accused of homosexuality doesn't have to prove the harm, it's *there*.

"Let me read what it says in *Selleck vs. Globe*," says Peyser, picking up a raft of documents. " 'Plaintiff, who is the father of celebrity Tom Selleck, brought an action against the publisher of a magazine featuring items about celebrities in the entertainment world. The article complained of was called "Tom Selleck's Love Secrets by his Father," and contained a number of statements attributed to Tom Selleck's father which disparaged and downgraded the romantic character and capability of his son.' I guess that's in the eye of the disparager. 'Plaintiff Selleck senior alleged that he never gave an interview to any of defendant's reporters, and never made any statements to anyone concerning his son's "love secrets." A cause of action was stated. The publication was held as libelous on its face.' So, in other words, there's a presumption of harm. You don't have to prove the actual damages. 'The content of the article, viewed in conjunction with the headline, clearly conveyed the impression that Mr. Selleck Sr. had granted an interview to the defendant in which he divulged for public dissemination matters which his son revealed to him in confidence. Although some of the statements attributed to Selleck Sr. were innocuous, some were not. For example, Selleck Jr. is "ill at ease with women," and he's "just not the person they think he should be." ' Well, what does that mean?

" 'Some readers could construe these matters to be of the type Tom Selleck would be expected not to divulge since they damage Tom Selleck's image as "TV's sexiest leading man," ' " Peyser's reading continues. " 'Since Selleck Sr. is not a celebrity who would benefit by publicity, the article was subject to the inference that he was paid to divulge his son's secrets to the *Globe*, thereby attributing to Selleck Sr. a Judas-like betrayal of his son.' So Selleck Sr. was injured by the suggestion that he was disloyal, and it's not about Selleck Jr. suing because it suggested that he was a fag or whatever."

So why did Tom Selleck sue? Was it worth all this trouble and cost to him? Peyser says it depends on the individual celebrity involved.

"Its become such a standard thing in our society, which is a very litigious society, for people to want to be able to say, for their 'honor' or whatever the issue would be, 'I'm gonna sue you.' And sometimes if they don't do that people will wonder why they aren't standing up for themselves. If there's evidence all over the place that Tom Selleck or whoever is in fact gay, and they bring a suit that is on that issue—which would be a true accusation if people involved have enough evidence—then the response will be you don't settle it, and make them prove the charges. If he can't disprove it—if it's a true thing to say—then you bring a malicious prosecution suit against him, and then he *really* gets it. You see, there's a complete difference between the public relations battle and what things represent in our society—the threat of a suit versus what you actually can and can't do within the legal process based on what the law is. Ninety-five to ninety-eight percent of cases settle out of court, so the fact that a case didn't go all the way through to the end doesn't necessarily tell you anything about its merits.

"The point I'm getting at is moving from where we are now to the point where we should be. As of now many people *do* care about sexual orientation, and many people will think badly of a gay person if their sexual orientation is known. So many gay people, for that very logical reason, don't want their sexual orientation disclosed. Everybody should have the right of privacy, and be able to control their own information. The press is always a very different thing because it has other duties and rights and protections. And when a person is a public figure or becomes a 'public figure'—even against their will, like that guy in San Francisco who was standing right there when the President got shot and the story got out that he was gay—it is very much a different subject. What we're grappling with here, not just in legal organizations but as a movement, is what we want to be saying to the court as to what should be a rule of evidence. Should we ask courts to consider this private information because it's special? Well, we don't want to say that, really."[64]

But what gays and lesbians want to say is quite different from what Tom Selleck wants to say. Moreover, his ability to both say things and have the words that others say about him accounted for puts him in a place apart.

"I am proud of my sexual preference as those who happen to be gay are of theirs," said Selleck in announcing a $20 million suit against the *Globe* in 1991. "There is not a man who has lived on the face of the Earth in my lifetime who can truthfully deny what is so obviously my choice; that is, that I am singularly heterosexual."[65] It was, however, quite a simple matter to pull the *Globe* to heel, as its article, " 'Gay' Stars Stop Traffic," had merely reported on a campaign staged by a group of anonymous gay and lesbian radicals, which put up posters in downtown New York proclaiming that Selleck, Merv Griffin, Jodie Foster, and other celebrities were "Absolutely Queer."

"By publishing the article, the *Globe* did not intend to express or imply that Tom Selleck is or ever was a homosexual, and the *Globe* apologizes to the extent that any statements made by the *Globe* editors concerning the article were construed to express or imply that Tom Selleck is or was a homosexual," the tabloid declared simply in "settling" with the star.[66]

"It didn't take long, however," writer and gay activist Larry Gross reported, "for word to leak out—through very reliable sources—that the undisclosed amount of the settlement was five dollars. Thus was honor saved."[67]

It was something of a surprise, then, to find "honor" put at risk six years later when Selleck was cast as a gay entertainment journalist reporting on the outing of a high-school teacher in the comedy *In and Out*. That someone once so sensitive to statements claiming he was merely unlike his screen image should change direction so radically was brought up by many members of the press—who characteristically failed to press Selleck about the situation in any detail.

"Listen, this is a great part, and that's all that counts. I knew all the tabloid stuff would come back up. But the movie isn't an answer, or any sort of apology [to gay people] for me suing a tabloid for saying I'm gay," Selleck tells *Entertainment Weekly* as part of their *In and Out* cover story. "That's nonsense. . . . No leading man in this business has ever gotten anywhere without somebody saying he's gay, and that's fine."[68]

"I haven't had problems with the gay community," Selleck declares to the *Advocate*. "The problems have been that there were some unethical journalists who felt a necessity to make people gay who weren't. I think that's reprehensible, as I do about any reporter who feels a necessity to lie or 'lawyer' the truth to further their own agenda."

So why did he take legal action against stories that even *sug-*

gested things indirectly, several individuals removed, as was the case with the piece involving his father?

"I was angry at individuals in the media for making up lies," Selleck explains. "I was very disappointed that there wasn't more public outcry and condemnation from the gay press about the kind of tactics used against me. 'Don't say anything about this. It will just draw more attention to it.' But I thought, What does that say about me? I don't believe in victimization. I got great peace of mind by doing something about it. And I knew some people would think of it as homophobic. Maybe as you live your life and you're a fairly decent person, people will get some sense of what the real truth is."[69]

"I'm surprised that people are surprised that I played this part," Selleck tells *The New York Times*. "If this came along 10 years ago, I still would have done it. This character's an interesting guy. The fact that he's gay is almost irrelevant. That's not enough to define a character. And he's very comfortable with his sexuality."[70]

But as Selleck certainly knows, no such part would have come along in 1987. For that was a year in which a major studio would have found the notion of a light comedy about gay sexuality unthinkable. A lot has happened in Hollywood in that ten-year span. It would be highly unlikely that any contemporary performer would spend as much time and money pursuing tabloid news items as Selleck did in the early part of the 1990s. Clearly, Selleck's feelings have changed. More important, Hollywood has changed. And squeamishness over inferences of same-sexuality are rather awkward when you're starring in a script by Paul Rudnick for a producer like Scott Rudin.

In the early months of 1995, the fourth estate was rocked by a "controversy" entirely of its own making. Jann Wenner, publisher of *Rolling Stone* magazine, and a figure almost as well-known to the public as Hugh Hefner, had left his wife for a man, a designer for Calvin Klein named Matt Nye.

"Wenner met Nye at a Christmas party in 1993, on the voguish French Antilles resort isle of St. Bartholomew," veteran celebrity journalist Jeanie Russell Kasindorf noted in *New York* magazine. "Nye is

the kind of husky, handsome, well-connected poster boy close acquaintances don't worry about calling 'a boy toy of the Velvet Mafia.'
He was accompanying the painter Ross Bleckner; he was the artist's
assistant and apparently his boyfriend. Spotting the young man
(Bleckner told one source), Wenner came up to Bleckner and said
'My, he's very attractive.' In other words, a bit of cruising that turned
into a crush that turned into an affair has turned into a business story
and a media phenom."

Items began to appear on "Page 6" of the *New York Post*, noting
the pair but not drawing any circles or arrows around them. Britain's
Daily Mail was more explicit. But the most complete "outing" came
courtesy of *Advertising Age*, which speculated on what the Wenners'
divorce would mean to a business in which they were both partners.

Wenner, claims Kasindorf, was upset by the attention. "In daring the world to write about him, by pursuing his affair so publicly—
even as he telephoned various media acquaintances (including the
editor of this magazine), seeking to keep his homosexual romance out
of print—Wenner may have thought he was protected by an unstated
policy deeming celebrity gayness the last taboo subject. But he was
done in by the press's increasing impatience with the have-it-both-
ways hypocrisy of it all."[71]

Advertising Age claimed the future of *Rolling Stone* inspired
their coverage. And the rest of the press turned to *Advertising Age* to
support their stories. "Do we need a 'business angle' to discuss the
liaisons of a straight celebrity?" *The Gossip Show*'s Gary Socol asks
rhetorically, recalling the Wenner brouhaha. "Certainly not. The
closet forces us to play by two very different rules."[72]

And the "rules" are getting more "different" all the time.

SIX

DEATH AND

TRANSFIGURATION

—

Y OUR FATHER WAS A MINISTER," OPRAH Winfrey begins softly.

"He wasn't a minister. He was one of the choir directors who's gay that no one ever talks about," a slightly agitated Anne Heche corrects her.

"And he was in the closet," Winfrey continues.

"So much in the closet that nobody ever talks about it," Heche retorts sharply. "He actually died in '83 of AIDS. It was not told even to his family until about a month before he died. He did not admit that he died of AIDS."

"So that was what kind of influence on you, Anne?" Oprah asks.

"Well, when you watch somebody who lives their life lying and then destroys themselves though a disease, you tend to look at that and go 'Now how can I do something different?' "[1]

Anne Heche was doing something very different on the *Oprah Winfrey Show* broadcast of April 30, 1997. She was "coming out," before a nationwide television audience, as the lover of stand-up comic and situation-comedy star Ellen DeGeneres.

That a performer largely unknown to the moviegoing and tele-viewing public, just on the cusp of a "high profile" career, would take such a step was utterly unprecedented. Stars with far sturdier profes-sional standing would never dream of following her example. What was especially fascinating to the industry was the fact that Heche had no prior history of same-sex alliances known to the press. She had, in fact, been linked to Steve Martin before meeting Ellen DeGeneres. And before Martin, there was George Clooney, who can be seen ob-serving Heche and DeGeneres from the sidelines in the uncropped version of the famous photograph in which the couple chat with Pres-ident Clinton. Yet in a curious way, Heche's candor was inevitable; less as a consequence of her father's life and death than because of the larger set of social circumstances that AIDS has created for every-one in Hollywood. For the most bitter of all ironies revolving around the international public health disaster known as Acquired Immune Deficiency Syndrome is that the segment of the Western populace hardest hit by it has won as a direct consequence an unexpected dividend.

AIDS has utterly altered the landscape of same-sexual life in America as nothing that came before it ever managed to accomplish. It has, in the words of writer Paul Rudnick, "made the closet obscene. . . . Gay people have been too busy battling disease and ignorance to worry about their hand gestures or manufacture a fiancée."[2] This could scarcely have been anticipated in the early part of the 1980s when a virus that, if at all known, was associated with obscure regions of "third world" countries suddenly began cropping up in New York, San Francisco, Los Angeles, and other major cities, among gay men and intravenous drug users. As the decade progressed, so did AIDS, spreading at in incredibly rapid rate amidst a same-sex-loving populace that had begun to challenge long-entrenched social prohibitions and was starting to stretch its legs into wider social and cultural arenas. Soon all gay and lesbian activist efforts would turn toward the epidemic, insisting an otherwise indifferent Reagan administration respond to it in some way.

Meanwhile, the pharmaceutical industry created AZT. Designed to slow the virus's spread among the already infected, AZT was manufactured and disseminated in relatively short order. Its toxicity, however, made it unsuitable for many. Moreover, it wasn't a vaccine or a "cure" of any kind.

As the nation's blood supply began to be monitored, it was expected the virus's spread via transfusions would be forestalled, preventing infections like that of Elizabeth Glaser (wife of actor Paul Michael Glaser) and Ryan White, a schoolboy who found himself facing the same social ostracism afforded gay men. Intravenous drug users, already ostracized, and having no political constituency or organization of any kind, were left on the sidelines as the media struggled to explain what up to now had been seen as the "shadow world" of same-sexuality. This was further complicated by the fact that as the toll of infections and deaths mounted, HIV's incursions into areas thought of as exclusively "straight" questioned how much of a dividing line separated homo from hetero sex to begin with.

Right-wing propaganda tracts like Michael Fumento's *The Myth of Heterosexual AIDS* tried to give the impression that all was as before. But such sexual apartheid didn't hold, as women infected by presumably heterosexual men joined an ever-growing "at risk" population. Elizabeth Glaser and Mary Fisher (the HIV-infected daughter of a high-ranking Republican Party supporter) did their best to illuminate the issue in a rational manner. But their calm, reasoned words mattered less to the media than the hysteria of Kimberly Bergalis, the

AIDS sufferer whose claims of sexual "innocence" were later contra-
dicted by fuller postmortem disclosure of her actual history. The record wasn't corrected in time to stem a nationwide panic that resulted
from her assertion that her dentist, a gay man who had died of AIDS,
had deliberately infected her.

Yet for all the attention the Bergalis case aroused, the media
found it didn't "explain" the epidemic in the "user-friendly" manner
the passings of Rock Hudson and Liberace provided. Their stories
proved irresistible to fourth-estate "sob sisters" long devoted to trag-
edies visited upon the rich and famous. Unlike ordinary mortals, Hudson and Liberace provided a touch of glamour to a visually
discomforting spectacle of skin lesions and wasting bodies. At the
same time, their life histories served to support media insistence that
AIDS was a "homosexual disease," and therefore heir to the shame
and secrecy the gay and lesbian civil rights movement had worked so
long to dispel. Now the old sad story of "hidden shameful lives" and
"strange twilight urges" was back in full force—with death as its
grand finale.

Or so it seemed at first. For ACT-UP, the leading AIDS activist
organization, far more vociferous than the "gay liberation" groups that
had come before, had seized control of the gay *Zeitgeist.* Perhaps not
so coincidentally, ACT-UP's founder was a former Hollywood screenwriter—Larry Kramer—whose credits include the 1972 musical version of *Lost Horizon,* produced by Ross Hunter.

A virus that attacks the immune system, and by so doing produces
skin cancer, pneumonia, dementia, blindness, and an overall
physical wasting and deterioration, seemed unimaginable to a sybaritic subculture where youth, health, and beauty were at a premium.
Hard to imagine, too, that a common denominator could be found in
lives as disparate as that of schoolboy Ryan White; tennis star Arthur
Ashe; veteran British character actor Denholm Elliott; famed ballet
star Rudolf Nureyev; feared attorney and right-wing political insider
Roy Cohn; experimental filmmaker and performance artist Jack

Smith; *Gunsmoke*'s Miss Kitty, Amanda Blake; and fashion designer/ Studio 54 habitué Halston. But there it was: AIDS.

The ongoing struggle to create treatments and find a "cure," and the emergence of an activist community—most of whom wouldn't live long enough to see their demands achieve results—has transformed American society in ways we haven't yet begun to deal with. In Hollywood, however, the impact of AIDS was obvious and immediate. Some of the brightest and most creative people to have ever worked in the industry were suddenly, irrevocably gone. Colin Higgins, screenwriter of the cult hit *Harold and Maude,* was just beginning a new career as a director of "mainstream" comedies with *9 to 5* and *The Best Little Whorehouse in Texas. Dirty Dancing* (1987), one of the biggest independent hits of all time, briefly threatened to revive the movie musical. Its director, Emile Ardolino, didn't live to see the telecast of his 1993 production of the musical classic *Gypsy,* starring Bette Midler. Director Tony Richardson had a long career already in British theater and film (*Look Back in Anger, The Loneliness of the Long-Distance Runner*) when the Oscar-winning success of *Tom Jones* brought him to America, *The Loved One, The Hotel New Hampshire,* and the television dramas that dominated his last years. Nestor Almendros's work on such widely varied films as *My Night at Maud's, Kramer vs. Kramer,* and *Days of Heaven* had won him near-legendary status among cinematographers. And that wasn't to mention *Improper Conduct,* his startling documentary protesting Castro's treatment of the Cuban people—gays very much included.

The four most important film programmers and historians in Los Angeles died within a few short months of one another, leaving an enormous void in their wake. Ronald Haver was director of film programs for the Los Angeles County Museum of Art. He was also the author of *David O. Selznick's Hollywood* and the story of the making of *A Star Is Born.* Douglas Edwards was director of special programs for the Academy of Motion Picture Arts and Sciences and a fervent supporter of archival research. Gary Essert and Gary Abrahams were the founders of Filmex, Los Angeles's long-running International Film Festival. They also instigated its successor, the American Cinemathèque, whose showcasing of rare foreign and domestic films has become a vital part of the Hollywood moviegoing scene. All four men were personal friends of long standing. And Essert and Abrahams were lovers.

And then—to name just a *few* more—there's Graham Chapman of Monty Python fame; Bronte Woodard, the screenwriter of *Grease* (and *Can't Stop the Music*); director-choreographer Michael Bennett (who might have guided his Broadway hits *Dreamgirls* and *A Chorus Line* to the screen); actors Howard E. Rollins (*Ragtime* and the *In the Heat of the Night* television series) and Ray Sharkey (*The Idolmaker, Willie and Phil*); Stan Kamen, head of the motion picture department of the William Morris Agency; producer David Bombyck (*Witness, Explorers*); Jerry Block, co-founder of Block-Korenbrot publicity; Warner Bros. executive Ashley Boone; Leonard Frey, the unforgettable Harold of *The Boys in the Band*; four other *Band* "boys" (Kenneth Nelson, Robert La Tourneaux, Frederick Combs, Keith Pretence), *and* their director, Robert Moore; and Robert Reed, the television stalwart remembered for both the serious-minded *The Defenders* and the all-fluff *The Brady Bunch*.

"Mr. Brady died of AIDS," Janeane Garofolo notes mournfully to Winona Ryder in the 1994 comedy *Reality Bites*, underscoring the fact that for the much-vaunted Generation X, AIDS had become a simple, ordinary fact of life. A fact in some ways less difficult to swallow was that two of the filmmakers to first bring the story of the epidemic to the screen would die of the disease. Bill Sherwood, whose low-budget 1986 hit, *Parting Glances*, launched the careers of actors Steve Buscemi and Kathy Kinney, was courted by the major studios but expired in 1990 before his would-have-been future projects escaped "development hell." Norman Rene, director of Craig Lucas's *Longtime Companion*, went on to helm two other Lucas-penned projects—*Prelude to a Kiss* and *Reckless*—before passing on. Neither film was gay- or AIDS-related. And this was scarcely surprising. For while there had been much discussion of major-studio AIDS projects over the years (the most frequently mentioned being Barbra Streisand's long-planned film of Larry Kramer's play *The Normal Heart*), nothing materialized from the "mainstream" save for *Philadelphia*.

Written by Ron Nyswaner, and directed (almost as if in penance for *The Silence of the Lambs*), by Jonathan Demme, this 1993 drama about a successful, but closeted, lawyer who sues his firm when they dismiss him once discovering he has contracted the HIV virus, won "mainstream" critical praise, muted gay criticism, and an Oscar for actor Tom Hanks. It lacked the emotional power of *Longtime Companion,* the insight of documentaries like *Common Threads: Stories From the Quilt* (1989) and *Silverlake Life: The View From Here* (1993), or the snappy irreverence of *Zero Patience* (1993), gay satirist John Greyson's musical take on both the disease and AIDS activism. But *Philadelphia* was seen by more people than all those films combined. Its success brought down the curtain it had seemingly raised on further studio-financed AIDS projects. For the difficulty in getting any serious-minded film made in Hollywood is only compounded when one manages to break through. "It's been done" is all any studio executive needs to say.

AIDS had been "done" in many forms, from the epidemic's very beginning. Theater set the pace with Kramer's *The Normal Heart* and William M. Hoffman's *As Is.* While the latter was a personal drama, the former was a fiery polemic. The plays, novels, poems, and essays the epidemic inspired generally followed either the Kramer or the Hoffman path. *Angels in America,* however, managed to bring the personal and the polemical together. Tony Kushner's two-part epic was at heart a love story, with the Reagan era providing a backdrop for a recounting of recent history. It seemed made for the movies. Yet even in 1991, when the play premiered, the issues it evoked were already part of a "long time ago in a galaxy far, far away" in an AIDS-weary public's mind.

Part of the reason for this was the proliferation of AIDS "personal dramas" on television. The first, *An Early Frost* (1985), centered on a young man disclosing both his sexual orientation and his HIV status to his family. It has been followed by such similar disclosure dramas as *Our Sons* (1991) and *In the Gloaming* (1997). The message from Hollywood was plain: If it was small-scale and "personal," it was "doable"—because it wasn't "controversial." Sadly, this controversy avoidance impacted *And the Band Played On* (1993), the dramatic rendering of Randy Shilts's highly problematic analysis of the epidemic's early years. In Shilts's book gay hedonism takes the brunt of responsibility for the disease, embodied by the quasi-mythical "Patient Zero," a wildly promiscuous French Canadian airline attendant whom Shilts portrays as the primary transmitter of the virus into the North American continent. (*Zero Patience* takes especial exception to the "Typhoid Mary" scenario "Patient Zero" evokes.) When this star-studded (Richard Gere, Ian McKellen, Anjelica Huston, Steve Martin, Alan Alda, Lily Tomlin) telefilm finally premiered, "Patient Zero" ended up playing a walk-on part. It was plain that the primary intent of *Band*'s makers was the avoidance of *anyone's* feathers being ruffled. The government, the medical community, the gay community, and an indifferent society were criticized, but *politely*.

As the epidemic's second decade progressed, AIDS-related plotlines proliferated on shows ranging from the family drama *Life Goes On* to sophisticated "adult" series like *L.A. Law*. The numerous organizations that had grown to deal with the care of those afflicted with the disease—AIDS Project Los Angeles (APLA) and the Shanti Foundation among them—had contributed to an industry-wide desire to promote "AIDS awareness." Red ribbons worn on the label became the symbol of this "awareness." By the late 1980s, no performer would think of going to one of the town's many televised awards shows without wearing one. But in the 1990s ribbons were viewed less as a protest tool than a fashion cliché. Likewise, the annual "Day of Compassion" on daytime television—where once a year programs are specially designed to highlight the disease and its prevention—began in a spirit of semi-provocation. But as AIDS issues became a daytime-talk-show mainstay, and HIV infection an increasingly common plot element in soap operas, such programming soon became less "special" than it once was.

With an industry currently retrofitting itself to reach a younger demographic market, perceived as being either untouched by or indifferent to AIDS, it isn't likely that films of either *The Normal Heart* (now no longer connected to Streisand) or *Angels in America* (pegged at one time as a project for Robert Altman, but now "in turnaround") are on the top of any studio chief's list of must-do items. And that's

not to mention the equally dispiriting fact that worthwhile independent works like *Under Heat* (a searing romantic drama written and
directed by Peter Hunt, who died during its editing) and *Green Plaid
Shirt* (journalist/filmmaker Richard Natale's love story—inspired by
the life and death of his lover, publicist Ed Pine) have been unable
to find distribution in an increasingly swollen independent film market. In a sense, it's all come full circle. Just as in the early 1980s,
when the epidemic was first impacting, as the century comes to a
close, no one wants to talk about AIDS.

I will go to my grave convinced that Rock got AIDS from contami-
nated blood during a transfusion," Tom Clark defiantly declares in
his memoir. "There is no other explanation in my mind. He was never
promiscuous. And he certainly wasn't Haitian."[3] Clark's insistence
may seem illogical from any objective standpoint. But in terms of the
Hollywood in which he had operated for so long it makes perfect
sense. Rock Hudson may have been gay, and he may have contracted
AIDS, but first and foremost Rock Hudson was a movie star. And
movie stars don't contract AIDS *the bad way*. It *had* to have been an
"accident" of some kind.

As absurd as it may seem on paper, Clark's attitude isn't atypical—not just of Hollywood but of the entire culture it serves. His
denial constitutes the flipside of the mass hysteria the tabloids provoked in the wake of Hudson's death, by printing specially blown-up
pictures of Hudson kissing actress Linda Evans from scenes they did
together on the *Dynasty* television series. There was ample evidence
at the time that AIDS wasn't passed on through casual contact. Yet
truth is useless in the face of fantasy—especially those engendered
by a former "masculine" ideal now "exposed" as not only homosexual
but *diseased*. Moreover, this wasn't just an example of the cynical
opportunism of the sensationalist press. For a not inconsiderable spate
of years, "sophisticated" Hollywood felt much the same way.

"Some in the industry now expect that there will be a rethinking
of the way sex is depicted in movies while others fear the possibility
of severe discrimination against homosexual actors," veteran industry

scribe Aljean Harmetz reported in *The New York Times* in 1985, making note of the Screen Actors Guild's claim that "open-mouth kissing" was a "possible health hazard" requiring actors "be told in advance if they will be asked to play such scenes."

> "I think there could be a purge against homosexuals," said screenwriter William Goldman. "A gay actor friend of mine who has lost 11 friend to AIDS says he is already feeling a backlash."
>
> Joseph Morgenstern, a screenwriter and newspaper columnist, added: "Gay actors are absolutely terrified by this, in the depths of despair. It's only my speculation, but I think a de facto blacklist may well emerge."[4]

For a while, it appeared that Morgenstern might have been right. "I make my money in an industry that professes to care very much about the fight against AIDS—that gives umpteen benefits and charity affairs with proceeds going to research and care. But in actual fact, if an actor is even rumored to have HIV he gets no support on an individual basis. He does not work." This stinging rebuke was lobbed by actor Brad Davis, in a written statement released to the press after his death in 1991.[5] Things hadn't worked out as expected for the leading man who first came to widespread public attention with *Midnight Express* (1977). He never found a role to properly showcase his somewhat opaque sexual appeal until *Querelle* (1980), Rainer Werner Fassbinder's baroque adaptation of Jean Genet's tale of murder and homoerotic longing filmed in a highly stylized set of a French seaport town. By that point, however, Davis's Hollywood profile had considerably diminished. Consequently, his need for work after contracting HIV was made even more complicated. Yet for all the particulars of his situation, Davis's postmortem protest rang true to anyone who knew anything about AIDS's impact on Hollywood.

"For the smallest reasons people don't use people," writer-director Gus Van Sant declared in an interview that followed the release of Davis's blast. "On a movie, everyone goes in for a medical checkup because the bond company isn't going to give the money unless the principals are in top shape. A bond company isn't going to risk $30 million on a guy who has AIDS. Davis wouldn't have gotten bonded, so he wouldn't have gotten lead parts."[6]

It had been clear from the mid-1980s on that rumors of AIDS infection had replaced those of drinking, drug taking, infidelity, or even homosexuality in Hollywood. Soon, female supporters of AIDS causes like Isabelle Adjani, Madonna, and even Elizabeth Taylor were rumored to have contracted the disease.[7] What was actually going on wasn't all that difficult to figure out. AIDS was a mystery. Putting a famous face to it seemed to some a way of explaining that mystery. But it was far from that simple.

"Asked how she thought her husband had contracted AIDS, Ms. Berenson shook her head and said haltingly: 'No. We don't really know. No. It's not worth it.' "[8] And indeed it wasn't worth it. For to try to explain how Anthony Perkins had contracted HIV would require an explanation of everything there was to know about him. And that was an almost impossible task. Anthony Perkins was, for the better part of his life, involved with members of his own sex in affairs of both long (dancer Grover Dale) and short (actor Tab Hunter, model Alan Helms) duration. Still, being attendant on the received psycho-analytic wisdom of the post–World War II period, Perkins wasn't "gay" in the sense that activists had struggled for decades to make socially viable.

In 1973, he married photographer Berry Berenson, the younger sister of model/actress/international bon vivant Marisa Berenson. They had two children and by all accounts were extremely happy together. Somewhere along the way, however, Perkins contracted HIV, whose incubation period it has been estimated can be as much as ten years. Still, "doing the math" fails to "explain" anything. Moreover, in Hollywood no explanation was required. For Perkins, like Davis, was someone about whom the town had long made up its mind. His career had been "over" for some time. For others, the struggle to survive—both personally and professionally—was on a different plane.

*   *   *

I t's not OK to be gay in Hollywood," *Who's the Boss?* producer Stephen Kolzak declares in a 1988 *TV Guide* story on the epidemic. "Gay men experience the increase in homophobia that is the result of the AIDS epidemic, just as much in Hollywood as elsewhere. They're not separated from the forces that exist in the rest of the country. . . . Gay people and lesbian people are the guests in a hostile host community. Sometimes that hostility is masked better than others."[9]

Kolzak himself was felled by the disease a few years afterwards. So was was his lover, writer and activist Paul Monette, who had himself lost a lover, Roger Horowitz, prior to meeting Kolzak. And following Kolzak's passing Monette would find happiness again with artist Winston Wilde, before passing on himself in 1995. It was a pattern of life, and love, and death that was becoming less and less uncommon among gays in Hollywood.

And among straights attitudes were fast changing as well. Gays weren't seen as colorful eccentrics anymore. They were people in pain who—often for the first time—had begun to speak about their lives. As a result, they could no longer be viewed solely in terms of "what they do in bed," but had to be looked at in light of what they did out of it as well. Moreover, this new forthrightness wasn't directed solely at straights; gays were speaking to each other as well. A major turning point was passed in 1992 when Bill Launch, lover of the late Howard Ashman, accepted his Oscar for the title song of *Beauty and the Beast* on the nationally televised awards ceremonies. Launch's first words, "Howard and I shared a home and a life together," spoke volumes. The truth was out: gay people had lives. Now there was no turning back—except to re-evaluate the lives of those we *thought* we knew.

G od, Tim Flack!" says producer and casting executive Joel Thurm, gasping at the very name of a former assistant who rose to became one of the most powerful and respected executives in television. "Talk about queens of England! Tim was that category of gay person who— well, let's put it this way: Tim was basically a drag queen. He never wore women's clothes, but he was so . . . *wild!* And straight men in the network's old boys' club aren't afraid of drag queens. Tim was the person who really made a difference for gays in television. No one will ever forget him. He was my assistant at one time at NBC. Then he went to CBS and became a vice-president. So did his assistant, Joe Voci.

"When people find themselves at an impasse," Thurm notes, "things can get very tense. Tim had this way of breaking that tension with humor—more often than not at his own expense. His favorite expression was 'I'd rather set my hair on fire!' That's why he rose so quickly from working in casting to working as an executive. He became one of the three people in TV who had the say-so that puts a show on the air—or keeps it off. And when you're that important, everybody—even the biggest homophobe in town—has to love you.

"When Tim was working with me in casting," Thurm continues, "we had a TV movie called *Mafia Princess*. Remember that one? The producers wanted us to go after Glenn Close. Tim and I just sort of looked at each other, because the script was not, shall we say, *Oscar caliber*. Tim suddenly asked, 'Have you ever thought about Susan Lucci?' And then he got up and *did* Susan Lucci—hand gestures and everything."

Lucci got the part.

Former CBS programming chief Jeff Sagansky (who has gone on to work as an executive with the Sony Corporation) was one of the many straights who truly enjoyed Flack's wild style. "The joke about Tim was that he was as funny as any of the shows he put on the air," Sagansky says. "He was instrumental in getting *Designing Women* and *The Nanny* on CBS. He believed in Fran Drescher long before she became hot. He loved larger-than-life women." There is a long pause before he adds, "I miss him."

"Tim Flack was the most flamboyant gay man I'd ever seen," says writer-producer Joe Voci. "He certainly gave me the encouragement I needed to come out. I mean, I'm *straight* next to Tim Flack. You know it's kind of sacrilege to say it, but Tim was funny right up until he died. His deathbed was a scream. There were all these people he'd worked with—including Carrie Fisher, whom he'd gotten very close to and with whom he'd done shows. Tim was running up and down the halls of the AIDS ward, doing impersonations of her mother, Debbie Reynolds. It was classic Tim."

"I think AIDS more than anything else changed things for people in this business," says veteran television writer Richard Gollance, whose credits include *Falcon Crest, Lifestories,* and *Beverly Hills 90210.* "When it became a matter of life or death, the reasons to stay closeted paled next to the anger and the grief and the frustration. You see, for a lot of gay people, show business is their whole identity. Their personal life tends to get short shrift. When gay men were suddenly getting sick and dropping dead left and right—accompanied by the shock of recognition that half of America not only didn't care but would just as soon have them dead—things changed. And when they let go and came out, and the roof didn't cave in on them, people felt safer."[10]

"AIDS resulted in a kind of a reaching out," says producer Laurence Mark, whose films *As Good As It Gets* and *The Object of My Affection* exemplify Hollywood's new nonsensationalist attitude toward same-sexuality. "We are all responsible for each other at some point. Before AIDS that fact could be ignored. Today it couldn't possibly be ignored. You'd feel like a fucking heel. It would be just the most inhuman thing to do, to ignore it, to assume all is well. So people didn't assume all is well. And then people realized that everyone is just like you and me. Gay became more accepted in an odd way. People cared. The town cared. And it forced people to come out—people who in no way would have come out prior to this. Suddenly it was like, 'Whoa, there are a lot of you!' That happened too.

"I used to never encourage folks to come out, ever. I *never* did," Mark confesses. "In the last six or seven years, I encourage everyone to come out. Everyone but actors. Because I do believe that for actors—it's not that they *shouldn't,* but it's a big decision. It's not just your life, it's your professional life. So it's: Be prepared. You know? People coming out to their parents—I think that's just a requirement now. Because it suggests that in not coming out you put a low value on yourself. 'Well, they know anyway.' Yeah, but let's have it acknowledged. Why not? Gay folks have also started feeling a little more entitled to a life. AIDS highlighted that. And because of that, gay people are living all sorts of different ways."[11]

And from these acknowledgments, gays in Hollywood began to discover that they had many straight allies willing to do more than simply lend a sympathetic ear.

"Tom Villard, who was on *We Got It Made*, a show in the eighties, had AIDS and was at risk of losing his insurance," publicist Howard Bragman recalls. "He needed to get a few days of work. And he hoped by coming out he could get them. He got help from Christian Slater's mother, Mary Jo. She's a casting person who has gone out of her way to help people with AIDS who need a few days' work for insurance and finding work for them. She did amazing things for people I can't even talk about, but she's one of the real quiet, dignified heroes of this movement."[12]

Quiet heroism wasn't what anyone had in mind when Hollywood Supports, an AIDS and gay-and-lesbian-issues support organization, was established in 1991 by two of Hollywood's leading moguls, Sidney Sheinberg and Barry Diller. Usually the trade press or the business pages would be the place to discover what these high-powered executives had to say about Hollywood. But it was the gay and lesbian newsmagazine the *Advocate* that was chosen for an announcement rostrum.

Diller had risen from the mailroom of the William Morris Agency to head ABC television, where he is credited with having invented the miniseries and movie-of-the-week formats. By the 1970s he had become chairman and CEO of Paramount Pictures. In 1984 he moved on to the same position at 20th Century–Fox. By the mid-1990s Diller left the studios for television, where through the QVC and USA networks he has assembled yet another base of operation. Diller has never formally acknowledged his sexual identity, and the *Advocate* interview was no exception to this rule.

"I have never given a personal interview in my life because I decided a long time ago that that was a necessary policy if I was going to claim some right to privacy and defend it as strongly as I do," he told the magazine. Still, he was anxious to talk about the impact a four-part piece on Fox Television on AIDS and homophobia in Hollywood, by journalist Henry Schipper, had made on him.

"This pointless acceptance of unfounded 'truths' about what an audience will or will not accept has got to stop," declared an uncharacteristically activist-sounding Diller. "We've got to start busting the myth that audiences won't accept gay material. We have no evidence of people running screaming from the theater because someone is playing a homosexual. . . . Actors are being told by agents and managers and PR people that there will be repercussions—in essence, that punishments will be incurred career-wise—for playing a gay role. The fact is that repercussions are mythological. People have to start understanding that."

As if to prove he really meant business, Diller went on to decry *Partners*, a much-criticized, stereotype-heavy comedy about a gay police detective, made on his watch at Paramount. "If the film had been done today, I would have deservedly been lynched," Diller said. "There was nothing really wrong with the idea, but the attitude of how the movie was made and how it was played was blatantly homophobic."[13]

Sidney Sheinberg, who began his career at Universal in the 1950s, didn't have a *Partners* in his past. As president of Universal Television, Sheinberg had green-lighted the production of *That Certain Summer*, the 1972 made-for-television drama considered a landmark for broaching the subject of same-sex relations in an unsensationalized manner. Megahits like *ET—The Extra Terrestrial* and *Back to the Future*, as well as *The Last Temptation of Christ*—the most controversial film to ever come out of Hollywood—were all made under Sheinberg's aegis. As for matters pertaining to AIDS and gay and lesbian causes, the studio chief was being honored that same year by AIDS Project Los Angeles for his work.

"My wife and I both have a great many gay friends, and it became something with which we can identify and sympathize," he told the *Advocate*. "I have friends who have died of AIDS. I doubt there is anyone in this business who hasn't."

As for the "blacklist" that many had charged AIDS had created, Sheinberg was diplomatically reserved: "There are a number of performers who, whether or not they have made public statements to this effect, are generally regarded by people as being gay. I'm unaware of the fact that these performers, both male and female, have been deprived of work in that regard."[14] Still, the very fact that Hollywood Supports was being founded bespoke a commitment to squelch any future troubles. And hiring longtime activist Rich Jennings to head the organization proved that both Sheinberg and Diller meant business.

"I had met Barry at an event for a gay and lesbian organization, as opposed to an AIDS organization," recalls Jennings, whose business-suited calm belies a commitment every bit as deep as that of more obviously fire-breathing activists. "It was at the home of one of the Disney people, two or three weeks before that news series ran on Fox he mentioned later on as inspiring him. We briefly talked about GLAAD [the Gay and Lesbian Alliance Against Defamation]. He was aware of the fact that fear in Hollywood was still really high, and that he as a leader should do something about it. This was an industry that traditionally had taken care of its own, and it wasn't happening with AIDS. He had already talked to Sid Sheinberg about the need for such a thing before he called us at GLAAD, and Sid had agreed to sign on and help fund it and chair it with him. He invited me to a meeting in Sid's office, with Jack Valenti, in early September of 1991. It was the Friday before Commitment to Life that year, which was the year Sid was receiving the award. Then came the news of Brad Davis's death, and his letter attacking Hollywood. Something was already in the works, but this led them to announce, quickly, that something was being put together. Since APLA was in charge of that announcement, it mainly referred to dealing with AIDS discrimination issues in Hollywood. But Barry's idea from the beginning was that there was a need for something that the industry sponsored that dealt with both sexual-orientation discrimination and AIDS discrimination. We wouldn't have had AIDS phobia but for homophobia, and the concern about that was a way to get in the door, for Hollywood and big business in general to deal with sexual orientation. But very explicitly they were both up front about it.

"Brad Davis's announcement and the negative publicity it resulted in for Hollywood certainly helped make AIDS a real priority for a lot of heads of studios. But Sid is tireless. I mean, he comes with ideas all the time. At one of the initial meetings we had he was talking about how they were pitching him and MCA to bring back *Dr. Kildare*, bring back the series that they still had the rights to, and he was saying, 'You got to update it. How about making him gay this time?' We didn't have the heart to say to him, 'Sid, you *had* a gay Dr. Kildare!' "

"When we first started, we sat down together and put down what our goals and objectives were, and high on our list was domestic partner benefits," Jennings continues. "That would be a way of sending a much stronger message than just adopting nondiscrimination policies, which we were also going to get companies to do as part of what the board members were signing on for when they agreed to be on the board.

"We opened the doors on January fifteenth of '92, initially sharing space with APLA on Sunset. I was the only staff person for two months until I could hire an assistant, and we were overwhelmed initially with media calls before we'd even had a chance to meet with human-resources people to figure out what programs were needed. We were also being told that APLA had 'AIDS in the Workplace' seminars that we could pull and use, and it turned out that program had not been happening for four years. We had to start from scratch. But a lot of calls came from people experiencing various forms of AIDS discrimination or problems with benefits, and there was no infrastructure to help people with that. Two years into it, about half the studios had someone in human resources or benefits go through our training program for facilitators. And some of them really became experts on the issue, really sensitive to what managers needed to do, how to handle things, how to act. They became AIDS czars for their individual companies. And now there's pretty much somewhat like that at all the major companies. Having the support of Sid Sheinberg and Barry Diller for doing it initially, and knowing that at least one major company, Universal, was going to instigate same-sex domestic

partner benefits, set the tone. We put together a task force of experts
to basically write a model policy that large companies, small companies, unions, anybody could use. It's really become a standard not
just in the entertainment industry but [in] high-tech companies as
well. That is a real achievement. We now have about sixty to seventy
'AIDS in the Workplace' facilitators based here and in New York.
We've got about fifteen in New York and they fly around the country
to entertainment workplaces all over the country. We've done over
twenty-five hundred 'Aids in the Workplace' seminars since we
started, according to the CDC. We're the most successful 'AIDS in
the Workplace' seminar programs in the country. Certainly the only
one that's industry-wide."

Part of the reason for the program's success, Jennings feels, is
the fact that straights in the industry were able to recognize the importance of the issue—in some cases, even in advance of the gays
and lesbians who would directly benefit from it.

"I found that at least for the first two years or so our primary
allies were heterosexuals," Jennings observes, "especially women who
were in opposite-sex domestic-partnership relations and were going
to be benefiting from the version of the policy that all the studios were
adopting which were for same-sex only. But they really got it right
away, that this was an issue of equality and benefits. There were a lot
of closeted benefits and human resources and other executives, so it
was really hard to get them to speak up on the issue. That was true
for the AIDS seminars as well. Half the time we were getting no's
from people we knew to be gay. In one tragic case it was a man who
was HIV positive—and probably had full-blown AIDS at that point—
who was in charge of employee training for one of the major studios.
He didn't want to have his name anywhere near AIDS seminars. And
so even though every other major studio was starting to bring us in to
train all supervisors and then the rest of the employees, he was standing in the way. So we had to go to the heads of the studio. Now I
would say that things have changed substantially. Once about a third
or so of the companies stated adopting these policies—I think that
people who were fairly out or felt comfortable anyway, were willing

to speak up about the need for these things and to talk it up—then we began to get a lot more support from gay executives. But it wasn't there to begin with.

"At an AIDS seminar you get positive response and feedback really immediately. You see shoulders dropping—tension draining off. Most people get comfortable with the information right away. You also see people who are challenging you with a lot of questions. We get a lot of questions about how to talk to teenagers, kids—other people in everyone's life. People walk away feeling like they know how to handle a situation. It goes beyond being supportive of co-workers, which is the primary reason we started up. And certainly it's helped people become more supportive of co-workers, and it's led employees infected with HIV to come out. Often people call us before, asking 'Is it okay' or 'I feel like I'm going to be facing some issues where I need some time off—who should I talk to and how much should I say?' Once the seminar has happened, it really clears the air.

"The sexual-orientation seminar is a different kind of animal. It's ninety minutes long—two hours for the LAPD. But it really highlights sexual orientation as a workplace issue. People think of the entertainment industry as being already pretty sophisticated on that subject, and many aspects of the industry are. But people when they think of the industry don't often think of the unions—the blue-collar people. And there are all kinds of others coming from all different walks of life. It's a challenge. Usually, for many people, it's the first time they've had an adult conversation about gays and lesbians, about being around people who are openly gay and lesbian at work. Some people have actually come out at those seminars. In some cases it's helped strengthen the move for a gay and lesbian employee group. That was one of our goals early on, to get some gay and lesbian employee groups going in the industry.

"The whole thing with Disney and domestic partnership was a long, complex effort involving working with people at various levels in the company," says Jennings, speaking of a situation that has grabbed the lion's share of headlines, thanks to the Southern Baptist Convention's demand to boycott the company over the policy. "Part of what helped there was finally getting some senior gay people to speak up about it. But again that's something that wasn't happening early on. Disney really has the biggest gay and lesbian group— League. We're not seeing too many more develop at other places, however. ABC has got one. Showtime's got one. So has HBO. There was one at MGM, but its leader left, and they've got domestic partner benefits, so there wasn't really much impetus for it anymore. And that's fine. There may be a need for some national umbrella sort of thing for other industries that people can belong to that can help them with benefits and issues.

"At the seminars we get everything from sophisticated crowds to others where some supervisors feel they know the issues, saying 'Oh yeah, we know all about that lifestyle.' We found out that many of them were just making a lot of assumptions and operating on stereotypes: 'I've worked with gay men before—oh yeah, they're great with the art work.' They were pigeonholing people instead of looking at them as whole individuals, and not realizing that even 'positive' stereotypes are a double-edged sword. If you've got a gay man who doesn't dress well, is he not even a good gay man if he doesn't live up to that stereotype?

"An African-American woman in human resources at a particular studio," said Jennings, recalling an incident he found especially interesting, "said she had a gay colleague, and that they had gotten friendly, and he had invited her to go out with him and his partner to a movie. She was sharing with us just how nervous she suddenly became because she didn't know if should she sit in the front seat of the car or not. She didn't know how much to talk to the guy's boyfriend, because it was all new for her. A lot of people have similar kinds of issues, because it's really been a recent phenomenon for gays and lesbians in the entertainment industry as well as elsewhere to be open about their orientation. We get a lot from Teamster types too: 'They've got AIDS!' And that takes us back to why we had a lot of 'AIDS in the Workplace' seminars in the first place.

"This industry has within it some of the most intense working environments and relationships imaginable. People can be on shoots for sixteen, seventeen hours a day—twenty-four hours a day in some cases. Animators put in incredible hours. And of course there are all these comedy writers working together who get to know basically everything about each other, coming up with a lot of material from their personal lives.

"Well, we've achieved domestic partner benefits at all the studios now," says Jennings, noting that in a few short years Hollywood Supports has seen the better part of its mandate enacted. "There are still some threats we're working with, but that's a lot less of a high priority than it was. Mainly where we'd still like to see it and where we're pushing it is a couple of the unions. SAG gives every indication that it will happen once they work out their issues over the AFTRA merger. That seems to be taking a long time. The bigger target, of course, now, that would cover the most people, would be the Motion Picture Health and Welfare Fund, which covers the vast majority of the union people and has so far refused to do it, and it looks as though it's the fault of blue-collar union representatives. We've tried to set up meetings and they've refused. We've met with the administrators and whatever, but we haven't met with the trustees, which we were able to do at the Writers Guild and Directors Guild, both of which are very complex efforts. It's a lot harder to do the union stuff than the company stuff, where you have one person in charge usually. But what we're finding out basically is that it's no issue anymore for the producers."

A IDS remains an "issue," however, in and out of Hollywood, as a cure has yet to be found. Still, the press and public response afforded such HIV-positive performers and personalities as diving champion Greg Louganis and actors Michael Jeter and Jim J. Bullock stands in contrast to what Brad Davis faced. Thanks to developments in treatment, the so-called protease inhibitors being the best known, the phrase "living with HIV" has come to replace "dying of AIDS" in public parlance. Yet for all this progress a loss of urgency has slowly descended over the epidemic in the public mind. The media by and large regard the new treatments as if they were a cure. With the ranks of its most dedicated members decimated by the disease, the glory days of ACT-UP and its social-activist sister organization

Queer Nation are clearly over. An obvious measure of a new media indifference can be found in the fact that *Time*'s seventy-fifth-anniversary issue, covering every major news story in the publication's history, didn't even mention AIDS in passing.

"It's still a fashionable charity," says Richard Natale matter-of-factly. "But I think the problem with what happened to AIDS has more to do with the gay community than it does with everyone else. I think the straight community took all this very seriously in terms of promoting fund-raising efforts, and certainly the gay community that's in charge of fund-raising realizes that even if there were a cure tomorrow there are more than enough people that have to be dealt with over the next twenty years in terms of their life spans to deal with. AIDS is a downer. Three or four movies have been made about it that people wanted to see—and that's it! Gay people want to see fluffy romantic comedies. They don't want to see 'that stuff' anymore."

As for the impact of protease inhibitors, Natale is similarly sober.

"It's true that the media has been treating them as if they were the cure. But so have people in the gay community, even though they're expensive and they don't always work. With some people it works for a period of time, then it stops. So it's a stopgap. It happens to be a better stopgap than the ones in the past, but that's about it.

"The other problem, I think, is there's a whole new generation of people with AIDS. The previous generation came from that sixties mentality where you go out and raise awareness and you protest and 'act up' and all that. This new generation comes from a totally different mind-set. They're very disorganized—or rather unorganized. They don't see being gay as a political statement. They don't see having AIDS as a political statement. So that there's that mind-set too. Hollywood is always in need of something new. AIDS is *old*. It's like the Vietnam War. They made a few films that paid lip service to it, and now it pops up in thrillers when you find people who were former Vietnam vets who are crazy. That's about where it is right now."[16]

For others, however, AIDS has engineered changes in their lives they're still trying to explain—as much as to themselves as to others.

"I was really in my closet for many years," says publicist Harry Clein. "The thing was, my closet had a glass door. I didn't know that at the time. People could look in. But even to my closest friend I didn't come out until probably around 1975. And we were both gay! We were just too frightened to tell each other."

Now in his mid-fifties, Clein looks back on the past with a mixture of amusement and regret that the AIDS epidemic has made more acute. Speaking in a soft, occasionally insistent voice, Clein easily conveys the impression of a man who's had a chance to take a long, hard look at his life. His many regrets are tempered, however, by the peace he now feels with himself.

"I guess the first time I felt uncomfortable about being hidden from the world was during the Anita Bryant thing in Florida in the 1970s when she was starting that campaign against gay teachers," Clein recalls. "You'll probably find that a lot of people will feel that that was a cutoff point. I started to really come out then. I was in Colorado working on a film with Alan Pakula, and I remember going down and telling his assistant—with great emotion—'I'm gay.' She said, 'I knew it.' It was generally the reaction everybody got. About that time I came out to my brother. Also when I got back here—this was about '76—David Mixner and Peter Scott were beginning their 'No on 6' campaign—the initiative against gay teachers here in California. I had time and I joined it. I guess that was when I became politicized."

Still, Clein placed limits on his new "political" leanings.

"I talked to a woman from the *Los Angeles Times*," he explains. "And I remember quite clearly saying to her, 'I will talk to you, but at this time I do not want my name to be used, and I want to see the quotes.' And she said, 'I don't know if I can do that.' And I said, 'I can't talk.' When it comes to my personal life, I want to see the quotes, not so they can't use it, but so I can see it's exactly what I mean. So I did the interview, and the only thing I remember about it is her asking why I didn't want to use my name. Times change. Now it's becoming more okay to be out. On the other hand, I don't know what it will be like ten years from now, because I know the political climate changes. I was near enough the McCarthy era to know that something you may do now is okay and accepted but ten to fifteen years down the line may not be. Anyway, the article appeared and all the quotes were great, and she kept her end of the deal—my name was not used.

"I went to New York and started working on *Starting Over* for Alan," Clein continues. "I got a follow-up call about an article about people in the industry. My name was given to them. I did agree this time that my name could be used. I moved that far in about six months! The article never happened, and boy, was I happy.

"Since then has been kind of a slow process, up until the last few years, which kind of speeded up. I used to go to the Unicorn bookstore on Santa Monica Boulevard and go to the place across the street and have breakfast with David Mixner and Peter Scott. And I heard them starting to talk about what they were doing in gay and lesbian politics. It was first time 'smoke-filled backrooms' were being used for political purposes rather than sexual purposes! In a sense I could now be welcome in political 'backrooms.' Peter's now dead. David has remained an acquaintance-friend I'm now seeing more than I have in the past. Because of Peter, I did APLA publicity for the first time. So they were the beginnings of my beginning to realize that one's circle could expand.

"It was about this time I had a relationship that went on for about eight or nine years," Clein continues, calmly. "I never lived with him. I was always afraid of that final commitment that a relationship would mean—that I would have to be gay to the whole world. Living with somebody would be the final unlocking of the closet to the world. He died in April of 1990. My father had died three and a half weeks earlier, so it was quite a wrenching time. And actually Joe and I weren't even lovers at the time of his death, because he had gotten so fed up with me that we had separated. Then he called me suddenly after about a year of our not seeing each other and said he'd just been diagnosed HIV positive and had been in the hospital. I had just finished a very traumatic relationship with someone else, so somehow we just became friends. That friendship grew into a strange kind of marriage-without-sex for the last two years of his life.

"He was my number-one relationship," says Clein, almost happily. "He was someone I *cared* about. For the most part, he was the person who went to premieres with me. A few people knew he was that important part of my life. But I never talked about him. I never referred to him as my partner. I never referred to him as 'my boyfriend' or anything like that. However, at his death, as he was sick, my staff knew about it. I didn't hide it. In fact, my assistant at the time—a man—would carry him into the doctor's office and wait. I used to do an event, leave and go to his house, and come back for the end of the event. The office knew what was going on, and when he died, we closed for the day and all of the staff came by. Someone from his family called and asked if I minded being put in his obituary as being his 'longtime companion' and I said no. So all these things made me cool out a bit more. I had a gay man working for me, and we became close and I would talk about it a bit, but that was it. I *still* never wanted to talk about this part of my life.

"Then this incredible temp came into my life," says Clein, brightening. "Young, good-looking. I fell totally in love with him, but we never had sex. He's now a good friend. He was in the process of coming out, and I began to mentor him. As I did that, all sorts of incredible things happened to me. I actually began telling him about all the things I had gone through. I was remembering things I hadn't even told my shrink. And what happened was we began to explore and do things. We went to see shows at Hi-Ways, the gay performance space. We went to all sorts of events. A lot of books on gay history began appearing at that time, and I started reading them. When the romantic infatuation had come to its end, and we had to figure out where we were going, I said, 'This is what I've learned from you. What have you learned from me?' He said, 'I've learned, working at your office, that I didn't have to be afraid.' It was the most wonderful thing to hear from somebody, since *I've* been so afraid all my life. I'd created an atmosphere where one didn't need to be afraid.

"Then, somebody I'd had a relationship with twenty years ear-lier came into my life again, and we became lovers for a year and a half. When we were first going together, he used to hide my photo when his parents came into town. But boy, he could make me laugh! For the first time I was feeling that there was someone I wanted to be with for the rest of my life, who tapped a part of me that had never been tapped before. I was beginning to just enjoy myself. That lasted about a year and a half. Every time his parents would come to town we'd still have these problems. It wasn't important for me to meet the parents, but I still didn't want to be in hiding. I had some ambivalent feelings about it, because I knew what it was like to meet someone's parents. I mean, I'd have *liked* to have met his parents just to know how their relationship with him works. So I began putting pressure on after that, because I felt this was wrong. Once we broke up right after his parents came to town, then got back together again. Another time his parents came out here and we broke up totally.

"By that time I was out to everybody and would talk about what was happening in my life," Clein continues. "I had a short relationship last winter. Everybody knew everything that was going on—male, female, it didn't matter. I was so open in talking about it. When it ended, I remember having dinner with this young woman producer. At one point she said, 'Are you married? Do you have children?' I said no. She went to the ladies' room and came back and I said, 'I'm gay.' And boy, let me tell you! She'd been ditched by her boyfriend. I'd been ditched by *my* boyfriend. We bonded. Men were dished that night like you wouldn't believe! I found that I was willing to *really* talk about a relationship—to be able to say 'my boyfriend' rather than 'this person' or 'it.' It's amazing. People feel closer. Several clients— women—fix me up with people.

"Back when I first came out here, the gay people I knew in the industry all felt they could achieve something professionally, and that it didn't matter what their sexual orientation was. I feel personally that they all felt they had to be in hiding, that no matter what their financial status—whether they were the head of the studio or what— that they literally could not ever achieve freedom in that regard. I don't think any of them thought that there was a 'lavender ceiling' professionally. Maybe they thought they may not quite get that high— to the tippy-tippy top where people who are gay are now—but they would get pretty high. It was never held against you that you were gay as a detriment to creativity. If anything, it was a bonus. But you *did* show up certain places with a woman on your arm.

"I went to the Academy Awards a few years ago, when *Forrest*

Gump won, and took one of my best friends with me. He looked
cute in his tuxedo. I went with him the other night to the Philhar-
monic, and I'd been invited to a party afterwards which was in San
Marino. Not showbizzy—very WASP. And you know something? I
sat at a table where there was husband/wife, husband/wife, hus-
band/wife—and then two men friends. It didn't faze me. In all honesty, the person who chose to go with me was really presentable,
fun to be with—so why not? He's someone I actually enjoy doing
all these things with. But I know people who've won Academy
Awards, where their lovers have stayed home while they went off
with someone else. It gave me great pleasure to watch the lover of
the lyricist for *Beauty and the Beast* stand up and accept the Oscar
for him in 1992. I think it's just wonderful that we are allowed [to
be]—and this is truly one profession where you can be—'out.' On
the other hand, to deal with the fact that I'm in my fifties, I spent
more time worrying I could lose a client not because I'm too gay
but because I'm too old."[17]

The peace that's come to Clein has been felt by others of his
generation. But some in Hollywood are still trying to sort things
out. This fact was made plain by remarks made by director Randal
Kleiser at a panel discussion at Outfest '97, Los Angeles's annual gay
and lesbian film festival. Working in the mainstream, Kleiser had
directed such megahits as *Grease* (1978) and *The Blue Lagoon* (1980).
But at Outfest, the film he wanted to talk about was *It's My Party*, his
very small-scale 1996 drama about an HIV-positive gay man electing
to commit suicide rather than face the final stages of AIDS. Holding
a party to say goodbye to his friends, he makes peace with the lover
who abandoned him when he learned of his diagnosis. Starring Eric
Roberts and Gregory Harrison, featuring a supporting cast including
Lee Grant, Bronson Pinchot, Marlee Matlin, and Olivia Newton-John
(all working for "scale" or less), *It's My Party* is easily the most serious
film Kleiser has ever made. More striking was the fact that it was
designed to deal with any number of issues *Philadelphia* sidestepped.
For that reason alone, its failure to find an audience wasn't surprising.

But at this panel discussion, the "failure" Kleiser wanted to highlight had to do with his own sidestepping in regard to the film's depiction of same-sexuality.

"I worked on studio films," Kleiser began, cautiously. "Then I did *It's My Party*, where I had some control. It was an independent movie. I wrote it. When I was cutting it there was a sequence at the beginning where the two lovers kissed. It was done in a very naturalistic way. But I cut it out myself, because I wanted to grab hold of the straight audience who had come to see this film, and not be turned off at the beginning by something they weren't ready for. A studio would have done so, but I did it myself."

"Did it work?" writer-director Paul Bartel asks. "Did your film reach a wide audience?"

"No, it didn't, unfortunately," Kleiser replies regretfully.

"Did you have any way of ascertaining whether it was viewed by a largely gay audience or whether it crossed over?" Bartel asks.

"It was a gay audience," Kleiser replies. "I think the subject matter was too down for a straight audience."

"What you're saying," writer-director Clive Barker breaks in, "is, 'I guess a straight audience is going to be turned off by guys kissing.' Well, I say fuck 'em!"

"They're going to be turned off by that too!" Bartel chuckles.

"Yes, and I have photographs to prove it," Barker adds playfully. "The issue is, if you're making a movie about gays anyway, and the subject of AIDS, as in *It's My Party*, are you going to make any 'converts'? Should you be concerned about putting up with their point of view?"

"You're coming on strong," says Kleiser. "It can be more of a seduction."

"Always?" Barker asks. "I guess I'm wondering if that is worth the effort—whether they're not just lost anyway. The person who is genuinely open to what you have to say is not going to be distressed by the sight of two men kissing."

"I want to find out more about why you cut that scene," says Nicole Conn, whose independently made drama *Claire of the Moon* can't be accused of shying away from depictions of same-sex affection.

"Well, I've worked for studios a lot," Kleiser explains. "I didn't want to create something that would turn off the audience."

"So you wanted to create something that would speak to the emotional content of the story," Conn says helpfully.

"Can you convert an audience without their knowing what the subject of the movie was?" Clive Barker asks. "I think people go to the movies because they know the content of the picture. And if they're predisposed to gay content, they're going to be predisposed to seeing two guys kissing. I know you don't want to blindside people, but this 'If we're gentle with them they'll come around'—I don't think they will. That was the subject of your movie right there. Love it or hate it, here are these guys—now get on with it."

"That's for your kind of film as opposed to *Philadelphia*," says Conn.

"Or *Batman and Robin*," adds Barker.

"I think in big studio movies today there's more opportunity to take those kind of risks," says Conn.

"There's *no* opportunity to take those kind of risks," Bartel declares. "The people who control those films and consider the material at every level—"

"Many of whom are gay, by the way," Barker breaks in.

"*Most* of whom are gay!" says Bartel.

"I really question how helpful those films are," says independent producer-director Sam Irvin. "They present a stereotype that may or may not necessarily be true. I feel very queasy about those kinds of films, going back to the *Philadelphia*s and whatnot—the idea of trying to convert the unconverted. But at the same time what you're saying I agree with. You shy away so much from any sort of real physical contact between these characters—whether they're wearing a dress or not—it really puts out the wrong message. It's like the filmmakers themselves are ashamed to show this on the screen, or feel there's something offensive about it. Denzel Washington and his wife had a much more passionate moment in *Philadelphia*, when they're in bed together, than you ever saw with Tom Hanks and Antonio Banderas."

"There was a long period when the studios were interested in

gay films about people dying of AIDS—as long as the gay characters
were portrayed as pitiful," says Bartel. "*Philadelphia* is an obvious
example, but there were others. I'm hoping that more and more films
are going to be made where there are gay characters and there's no
particular point being made that they're gay. The world is full of gay
people and they get along with straight people and they're side by
side, each do their own thing and they don't offend each other."[18]

R ight now there's this lull," says Outfest director Morgan Rumpf,
noting the problems Kleiser, like so many other filmmakers, has
faced in dealing with AIDS in what can only be called the post-ACT-
UP era. "Films are always one or two years behind what's going on—
particularly now with AIDS and the success of protease inhibitors.
There are all these questions and concerns: Where are we going now?
What does it mean to be living with this disease? Those films aren't
there yet. We see films coming out right now like *Alive and Kicking*,
which is a wonderful film about an HIV-positive man. Still, you leave
it thinking, Oh, but that's not really reality anymore.

"We know how people are dying—we've watched them die,"
Rumpf continues. "What it means is, the questions we're asking as a
community right now are different from what's being reflected onscreen at the moment. There will always be new issues for the gay
community. It's not like, 'First we'll do the coming-out stories, then
the AIDS stories, then the protease-inhibitors stories.' There will always be something new and fresh on the horizon."[19]

The question remains as to whether anyone will be ready to
deal with it. The example of the *Nothing Sacred* television show can
scarcely be heartening in this regard. This series, about a Catholic
priest as much at odds with himself as with his church over questions
of faith, became a lightning rod of controversy when it debuted in
1997, rousing the ire of conservative Catholic groups. Then there
came what would have been the show's eleventh episode: "HIV Priest:
Film at 11." Written by Richard Kramer (*thirtysomething, Tales of
the City*) and Bill Cain, the show dealt with the plight of a Catholic
priest being forced to reveal both his sexual orientation and his HIV

status. The fact that AIDS has created a major crisis in the priesthood is scarcely unknown—despite the fact that the church has done everything in its power to hide it. "HIV Priest: Film at 11" would have had a hard time making it to broadcast under optimum circumstances. But as it was tied to a low-rated series already under political pressure for daring to deal with abortion, loss of faith, and other issues, ABC programming chief Jamie Tarses found little difficulty in declining to run the show—despite excellent reviews from those in the press who managed to see a preview.

"Had the episode been the second broadcast in the series, as planned, it would have, I believe, established *Nothing Sacred* as remarkable and remarkably sympathetic to Catholicism and the priesthood," said Father Andrew Greeley in a *New York Times* op-ed rave. "Yet ABC strangely shares the stereotype of those Catholics who would drive it off the air in their own hardball bid for power. Catholics are seen as defensive to the point of paranoia, so uncultured they cannot see the context of a story but fixate on a particular incident, and obsessed by political attacks that lurk everywhere. That picture is simply no longer true of most Catholics, if it ever was."[20]

With *Nothing Sacred* canceled, there is little chance that "HIV Priest: Film at 11" will ever be televised, unless the Lifetime cable channel picks up the series and plays it in reruns. But that's television. Meanwhile, the epidemic continues, people become infected, become ill, seek treatment with varying degrees of success, try as best as they can to live their lives—and die.

GOING PUBLIC

—

I 'VE BEEN GAY ALL MY LIFE,'' DAVID GEF-
fen remarks matter-of-factly, "and I can tell you I've never had

a hard time being gay and trying to have a career. Being an agent, or

a manager, or a record-company executive—gay was never an issue.

Not in the sixties, not in the seventies, and not since. And I think it's an excuse for a lot of people who don't have a lot happening in their own lives to say that the reason it's not happening for them is because they're gay. I've never come across a serious problem. I'm sure other people have, but I have not. And I've never seen with any of my friends that it's been a problem. But I'm sure there are many people for whom it is."[1]

The entertainment entrepreneur isn't being flip. Delivering his words in a calm yet forceful manner, he has clearly given a lot of thought to what he's saying. For unlike the studio chiefs of yore, whose lives rarely roused the interest of a public too bedazzled by the stars to care, Geffen has emerged from an era that has anointed all manner of businessmen and -women with the half-coveted, half-despised label of "celebrity." In that "celebrity" spotlight he has been linked in the past to Cher and Marlo Thomas. Outside of it, however, his sexual orientation has been well known—from his earliest days as a record producer—to be directed toward other men. But there's an enormous difference between the availability of such knowledge within the entertainment industry and its being brought to the full light of public (which is to say by definition heterosexual) attention. And this in turn relates to the fact that media moguls like Geffen have, over the past two decades, become figures almost as alluring to the public fancy as the stars they package and sell.

With gay and lesbian issues exploding across the American cultural landscape in that same two-decade span—with such notable pop-music figures as k. d. lang, Elton John, and Melissa Etheridge taking the lead—David Geffen's coming out would seem to have been an inevitability. But as late as 1990, an "I'm not interested in saying" was Geffen's reply to a point-blank query about his sexuality by columnist Michael Musto.[2] It was a curious time for Geffen. He had been working to raise money for AIDS causes for years. Then his record label's leading band, Guns N' Roses, offered to play a benefit for the Gay Men's Health Crisis in New York. When objections were raised to the lyrics of one of their songs, "One in a Million"—which indicted "faggots" who "spread some fucking disease"—the band withdrew from the benefit. Clearly "business decisions" that had once been ignored were now being closely scrutinized by a gay and lesbian community energized by the AIDS crisis. In his "Gossip Watch" column in *Outweek* magazine, Michelangelo Signorile went so far as to declare war on Geffen, Barry Diller, and Merv Griffin—demanding these media moguls come out out of the closet in solidarity with other gays and lesbians nationwide to deal with the twin crises of AIDS and homophobia.

"Here is a horrifically wealthy man in a position to move mountains for us," Signorile said of Geffen, invoking the wish of millions that some privileged figure could rise up and magically solve all problems.[3] On the evening of November 18, 1992, at the annual "Commitment to Life" benefit for AIDS Project Los Angeles, Signorile got part of what he was asking for—to the extent that David Geffen came out, in public. It's something that Barry Diller has never done, despite his wholehearted financial support of gay and AIDS causes. And it's something that Merv Griffin would never do under any circumstances whatsoever. By enunciating four simple words—"as a gay man"—Geffen closed the door forever on what the media had so long insisted on calling "speculation" about his "private life."

He wasn't, however, doing this in order to please Michelangelo Signorile. "I could not face an audience for APLA, a third of which were dealing with HIV and AIDS, without acknowledging that I was a gay man," Geffen explains. "It's not something that I've felt, as an adult, ashamed of. And beyond that, I don't feel people have to make these kinds of statements." As for his public past, Geffen is similarly straightforward—and unapologetic. His heterosexual experiences were simply one part of his life.

"During different periods of time in my life I've been interested in being with women—for whatever reason. A lot of that was because I never had the experience. Most young people really haven't got a clue about what's going on inside themselves. I used to think, when I started having my first gay sexual experiences, that I could give them up at any time. Then after a few years you realize, no—you can't.

"You see," the fifty-five-year-old DreamWorks Studio cofounder continues, "when I was twenty-five years old, and had my first sexual experience with a woman, I thought, Oh, this isn't so bad.

But it just wasn't as hot for me as having sex with men. It was as simple as that. I had a cancer scare in 1976, and I thought, Well, life is short, I might as well do exactly what I wanted, and I have done so ever since. Other people's desires for me to make statements about my sexuality never meant much to me one way or another. But I'd gotten lots and lots of letters from people—young gay people who some way or another look up to me as a role model. And I felt that if I was going to end up as a role model—and I didn't *want* to be, but I felt if I was *going* to be—I had a certain level of responsibility. So from that point on, having acknowledged that to myself and saying. "This is the way it is,' I felt that I should do it—extend something to young gay people, who have very few role models. A lot of people feel you can't succeed if you're gay, and I think I'm a testament to the fact that that's nonsense.

    "Shame and self-loathing and low self-esteem is something that gay people share with straight people," Geffen continues. "It's a part of growing up. It's not a part of being gay or straight. There are infinitely more straight people suffering from low self-esteem than gay people. I think that it's something that comes with being a human being. Gays have, as part of their story, low self-esteem and self-worth. But if you're straight there are other issues that can create those same problems. That's why I abhor people like Michelangelo Signorile, who are seriously damaged people, who have made their lives about these kinds of things—who make their living being professional homosexuals."[4]

W hat you've got to remember about the 'Commitment to Life' speech," Richard Natale points out, "is that it happened *after* he sold Geffen Records to MCA, and got around $750 million in stock. He was finally in the 'Fuck you' position. So for him that became the threshold—the 'Fuck you' threshold. He had the wherewithal for his social conscience to take over. He was no longer building an empire. He *had* an empire. And there was nothing to endanger his empire, because it was safe. He had sold the company and received the stock and there was nothing that was going to negate that. So there was no danger in all the work that he had done being sabotaged by someone else."[5]

Still, Geffen's strategic "safety" didn't lessen the impact of what he was doing at the APLA benefit. He was, if only rhetorically, putting his entertainment-industry status position to one side and identifying himself as a member of a group toward whom no across-the-board social privileges had ever been extended. At the same time, Geffen's statement didn't in and of itself magically alter the dynamic of the AIDS epidemic or the problems gays and lesbians face nationwide. It was simply a *contribution*. It was welcome. The Geffen Foundation, which he established to assist AIDS charities and the arts, is another contribution, and it has also been welcome. But the rich and powerful, after all, have limits—even though we'd like to think they don't.

In an interview he did with the *Advocate* shortly after the APLA event, Geffen spoke of the impact of AIDS by making mention of the Rolodex cards he'd saved containing the addresses and telephone numbers of all those he knew who'd died of the disease. "I now have a rubber band around 341 cards," he declared. He also recalled the first time he walked into a gay bar in Los Angeles—the Red Raven, where everyone in the 1950s kept their hats on. In the sixties, when Geffen arrived, "people told me right away, 'Don't touch anybody, because if you actually put your hand on someone's shoulder you could get arrested.' "[6] It was an experience any number of gay men of his generation could recognize and identify with.

In 1993, the *Los Angeles Times* reported that within weeks of the *Advocate* interview, Geffen became a "[leader in] the fight for gays in the military—even pushing the issue in discussions with his new friend, President Clinton—and intensely monitoring developments on CNN like some foreign head of state." The article also noted that Geffen's financial clout had increased, making him "Hollywood's richest man . . . when Japan's Matsushita Electric Industrial Co. bought MCA for $6.59 billion. As the owner of 10 million shares of MCA stock—the payment for his company—Geffen realized more than $700 million from the sale."

"But I, unfortunately," the mogul told the *Times*, "am not a private person. I have become, by virtue of my success and other things, a public person."[7] And so, because he was now so thoroughly "public," David Geffen became a subject of gossip and rumor in a new way. One might have thought such comments might have lessened as his sexuality—the factor most likely to inspire idle clucking—was now a simple matter of fact. But another factual matter came into play via Geffen's standing as one of the richest and most influential men in show business: what does the gay man who has everything want? According to a story making the rounds in 1994, it was Keanu Reeves. And not just a simple love affair—a marriage!

The "rumor" of a Geffen-Reeves alliance first appeared in print as an item in the British tabloid the *Daily Mirror* (August 30, 1994), which reported that the pair had been "painting the town red at parties and going on wild shopping sprees . . . giggling like schoolboys as they tried on mounds of $500 shirts" at Barneys men's store in Los Angeles. This mildly malicious but otherwise silly squib spread to France by December of that year, by which time it took on a far more bizarre cast. According to *Voici* magazine, Reeves and Geffen had been wed in "the first gay marriage in the history of show business," at a Los Angeles restaurant. Performed by a rabbi, the ceremony was allegedly witnessed by such luminaries as Steven Spielberg, Cindy Crawford, Claudia Schiffer, and Elizabeth Taylor. Other variations of the story, making the rounds verbally at that time, had it that the wedding took place at a European resort or on the beach at Geffen's Malibu home. Elizabeth Taylor's presence was the one consistent element in all three incarnations of the tale. Thirteen days after the *Voici* story, news of the "wedding" hit stateside via the *Hollywood Reporter,* where a credulous George Christy featured it in his "The Great Life" column. Clearly things were getting out of hand, for after numerous personal denials, Geffen announced to *Time* magazine (March 27, 1995) that not only was the "marriage" bogus, but he didn't even know Keanu Reeves (who has no known history of gay affairs). The actor did likewise in (of all places) the July issue of *Out* magazine.[8]

"Here I am," an unamused Geffen recalls of the uproar, "with people calling me up and saying, 'Wow—you and Keanu Reeves!' A guy I've never met! Also, about my buying him fifty thousand dollars' worth of clothing at Barneys! Let me assure you, Keanu Reeves can afford to buy that himself! He makes millions of dollars a picture. Frankly I've never seen him wear those kinds of clothes. And having been the focus of that kind of rumor, you understand them.

"I know where it comes from," says Geffen angrily. "It's *gay people*! It's gay people that make up these stories about Richard Gere and gerbils!"[9]

Exactly who starts rumors and why is open to question. And it's easy to think of far worse fates than being "married" to Keanu Reeves. As "urban legends" go, it's benign compared to allegations of Richard Gere having carnal knowledge of a gerbil, and far less absurd than seventies-era reports of Rock Hudson's "marriage" to Jim Nabors. But what was at play in this new phantom-nuptials story was rather different. For as an "out" gay man, David Geffen was no longer subject to "rumors" about his sexuality as he had been in the past. At the same time, with him universally acknowledged as one of the richest and most influential moguls in Hollywood, his life had come to inspire interest as never before. And so the question hovers in the cultural air: how does such a man "really" live? The "marriage" story provides an answer in parody form, neatly conflating the "scandal" of sexual identity with the allure of power. If David Geffen is "out," and rich beyond one's wildest dreams, then he can have anyone he wants—say, Keanu Reeves. After all, hadn't Keanu played a male hustler in a film by an openly gay writer-director? Wouldn't marriage to a mogul boost his career—much like actress Norma Shearer's to MGM production chief Irving Thalberg? It all made—perfectly silly—sense.

But in many ways "marrying Keanu" was no less idiotic than a reality-based cover story in the August 1997 issue of *New York* magazine, glibly entitled "Boys on the Side." "The boldfaced respectability upstairs contrasted notably with the anonymous gym rats frolicking below," the article notes of a Fire Island house party.

> But the attention of both tiers was fixed firmly on the young man in cutoffs and tank top at David Geffen's side. He barely uttered a word that afternoon, but no one

seemed to mind: He was, without question, *the* best-looking man at the party, blond and in his mid-twenties, with a winning smile and pale blue eyes. When he excused himself to fetch Geffen a Bud, another guest sidled up to the billionaire.

"Your date is spectacular," the guest said.

"At these prices," Geffen replied, smiling, "he'd better be."[10]

"That was really a despicable article," a livid Geffen blurts out the minute it's mentioned. "It was all a lie. First of all, I have to tell you that the last time I was at Andy Tobias's house for a July 4th party was four years prior to that article. I wasn't there with Juan. And if I was, I certainly wouldn't say about him 'not at these prices.' That's a very shitty thing to say about somebody, and I assure you that if anybody was going with me I would have treated them incredibly respectfully. But the article was written by guys who are gay who really want to in some way demean other gay people."[11]

What the article also underscores is that the confusion about the place gays and lesbians are coming to occupy in the culture isn't troubling to heterosexuals alone. The "coming out" of stars and "celebrities," once seen as the answer to all manner of societal ills, has created troubles of quite another sort. For the culture has yet to reach the stage where sexual identity is a simple fact of life. It's still a "cause" to be either embraced or rejected. Moreover, it doesn't know what to do about gays and lesbians who, whether they like it or not, embody this "cause."

These days if a huge star comes out, it can't help but be a political statement," publicist Howard Bragman declares. "I go back to the research. People who know gay and lesbian people are two-to-one more supportive of gay and lesbian rights. People who don't are two-to-one the other direction. And if you look at the record—every gay show, every kiss episode, they go through the fucking roof. I don't see where it's hurt people. So all we gotta do is make sure people know that Ellen is a lesbian. Excuse me: Ellen her *character*, not Ellen DeGeneres."[12]

Bragman was making this remark with tongue somewhat sarcastically in cheek. For it was March of 1997—a full month before Ellen DeGeneres *officially* came out as a lesbian. And Bragman, like everyone else in Hollywood, had already lived through seven months of a public-relations charade in which we were asked to believe that the character of Ellen Morgan on the *Ellen* show supposedly occupied a separate and unique sphere from Ellen DeGeneres, the actress who played her.

From the minute she arrived on the scene, no one in Hollywood had any reason to question Ellen DeGeneres's sexual identity. And neither did any halfway intelligent member of the fabled "general public." But thanks to a long-standing practice of the so-called legitimate press, even the most casual broaching of the actress-comedienne's sexuality would be considered "an invasion of privacy" until DeGeneres had offered up such information herself. This unwritten law became harder and harder to follow after it was learned, in August of 1996, that plans were afoot to transform a show whose central character was most notable for her lack of interest in men to one where she showed a decided interest in women. Clearly DeGeneres's own sexuality played a role in these unfolding events, but getting an answer as to how and why was, for many months, harder than keeping the Mir space station in working order.

"We don't comment on rumor and speculation," a spokesperson for Walt Disney, the owners of *Ellen*, told the *Los Angeles Times*, conflating a fictional character's story arc with "gossip" about the performer playing her.[13] DeGeneres herself didn't help matters, making a series of television appearances in September 1996 on *The Rosie O'Donnell Show*, *The Late Show with David Letterman*, *Late Night with Conan O'Brien*, and *CBS This Morning* to promote her new comedy CD. Each appearance turned into a rhetorical standoff as each host (with the exception of O'Donnell) ever-so-gingerly tried to question what was going on—with her character and herself—to a smiling but impassive DeGeneres. For her "coy deflection" of Letterman's perfectly reasonable inquiries, DeGeneres won a "Cheers" accolade from *TV Guide* magazine, which apparently found the closet more admirable than candor.[14]

In October at a Museum of Television and Radio event celebrating the *Ellen* show, DeGeneres continued to dodge the issue, claiming a big but unspecified change in an upcoming show would be "a risk, but it is a risk I would be willing to take." Taking note of the adoring atmosphere surrounding the event, journalist David Kronke remarked, "Substantive questions of a timely nature were not invited, but repetitive inane gushing was."[15]

"The whole thing is speculation that's been overblown. It's never been substantiated. This is a rumor," *Ellen* show spokesman Michael Di Pasquale told *The New York Times* at the time of the museum event.[16] But it became harder and harder to keep this sort of "lid" on the story when DeGeneres began to make further public incursions into gay and lesbian territory, such as her appearance in February 1997 at a Los Angeles Gay and Lesbian Center Awards dinner honoring k. d. lang.

"I am very proud to be here," DeGeneres told the nearly one thousand attendees, going on to note of lang, "I think I was as surprised as anyone when I found out two days ago that she is gay," although there was the chance that "it might be a phase. When you have a phase and stick to it, it becomes a way of life, which is my motto. I hope to do the same."[17]

Clearly this wasn't the sort of public appearance normally associated with employers of the supremely powerful press agent Pat Kingsley. Boasting a client list that, besides DeGeneres, includes Tom Hanks, Demi Moore, Arnold Schwarzenegger, Holly Hunter, Al Pacino, Ralph Fiennes, Emma Thompson, Tom Cruise, Whitney Houston, Lily Tomlin, and Jodie Foster, Kingsley has come to embody modern public relations. A familiar face to anyone with any interest in show business, Kingsley is invariably seen hovering inches away from her top clients on entertainment news shows featuring clips of the stars at the premieres of their latest films.

"She was the first to demand cover stories, the first to elevate publicists themselves to the rank of star," the *Los Angeles Times* claimed of Kingsley, going on to note how she succeed in "keeping

Tom Cruise virtually beyond the reach of the press."[18] This power, and its selective application, earned Kingsley the disdain of one *Times* reader who observed, "Undoubtedly tabloid coverage isn't dependably accurate, but at least there's a degree of honesty about it."[19]

Honesty was, in fact, what was called for with the *Ellen*/Ellen situation. But it wasn't easily achieved. News of the character's coming out leaked out the moment DeGeneres made the decision to pursue it. A script hadn't been written, and plans hadn't been made to present it to the public. Consequently, the whole seven-month period between news of the announcement and broadcast of the show was a mad scramble on the part of DeGeneres, her representatives, and ABC television to get control of a story that was spinning far out of anyone's control. Kingsley, normally in the position of withholding material rather than offering it, turned at one point to Howard Bragman for counsel, as he had served as publicist for many gay and lesbian performers seeking to come out to the press. This would involve, among other things, interviews with gay and lesbian press outlets—a perfectly reasonable method for solidifying one's "base." Kingsley disagreed.

"Everybody wants to be supportive," Bragman said of the media-relations quandary, "but talking to the gay press isn't a political act."[20] But it apparently was political, in Kingsley's view. For while Ellen (and *Ellen*) seemed to be everywhere from the fall of 1996 on through the summer of 1997, she kept a conspicuous distance from the gay and lesbian press. It was therefore no surprise that *Time* magazine, *The Oprah Winfrey Show,* and *Primetime Live* became her forums for fielding what had become both a personal and professional issue.

Yet even if DeGeneres had used the gay and lesbian media as a platform, there's no saying it would have made things go any smoother. This was clear as far back as October of 1996, when a panel discussion entitled "Out on Hollywood," featuring performers whose sexual orientation had been formally disclosed far in advance of DeGeneres's, was held at the Walt Disney Studios. Mitchell Anderson of *Party of Five;* Lea DeLaria, the stand-up comic, who recently had scored a personal triumph in *The First Wives Club;* Dan

Butler of *Frasier* (and the semiautobiographical one-man show *The Only Thing Worse You Could Have Told Me . . .*); performance artist and character actor John Fleck (who had been embroiled for several years in controversy over National Endowment for the Arts support of his work); comic actor Scott Thompson of *The Kids in the Hall* and *The Larry Sanders Show;* and rising comedy performer Carlease Burke—all spoke of their personal experiences at length. But Ellen DeGeneres remained a perpetual touchstone.

"Who doesn't know she's a lesbian? Ray Charles?" an exasperated DeLaria asked.

"Oh, he knows," Scott Thompson countered facetiously. "He called me about it. He can tell from the sound of her voice."

"Look, I've been trying to be sympathetic about all this," said DeLaria, suddenly shifting to a serious tone to talk about the problems DeGeneres faced as a performer thrust into a situation that didn't appear to be of her own making.

"Oh no," Thompson countered. "*She* started it all."

"Oh, in that case to hell with her!" said DeLaria, resuming her normally sarcastic manner to the delight of the assembly.

Ellen and Ellen had obviously touched a nerve in this audience, which was largely composed of gays and lesbians in the entertainment industry who had themselves struggled with the question of how "out" they might allow themselves to be. Some felt, things being as they were in Hollywood, that DeGeneres might not come out at all. Some had personal stories of how producers, agents, and casting directors known by all to be gay or lesbian had refused to give work to performers more "out" than they were.

"They won't hire you for a gay role," said Mitchell Anderson. "They won't even give you an audition. They think it's too much of a risk." The actor went on to speak of an even more curious circumstance. At the GLAAD media awards of the previous year, where he decided to formally come out in response to a reporter's query, many of Anderson's still-closeted actor friends "sank into their seats" during his speech. For it's one of the everyday absurdities of Hollywood that performers who are known to be gay or lesbian, support gay and lesbian causes, and attend gay and lesbian events can still insist on being regarded as sexually "private."

As if inspired by Anderson, Lea DeLaria resumed her serious mode to speak of a related issue—the curious way the larger gay and lesbian community has come to regard those in Hollywood. At the top there are the "straights who like us," next come the "closeted gays with power that we'd like to come out but probably never will. Then *way* below them are all the people who actually have come out"—a group whose members clearly didn't extend far beyond the panel.

As for Ellen DeGeneres and her relationship to others in the industry struggling with same-sex issues, Scott Thompson summed things up simply, if bitterly: "Ellen's coming out is redundant. At this point there's no bravery in the act at all. She's ruined it."[15]

And this was in October, a full six months before the Kingsley-engineered media onslaught was pushed full-throttle. The ambivalence, even hostility, of these panelists wasn't difficult for any gay or lesbian in Hollywood to understand. For years knowledge of the disparity between "private life" and "public image" had built up bitterness and resentment among those willing to take risks. Throughout the 1970s there had been any number of "false alarms" that well-known performers (including Rock Hudson) would be coming out at any moment. And who was this Ellen DeGeneres person, anyway? A stand-up comic who specialized in "observational" humor so mild as to make Jerry Seinfeld seem in-your-face confrontational. Her show (which began its life as *These Friends of Mine*) was likewise low-key, featuring characters whose personal quirks barely rose to the level of the mildly eccentric. It never featured political humor of any sort. All it had going for it was a pleasant, self-deprecating leading woman whose sole curiosity was an absence of any romantic life. If nothing else, "going gay" would give her one.

Y ou can make a very strong case that it's a more political act for your character to come out than for you to," says producer Nina Jacobson, commenting during the seven-month "grace period" be-

tween the "leak" about the character and the "Yep" of its star. "On
the other hand, I find it so interesting that every article that you read
is just about this crazy idea that there's this character that's going to
come out. There's no reference that I've found once in any of the
coverage, and certainly not coming from her, that 'the reason why this
is meaningful to me is because I'm gay.' I admire her for saying, 'I
find it weird to play a straight person and it's so implausible.' But
she's an actor. Actors play all sorts of things. But it's so amazing to
see 'Fight the war on this front, but not on *that* front.' I think about
how ambivalent I felt about coming out for the first time. There's this
crucial role internalized homophobia plays in our psyche, in our
lives."

Jacobson, a production executive who began her career at Universal Pictures before moving on to DreamWorks, and then to Walt
Disney Pictures, has given a lot of thought to this process, both personally and professionally. To that end she helped in 1996 to co-
found Out There, a support group for gay and lesbian professionals
in the entertainment industry. Working in tandem with other organizations involved in both same-sex issues and "progressive" politics
in general, Jacobson sees *Ellen* (and Ellen) as part of a larger picture.
And so does her Out There colleague, DreamWorks producer Bruce
Cohen.

"I hope all of what's going on with *Ellen* has to do with theat-
ricality and dramatic impact," says Cohen, chatting with Jacobson in
DreamWorks' hacienda-style suite of offices on the Universal lot.
"Once she comes out as a person, there's no Nielsen interest in her
character coming out. We know she's gay, she's playing herself, it's
the same name, the show's named after her. Put two and two together
and you have four. The fun of it is the character coming out first. I
think it's a done deal. They create their whole season in advance. No
one makes that up at the spur of the moment. It got leaked either by
accident, or on purpose—to test the waters so it wouldn't be a huge
shock. I think Disney got cold feet and wanted to know what the
reaction would be. By now they should know who'll jump and shout.
They've been through this before with the Baptists years ago over the
animated features, and gays and lesbians going to Disneyland. Re-

member when the Baptists made their announcement that there was to be a boycott of all Disney services 'excluding the parks,' and the next day they announced that they were calling for a conversion of the Jews?"

"We are a group of people who can afford to be 'out' in every way: professionally, financially, and politically," says Jacobson. "There are so many people in so many walks of life who simply *cannot.* Look at the state of the nation. It's incredibly homophobic. It's not an imagined ill. All you have to do is look at the debate on gays in the military or gay marriage or simple employment discrimination to see just how many people *really hate our guts,* and how okay it is still to *really hate our guts.* Then we say to Ellen, 'Look, prove that it's not a problem, because otherwise what good are you?'

"Things have been moving forward," notes Cohen. "But if anything has gone backwards it's the fact that stars of twenty or thirty years ago had a much clearer idea of what was expected of their public lives than they do now. I've heard a lot of them say, 'I give my talent, my looks, I'm paid my money, and I'm entitled to go home and have my life.' "

"I feel a lot of sympathy with the stars that don't come out," says Jacobson, "because on a very personal level, there are still your own feelings of shame and ambivalence to deal with. No matter how much you say you're okay with it, you do internalize the loathing of a nation. You work those things out in your life eventually, but you can't grow up in a homophobic or racist culture without internalizing it. Just read the paper and watch the news. And *then* you turn around and say to these performers, 'Get over your feelings, get over everybody else's feelings, and put your career on the line.' We're in a business that chews people up and spits them out daily, where yesterday's phenomenon is today's has-been. 'What's your problem? Go for it!' just won't do."

"I actually take a bit of a more militant position," says Cohen. "If we accept as truth the idea that coming out is a fulfillment of your total self—to fulfill your potential and be the person you're capable of being—then if you're living your life and not coming out, it is harming you in profound emotional and psychological ways and will continue to do so. So even if you're a movie star, the downside of not coming out is so much scarier to you as a person, and to what's truly important to you, I don't think it's an even exchange. Every day these people spend in the closet only exacerbates their self-loathing. I hurt for them, and want them to burst through. 'This might ruin my career' can't be worse than what you're doing to yourself."

"But to play devil's advocate," says Jacobson, "would you say that to the middle-class bank manager in the Midwest who will quite possibly be fired by her boss?"

"No," Cohen replies, "and it's one of the reasons why gay people do lead these very productive, creative sort of lives. We were forced to deal with ourselves whether we wanted to our not."

"Still, I think that when you get to be someone on the big star level and you're her agent, you don't tell her, she tells you," Jacobson declares.

"I've got to believe there's creative blockage as an actor," Cohen insists. "To not be able to fully express who you are as a person cannot be good for you as an actor. I can't believe that it doesn't hurt their performances on many levels."

"Nobody wants to live this way," says Jacobson bitterly. "Nobody wants to live clouded in shame and secrecy."

"But there are a million games in Hollywood," Cohen reminds her. "And this is just one of them."[21]

The "game" came to end in the April 14, 1997, issue of *Time*, when Ellen DeGeneres confessed, "When I decided to have my character on the show come out, I knew I was going to have to come out too."[22] But no sooner had one game ended than another began. For as is common with all gays and lesbians, Ellen DeGeneres was forced to run a gauntlet of questions lobbed by a culture that persists in claiming ignorance of persons whose presence they've been aware of since the dawn of time. The difference with DeGeneres was that she was running this gauntlet in public—worldwide.

"I know what it's like to try to blend in so everybody else will think you're okay and they won't hurt you," she told Diane Sawyer on the *20/20* broadcast scheduled in tandem with the coming-out episode of *Ellen*. "I decided that this was not going to be something I was going to live the rest of my life being ashamed of."

"Ashamed of what?" Sawyer asked her, as "sincerely" as she knew how.

"You're kind of bombarded early on that you're supposed—if you're a girl—to meet a nice guy, get married, have kids, and be accepted," DeGeneres explained.

"The girl next door," said Sawyer helpfully.

"I'm the girl on the other side of you," Ellen replied.[23]

The questioning continued on *The Oprah Winfrey Show*. The difference this time out was the fact that DeGeneres wasn't alone. Right alongside her was her lover, actress Anne Heche. An up-and-coming leading lady, who had just been brought to public attention through her performances in the modern gangster melodrama *Donnie Brasco* and the disaster epic *Volcano* (the political satire *Wag the Dog* had been shot but not yet released at the time of the *Oprah* appearance), Heche had come into DeGeneres's life only a month or so prior to the *Time* magazine cover story. Signed to appear opposite Harrison Ford in the romantic adventure comedy *Six Days Seven Nights*, Heche was on the cusp of a major career. And now, as conventional Hollywood wisdom would have it, she was going to put that cusp in peril through an undisguised affair with Ellen DeGeneres.

"How did you meet Ellen?" Oprah asked excitedly.

"Oh, I saw Ellen across a crowded room, not knowing anything at all of how I was drawn to her," said Heche, perhaps unconsciously evoking Rodgers and Hammerstein's "Some Enchanted Evening." "I was not gay before I met her. I never thought about it."

"That confuses me," said Winfrey, echoing the sentiments of a million viewers.

"Nobody could have been more confused than me," Heche replied, "but it was clear from the second that I saw her that this was more powerful than anything I could have controlled. . . . I fell in love with a person. I don't think it was an immediate sexual attraction. I just thought, 'Wow, you are the most incredible person I've ever met and I want to be with you.'

"I've never been in a closet," Heche continued. "I have nothing to hide. I live my life in truth. This was just a natural progression. . . . I don't have any fear about this. This was the easiest thing in my life I've ever done."[24]

This "ease" stood in marked contrast to the difficulties DeGeneres had spoken of to Diane Sawyer, particularly as regards the fact she was forced to move out of her father's house as a result of her sexual status.

"The woman he's married to had two daughters, and they asked me to move out of the house," a saddened DeGeneres recalled. "They just thought it would be better for me to live somewhere else. I've never really, like, acknowledged that, but that was bad. They loved me and I loved them and they didn't want me in the house."

"Have you talked to them since?" Sawyer asked.

"Oh yeah," said DeGeneres, brightening a bit. "They love me and I love them, but that's what they felt at the time. They just didn't want that to be around her little girls. So . . . You know I was raised surrounded by heterosexuality, as most gay people are. That's where we come from—all you heterosexuals out there. And it doesn't change anybody. It's not contagious. Nobody in their right mind would choose something that's so *hard*. You're not only a minority in society, you're a minority in your own family. If you're black, your parents can say, 'Hey, we're black, and this is kind of hard sometimes, but that's who we are.' If you're gay, your parents are not saying, 'Good for you.' It's 'How did this happen?'"[25]

I do think that the reason Melissa Etheridge and k. d. lang have soared is that they love being the big dyke," observes Jenny Pizer of Lambda Legal Defense. "It works for their performance persona, k. d. lang has said her role as an out lesbian is as it had been before, but it works better. She wants every person in her audience to be utterly taken with her. I think it's much harder for a gay man to do that, because many men find the idea difficult—being attracted to a gay man the way straight men can be attracted to a lesbian. Straight men pursuing lesbians is a stock *Playboy* fantasy. The lesbians are lesbians until the guy jumps into bed and they're actually more interested in him."[26]

And that, in a nutshell, is the situation that has come to revolve around Anne Heche. She is now, as the whole world knows, a lesbian. Outside of her role in Donald Cammell's HBO telefilm *Wild Side*, her onscreen image has had nothing to do with same-sexuality. Moreover, her past heterosexual liaisons were matters of public record. Few can claim surprise at the mixture of nervous panic and prurient interest Heche's "confession" has evoked. Was she "really" a lesbian, or just "experimenting"? She didn't "look like a lesbian"— save for the *faux* lesbians of commercial eroticism. No wonder, then, that rumors of a breakup with DeGeneres immediately followed the couple's television interviews. No wonder, too, that months later stories as unfounded as the breakup rumor made the rounds that linked Heche with actor Vince Vaughn. No similar rumors were advanced about DeGeneres.

It is a dearly held Hollywood belief that it's easier for female performers to come out as lovers of their own sex than it would be for a man—the success of Rock Hudson's "Don't ask, don't tell" to the contrary. This certainly isn't true of someone like Ellen DeGeneres. From the moment of the first hints that an announcement might be in the offing, she faced a hailstorm of criticism from all sides. And it hasn't been true of Anne Heche, either. For while her overall presentation of self may place her well within the range of "acceptable" feminine imagery, she is clearly barred forever from "mainstream" wife/mother/girlfriend roles. This may turn out to be a blessing in disguise, as such thankless parts involve little effort and yield only minimal screen time. But while she may be offered far more interesting movie roles, particularly in the independent film arena, interest in Heche on the part of the moviegoing masses isn't likely to reach the Julia Roberts level. From the moment she appears onscreen, Heche presents a puzzle. Who is she? What does she want? Can I "identify" with her? Such questions cannot help running through even the most sophisticated viewers' minds. And Hollywood is supremely aware of this fact.

"Harrison, director Ivan Reitman, and I all found out about

Anne's homosexuality before we hired her and it made no difference to us," Roger Birnbaum, chairman of Caravan Pictures, which produced *Six Days Seven Nights*, announced when the film's shooting began. "Harrison had veto power over casting and he was immediately supportive. If Anne did something heinous, that might interfere with the public's ability to accept her in the role. The only thing she did was love another human being. . . . I can't imagine why it's an issue."

But it was enough of an issue that the film's casting director, Michael Chinich, visited Heche's representatives at the Endeavor Agency and discussed her relationship with DeGeneres. "Given the filmmakers' discomfort with the situation," the *Los Angeles Times* reported, "her agent, Doug Robinson, and manager, Julie Yorn, suggested she keep things under wraps until negotiations were complete.

One highly placed agent defends that course of action. "Heche's career is ascending to the skies," he said. "Her managers felt a responsibility to advise her about the potential ramifications of this very public announcement so she could make a smart analysis of her options. Though they were supportive of her choice, she regarded the advice as less supportive than she had hoped."[27]

"Several executives at these companies are known to be perplexed and dismayed by the publicity involving Ms. Heche," noted *New York Times* film-industry scribe Bernard Weinraub.

> It's highly improbable that Ms. Heche will lose her role in the film. But the question Ms. Heche and her agents face is whether studios will cast her in future romantic roles or turn to other actresses of similar talent and beauty.
>
> Even before she revealed her relationship with Ms. DeGeneres, Ms. Heche called attention to herself by dismissing her longtime agent, Doug Robinson, of the Endeavor Agency, and her managers, Keith Addis and Nick Wechsler, last week.
>
> People close to Ms. Heche said that Mr. Robinson, Mr. Addis and Mr. Wechsler had told her that they supported her but asked her to understand the ramifications

to her career of publicly proclaiming her lesbianism. Ms. Heche dismissed them and hired Ms. DeGeneres' manager and agents at the Creative Artists Agency.[28]

And so Anne Heche found herself—no doubt appropriately—represented by Bryan Lourd, the father of Carrie Fisher's child, who left the actress/author for another man.

"No one would have had a problem if Madonna and Sharon Stone met at the *Vanity Fair* Academy Awards party and started a torrid affair," writer-director Lizzie Borden observed of the "scandal" of the Heche/DeGeneres alliance. "Guys seem to be upset because the bedroom door has been slammed in their face."[29] Indeed, while Heche might well have inhabited a straight man's fantasy of lesbian sexuality, DeGeneres would have no place there. And this in turn brings up the issue of exactly how Ellen DeGeneres's lesbianism fits into gay Hollywood history. She's not an exotic like Garbo, Dietrich, or Nazimova. Nor is she a gamine of the Janet Gaynor, Mary Martin, or Helen Hayes variety. And while a performer with physical comedy skills, she stands apart from the wild gawkiness of a Nancy Kulp or the composed oddity of a Beatrice Lillie. More important, the Hollywood in which she lives no longer looks away from her offscreen affairs as was the case with performers as varied in temperament and personality as Claudette Colbert, Agnes Moorehead, Judith Anderson, Barbara Stanwyck, and Jean Arthur. Unlike her lover Heche, DeGeneres isn't a figure of "mainstream" sexual fantasy—which may very well be more of a blessing than a curse.

"Poor Ivan Reitman! Duped!" says journalist Matthew Gilbert, of the *Six Days Seven Nights* director's widely reported upset over Heche, which saw Reitman claiming, "It will do the movie some harm, and that makes me nervous."

"If there is a fact in the matter," notes Gilbert, "it is that moviegoers have been buying homosexuals in heterosexual roles for decades. There are the infamous cases, such as Rock Hudson and Montgomery Clift, and then there are the many, many more unknown cases, some of whom are still topping the weekly gross charts. Movies are all about illusion and story, after all, and acting is all about pretending. Rock Hudson convincingly played a heterosexual man in seventy motion pictures, a good number of which revolved around romance. For an actor, acting almost inevitably involves taking on the identity of someone other than oneself. Did it harm *Fatal Attraction* that Glenn Close had no experience as a rabbit-boiling, obsessive, lover-stalking psychopath?

"Even Reitman says that Heche gave a 'very sexy' audition with Harrison Ford, though it was when he 'wasn't aware of her homosexuality.' Now Reitman feels compelled to do damage control for *Six Days Days Nights,* saying about Heche, 'I don't think she is a homosexual, by the way. I think she is probably bisexual. She's gone out with all kinds of guys.' "[30]

In other words, it's all right to be a lesbian as long as you're not a lesbian.

I've always had this very simple theory of why most current stars don't come out," notes Howard Bragman. "It's because it doesn't help the financial system. A publicist gets their money every month, an agent gets ten percent, a manager gets ten to fifteen percent, a lawyer gets five percent. Nobody wants to shake it up. If you've got a superstar who's a twenty to twenty-five-million-dollar-a-year business, nobody wants to say, 'Oh, it would be good for you to come out!' There's a talent agency making two and a half million, there's a business manager, personal managers, a personal assistant, a publicist, a wardrober. Nobody wants to kill the golden goose.

"I didn't come from a PR firm that only had 'A' stars and was protecting their image," Bragman continues. "I came from a PR firm where for the most part we had to develop our stars. The clients we have here are clients we've had to build our relationships with. And there's a corollary to the whole coming-out thing. And the interesting thing from the PR point of view is you can take somebody who's not particularly newsworthy, à la Dick Sargent, and by coming out he's *very* newsworthy. It's still that way. Mitchell Anderson, who's featured player a Fox show, wouldn't have been rating magazine covers. Now he's on the cover of the *Advocate.* Covers are far more important than the circulation of the magazine. It means you've reached a new plateau. And magazines being marketed the way they are, many more people will see the cover and read the image than will buy the magazine.

"I think the first thing you have to realize is ten years ago gay and lesbian wasn't a story. It was different than Mitchell Anderson coming out—a young, attractive leading male. It was something to deny: 'Oh my God, we've got a problem!' The whole mind-set has changed. To give you a little historical perspective: It was around the time of AB101, the anti-gay-and-lesbian-teacher initiative, and there were all sorts of protests. David Smith, who was doing publicity for the Gay and Lesbian Center, called me and said, 'Listen, we have National Coming Out Day. I have Sheila Kuehl and Dick Sargent speaking, would you help me?' I said sure. I knew Sheila, and I hadn't known Dick before, but I'd seen him around town. They were on *Entertainment Tonight* talking about being out of the closet. The good news was in both their cases they were on to other careers, so neither was depending on their Hollywood careers. Dick's response at the time was, 'You know what? I don't see how it's going to help anybody, but if it can make a difference I'm there.' Everybody worries about the negative. But we had one negative piece of mail, from [right-wing activist] Lou Sheldon. Other than that we had thousands of letters from gay people—young people who watched *Bewitched*, older people. The message was, 'We loved you before, we still love you—what a courageous thing you did.' And you know, even when [Dick] passed away a few years after that, he went to his grave knowing he had made a big difference. I asked him and Elizabeth Montgomery to be grand marshals at the gay pride parade in West Hollywood, and you would have thought that he had flown to the moon! It was a community so starved for role models, and so starved for positive affirmation.

"Usually there's a precipitating reason for coming out," says Bragman, speaking of the process in public-relations terms. "Mitchell Anderson was the exception rather than the rule. He came out all of a sudden at the GLAAD dinner and I called him the next day and said, 'Whoops!' I've always had the standard offer for any legitimate actor that wants to come out: I'll help them through it. It's not about money, it's about the process. Tom Villard came to me through a friend and had a specific need related to his health. In the case of Dick Sargent it was a political agenda. Rebecca Armstrong, who was a *Playboy* Playmate of the Month, we put on the cover of the *Advocate*—which helped her sell the rights of her story to a movie. Dirk Shafer, the *Playgirl* Man of the Year, who made a movie about his experiences, was the same way. It was a nice tidy article that you could give to a studio, because studio executives love reading a great article so they can say, 'This will make a fabulous movie.' Everybody has a slightly different reason.

"I think the most important thing to put forward is what I put forward in my own life: I'm a gay publicist, but I'm not *the* gay publicist. 'Oh, he's the fag publicist!' I've heard that remark about me for many years. I look at the way Sheila Kuehl ran for office. She didn't win because she was a lesbian—she won because she was the most qualified person for the job. She happened to be a lesbian, and used that to hone her political skills, but she had a much broader base than that. If somebody came to me as an actor who could play fey and that was about all they could do, I don't know if it would be that interesting. I'm looking for a talented person, not just someone trying to make a political statement.

"There are six networks and 120 shows on the air," says Bragman apropos of *Ellen*. "You've got twenty-two minutes to tell a story each week. The NAACP was upset about the characterization of blacks. The truth of the matter is being gay is a quick stereotype. It means you're a little more flamboyant, you're a little wittier. It's a shorthand people understand."[31]

But getting people to understand in the rest of the media is another matter.

"One of my first experiences in writing about gay issues was I guess in 1991," recalls Mark Miller. "It was about Pete Williams, the assistant to then-Secretary of Defense Dick Cheney. I was working on that story for *Newsweek*, and there was the *Advocate* outing him. I thought we should have named him, because we were dealing with the case of a gay high government official fronting for a policy that was against gays. This was compelling. I made the argument that if we'd known he was secretly Jewish and they were expelling soldiers because they were Jewish we would certainly have revealed that in the magazine. Why was this different? Because of the Gulf War, it was clear that he had access to the most sensitive documents, and was a trusted advisor to the secretary of defense. He had helped put to rest the idea that this was a security risk. And here was the military throwing people out of the service after the Gulf War was over because they were gay. So obviously for a number of reasons I thought we should name him, although I did subsequently become friends with him, and he's such a sweet guy. He was tortured a lot by what Michelangelo Signorile had written about him. But at *Newsweek*? Well, we got to the point where we had this conversation at the highest level. And I considered it something of a victory that we could at least have a rational discussion about it. Because the first reaction was, 'Oh my God, we could never do that, because it's such an invasion of privacy! It's so terrible!' But at the end we were talking about the real issues. I was overruled, but they were finally beginning to deal with the question: 'Why do you think there's such a stigma attached that to name him as gay is too horrible to be contemplated?' So they became more open to that. And I think the magazine has become more open to discussion than they were then.

"*Ellen* was a very illuminating thing," Miller continues. "The editors were loath to deal with it. We were in a difficult situation because *Time* had the interview. Everything I needed to know was that she was going to come out in this interview. But in the end, the thing that was lost on these people in New York—these straight editors—was that she wasn't really closeted. It was difficult for them to comprehend that in L.A. she wasn't in the closet. She had girlfriends, she went out to clubs, people saw them out. I would run into her at the Hush Puppies store with her girlfriend. But these editors in New York didn't really understand that, and didn't really understand that there's a blurrier distinction to being in or out of the closet than they were willing to concede. They thought, 'Oh, she's entirely in the closet. No one talks about it. No one knows.' I showed them that this wasn't true, but they were *still* loath to say she was gay until *she* said it herself. Our story came out the same time the *Time* story did. And

I know they were quite reluctant to do some of that stuff at *Time*. They don't really do many lesbian or gay things. Or rather, they're like *Newsweek*—doing them once every few years, and they're huge sellers. Ellen was one of *Time*'s biggest sellers—which really surprised them.

Newsweek may have been surprised by the Ellen cover sales, but they soon got over their loathing to detail the sexual lives of the rich and famous. In fact, by the spring of 1998, the magazine had become the major conduit of unconfirmed allegations concerning President Clinton's presumed extramarital affairs. Of course the fact that Clinton is heterosexual may have had something to do with the newsweekly's lack of shyness.

"The thing that interested me about Anne Heche," says Miller, turning to what's proven to be the most talked-about aspect of the Ellen story, "was the reaction of gay people. What she said on *Oprah* didn't fit our very carefully scripted-for-heterosexuals story of how we became gay. People were running around saying, 'My God, she's confirmed every straight person's worst nightmare! That they will see someone across a crowded room and become gay!' I don't believe her story. But I do object to this idea that because she was disturbing our carefully created script we had to turn on her."[32]

Anne Heche had opened a hornet's nest of controversy. But it was bound to have happened, one way or another, given the industry's record of sweeping same-sexuality under the rug, and efforts of gay activists to send that rug to the cleaners.

I started as a secretary and I kept getting promoted and within three years became a junior publicist," independent publicist Kim Garfield recalls of a career that began at MGM. "I worked specifically with the national magazines, trying to get photo layouts or interviews for national magazines for our stars. The stars would come in to New York for publicity, interviews, photo shoots on their movies that were coming out. Each publicist had a specific area: national magazines, newspapers, fan magazines—one guy just did column items. It was very, very categorized.

"Dore Schary was the head of the studio when I got there. Howard Strickling was the PR head. Howard Dietz, of Dietz and Schwartz, was the vice-president of publicity of the New York office. That was in the mid-fifties. And that was a time when you kept your sexual proclivities a very closed subject. It was *never* discussed. I had two separate lives—my work life and my personal life. At work I tried to be like a woman; at night I would go with my girlfriend to the lesbian bar and carry on and let loose and feel free and be myself. I *did* feel the need to make up boyfriends. I handled myself as a straight woman. If I developed a crush on one of the women, I kept it to myself. Almost from the beginning. And all the way through the sixties."[33]

Garfield worked for years with producer-director Jerry Wheeler trying to get a film version of Patricia Nell Warren's gay love story *The Front Runner* off the ground. Leading man after leading man turned the part down out of fear of the perceived repercussions of playing a gay character. Wheeler went to his grave without having made the film, and not knowing that in a few years' time actors would be lining up to play gay characters—and win the Oscar nominations that almost invariably come to such roles.

For lesbians, however, things were rather different. For while serving as figures of pornographic fantasy for heterosexual men, less sexually conventional women-loving women—like Ellen DeGeneres—remained largely despised or ignored.

"Men have such a different perspective on being gay," observes Jill Abrams, a twentysomething producer for CNN's *Showbiz Today* program, who was the reporter whose questioning of Mitchell Anderson led to his otherwise unplanned public coming out. "I know gay men have had to deal with a lot of death. The lesbian experience is so different. History always seems to be more about men. It's been a *lighter* experience for me, because men—straight men—treated me well. It's been a positive thing for me in many ways. Its only been horrible when it comes to my parents. As far as the work goes, as long as you're attractive and appealing—as shallow as that sounds—it works in your favor. Straight men can come on to you and know you don't want them that way, so it's easy to cut them off dead. I'm not talking about sexual harassment, just flirting. We can have all the fun we want, knowing it's not going to turn into a real sexual affair. With straight women who are confident with themselves—they've been intrigued by lesbian women.

"This is a very wealthy town, filled with people who are very attractive and *groomed*. People are making a nice living and getting a lot of stuff for free. Being a lesbian is a kind of a spark for people. They want to know things. They ask questions. I think I've educated a lot of them, because they have all the stereotypes. It is changing for us. I think we have better images—like on *Friends*.

"You know," Abrams continues, "it's interesting too how we reward attractive people. My mother called me recently and told me she saw a *Jenny Jones Show* about lesbians. There were two couples on the show. One couple was very butch; the other was this gorgeous, very fashionable-looking couple. Everything the gorgeous couple said got applause and screaming. When the other couple got up to speak, people were *booing* them. They weren't any less nice than the other girls, or any less intelligent. Now my mother made this observation about this, and she's not very open-minded. It's like a lot of things. Look at musicians today—don't you just know there are terrific singers who are eight hundred pounds and they're never going to make it 'cause no one wants to look at them."[34]

And then there are those gays and lesbians the public has found itself looking at in far more subversive ways. Like Dan Butler of the hit sitcom *Frasier*.

"I'm in my own skin," says Butler, who came out even as public attention for his portrayal of the relentlessly heterosexual "Bulldog" Briscoe was rising. "I don't put that much emphasis on it. It's sort of a nonissue to me. When I first did my one-man show, *The Only Thing Worse You Could Have Told Me . . .* , everyone wanted to characterize it as coming-out play, whereas it really wasn't that to me. That became a tangential thing on its own, which was a lot of fun, but there were a lot of other elements involved. I'd never performed my own work. I'd never done a one-man show, and enlivened it through the processing of an issue. My journey as an actor has always been 'Where do you put me, anyway?' because I'm sort of a character actor. I don't think when you meet me you say, 'Oh, you should play *this*. To blend in the gay aspect—other than it being fun and ironic that I happen to be playing this very heterosexual role on a national television sit-com—was great. With humor you can get people unstuck about the way they view things, and start thinking for themselves.

"The bottom line with *Ellen*," Butler continues, "was that it lived up to its buildup. The coming-out episode was a terrific show. It was very well written. And it was very moving seeing someone parallel their own real-life issues on a situation comedy. But it's also not to take credit away from all the people who have been out and have been silent groundbreakers, like [activist/actor] Michael Kearns and Amanda Bearse. I think it should just lead you to investigate your own history. Like this film with Ian McKellen about James Whale. It's not a happy part of this character's life that the story deals with, but this guy was living in Hollywood in the 1930s and was an influential director. It took amazing courage to live his life the way he did.

"I like looking at the big picture. It's hard for me sometimes to stay with just gay issues. That bores me. What moves me is that it is a part of a whole. It's a human-rights issue. And I think we can get snooty and selfish, since we've had to go through this whole battle with AIDS, and being denied civil rights. But it is part of a larger picture. Look at Lea DeLaria. What moved me about her story was how people will still go after their individual, unique dreams. There are so many stumbling blocks, personally and professionally, with this issue, that you can either use it as a freeing process or a scab that will never heal that you can always be angry about. Sometimes that may be true. It depends on where you choose to put your focus. And sometimes it's bullshit, and you're just using that as an excuse to hold yourself back."[35]

Butler's reference to DeLaria brings up the importance of a story that passed below the radar of the major media while Ellen still had her closet door half-open. A stand-up comic whose rowdiness might be likened to a that of a considerably more macho Don Rickles, DeLaria had been something of a legend in cutting-edge stand-up circles. Her appearance at the National Gay and Lesbian March on Washington in 1993 drew gasps from the activist community as well as heterosexual onlookers when she saluted Hillary Rodham Clinton

as the first First Lady she ever wanted to "bang." Yet she had also
charmed spectators on *The Arsenio Hall Show* in a televised appearance made around the same time. Wild, freewheeling, and utterly
unapologetic about her sexuality, DeLaria stands in polar opposition
to the sweet-natured DeGeneres. Yet in a small but pivotal role in
the "mainstream" comedy hit *The First Wives Club*, DeLaria managed
to break through as never before. For her screen success not only
underscored the fact that the mass audience could appreciate her
style, it set her on a new-show business trajectory, toward the Broadway stage.

"I think for me it's just a really mixed bag, because I was
mainstay and a standby in the queer community before I ever got to
Hollywood," said DeLaria over afternoon coffee in the popular West
Hollywood lesbian hangout Little Frieda's. "Everyone knew I was gay
when I got here, and that's a little different than Dan Butler, Amanda
Bearse, or Mitchell Anderson, who said, 'I have my career, now I'm
coming out.' My career has *always* been wrapped around my being
out. Right now what's happening with it is very difficult. It's hard to
make that crossover from that edgy gay world to this 'mainstream' one.
It's *very* difficult. The reason it's more uphill for me than [for] others
in my position is because I wasn't entrenched in a career when I came
out. I didn't have a regular role on *Frasier* like Dan Butler has, and
be able to say 'Nyah nyah nyah. Oh, and by the way, you cast me as
the sickest heterosexual man you can think of—and I'm a big fag!'
That is *so* cool! Ian McKellen comes out—and gets knighted! How
fabulous is that? But see, I could never do that. It's been a fight for
me.

"Toss out the names of openly gay actors and actresses in Hollywood," says DeLaria, working up an activist froth. "Can you do it
and take up more than five fingers on one hand? It's really hard. There
are plenty of people out there who say, 'Well, everyone knows I'm
gay. Do I have to bring it up?' Well, it's a matter of politics. I find I
have this very mixed pro-and-con view towards it. My personal integrity—from where I am, and who I am, and my choices as an individual—say, 'How could I do anything else?' Look at me. I mean, I'm
not going to walk up on stage and talk about my boyfriend, and every-

one in the audience is gonna buy that. I couldn't look any dykier if I walked out on stage eating a vagina. And *then* talk about my boyfriend?

"I've always been out. That's where my brain has been and my personality is and the choices I've made. But it's hard to be out in this society—in Hollywood or anywhere else. And I think it's ridiculous to say that it isn't."

Still, DeLaria finds the whole subject of "outness" an irresistible opportunity for comic observation.

"Why were people so 'surprised' about Rock Hudson?" she says, laughing. "Oh, puh-*leese*! We always knew Rock Hudson was gay. Why? Because he was a friend of Elizabeth Taylor's! I've decided to tell people when they're coming out not to tell their parents that they're gay. Just say, 'I've become a very good friend of Elizabeth Taylor's.' Because every man she has ever been linked with has come up gay. Malcolm Forbes was the last straw. That did it for me on that score. They've found the gay gene! It's Elizabeth Taylor!"

DeLaria is equally attentive to her own image as a very out, very butch lesbian—and the perceptual problems this creates both within and without the gay and lesbian community.

"There's a moment in *First Wives Club* that could be viewed as pretty negative in the dyke-bar scene. The characters make a statement about women, and then they do a pan shot of all these tough and masculine butches sitting at the bar, which makes the butches the butt of the joke. I don't particularly find the masculine-woman concept so funny in and of itself. I know plenty of different kinds of women, so I can make a mannish woman *be* funny, like I did in *The First Wives Club*, without being offensive. That's my mission right now. I'm usually offered very offensive roles. Sometimes I turn them down, and sometimes I take them. I knew I could take that part in *The First Wives Club* and make it funny without being offensive to butch dykes."

What surprises DeLaria is the fact that the part ended up in the finished film at all.

"Who knew? I mean, *who knew?* I had been edited out of the Steve Martin *Sgt. Bilko,* so I went in thinking about this one, I'll just take my money and run, 'cause I'm probably gonna get edited out.

Even though I knew this part was different and it had been written for me. They said, 'We want Lea DeLaria to do this and no other person.' *That* was different. So in a way I knew that there was *less* of a chance of my being edited out. But as it went longer and longer in postproduction, I began to wonder. Heather Locklear lost her lines and Jon Stewart was cut. I thought, I'm in trouble here. What a relief when half of what I filmed that day made it into the final cut!

"*First Wives Club* has just been like bam! Instant recognition everywhere," says DeLaria, delighting in her success. "I've had such an interesting amount of press in such a wide variety of places. I would say I'm more famous than I am rich. More people know me than I have money in the bank. Does that make sense? I always say for me it's been a long time getting to the *middle*. I can't even imagine what it would be to be like for—let's say k. d. lang. Knowing what I have to go through, I can't even envision what it's like for people who are instantly recognizable wherever they go. That's why you can be out easier anywhere else than you can in Hollywood.

"I'm constantly amazed at how obsessed we are over who's out and who's not," DeLaria continues. "We spend an awful lot of time pointing our fingers at Hollywood instead of working on trying to change the society. There are all these different images of what straight people are like: *Roseanne, Grace Under Fire, Home Improvement. Melrose Place* is like the camp idea. But the reality—the only one that a lot of straight people have of gay people—[is] the images that Hollywood and TV give them. They have boxed us into certain criteria that's either ruled by some sort of 'political correctness,' or is the limp-wristed faggot in *The Rock*, which to me was terribly offensive. This is a character in a part that was written to be played very simply. It was a funny part. It did not have to played like a screaming queen with a lisp to make it funny. So the second we take this part that was funny and make *it* the joke—the limp-wristed screaming queen—*that's* when it becomes offensive. That's the difference between that guy and Scott Thompson's Buddy Cole character. What makes Buddy Cole funny is the things that he says, not the way he acts. His comments are completely outrageous. How many faggots do we see who come out of Hollywood who *aren't* limp-wristed screaming queens? That disturbs me when that's just about the only gay character we see. The last butch gay character to come out of Hollywood was Alex Karras in *Victor/Victoria*. Let's show who we are!

"Or," says DeLaria, changing direction in mid-thought, as she often does, "are we so far in the other direction that we're boxed into this 'politically correct' thing so that we can't move? We are becoming a mirror image of straight people now. It's as if we have no culture, no way of doing things, dressing, or looking that's all our own. If you look at these high-profile shows that are supposedly by our friends— everything from *Designing Woman* to the *Friends* episode they just aired with the lesbian wedding—they're being run by gay people who have boxed us into the 'We are just like everybody else' category. It's not real.

"Straight men fuck women," DeLaria continues philosophically. "Men are here to screw and screw, to spread their seed. It's biological. Women are just the opposite. Women are taught to cleave, cleave, cleave, cleave, cleave. Nest, nest, nest, nest, nest. Children, children, children, children. It's biological as well as sociological. So when straight men fuck, they are fucking these women who have this other thing going on. That's why it's harder for them to get laid. Whereas when two gay men go for it—boom! That also explains the whole concept of lesbian fusion. A lot of lesbians meet each other, go to bed, get married, and don't even know each other's last names."

DeLaria laughs heartily, but turns serious when she thinks about her upcoming plans. George Wolfe of the New York Shakespeare Festival wants her to come to New York to appear in a revival of *On the Town*. DeLaria is excited, but ambivalent.

"God knows where I'll be," she says. "It changes for me daily. Bang. I get a phone call from a record guy who wants to offer me a deal. Great. Thank God I have a manager, an agent, a publicist, or I would have left here two years ago, moved to Provincetown, looked at the pretty water, read, and been really happy. Written plays and movies and books and been completely happy. Because this town is too much, too much!"[36]

And so, leaving the too-muchness of Hollywood, DeLaria goes to New York, where she triumphs in the revival of *On the Town*, staged in the open air of Central Park in the summer of 1997. Taking on the role of man-crazy cab driver Hildegard Ezterhazy, DeLaria stops the show. "Ethel Mcrman with attitude," raves *The New York Times*. In the spring of 1998, DeLaria grabs notice once again as Marryin' Sam in an "Encores!" series concert revival of the musical *Li'l Abner*.[37] She goes on from that to tour in *Chicago*. In short, as far as Broadway is concerned, there's no limit as to what a singing, dancing, wise-cracking, and very butch lesbian can do.

Hollywood is another story.

I can show you chapters on homosexuality in my parents' books in their living room," says Steven Dornbusch. "I knew and I read those and I knew that they had something to do with the choices I had to make. I *knew* it had to do with me. And that didn't make me any more comfortable. The stuff I read wasn't any help. There wasn't much truth in it. Thirty years ago, I knew what it was. Sixty years ago maybe I wouldn't have. There is a price to be paid for an educated population when we have twisted, hypocritical sexual values."

A grip and union activist in his early thirties, Dornbusch is as far from the average heterosexual's conception of a gay man as it's possible to be. But from a gay perspective, his rough-hewn features, muscular forearms, and louche demeanor wouldn't be out of place in a Tom of Finland illustration. To his co-workers, however, few of whom are aware of his sexuality, its revelation would be decidedly out of place.

"I don't socialize with grips," say Dornbusch calmly. "But what is our life like? It's a macho thing. It definitely a macho thing. There are few women. Maybe there's twenty or thirty in the union. I believe there are fourteen hundred, fifteen hundred members in the union. But only a certain kind of woman can handle being a grip. I don't mean the work, physically. It's the vulgarity that goes with it. People who are macho with bad tempers can't handle it, either. They don't get chosen for good steady jobs. If you want to do well, you have to know how to keep your mouth shut just like in any other business. You've got to learn how to cooperate. You can't exchange blows. And there's definitely a mystique about being a grip. Women grips? I don't know most of them, so I won't make any finite remarks, 'cause it wouldn't be fair. But some of them are lesbians and some of them are not. Lots of them are. Personally, I prefer to have some women around.

"I have to be very careful to decide who I want to deal with socially as a gay man," Dornbusch continues. "But I don't want to go to a fuckin' straight club to socialize. I just don't do stuff like that. I am single. I don't mind putting in the long hours. Being a grip is a terrible stress on family life. Grips are a tremendously divorced group, even compared to the regular population. But I'm suspect as a gay man, simply because I've never been married. I don't lie about such things. 'Are you married?' No. Five days later: 'Have you ever been married?' No.

"Being gay—it's all seen as a threat," Dornbusch continues. "When grips talk about it, it's all about sex—about butt fucking, about AIDS. It's stereotypical, superficial, ignorant talk. Not that everything people say is false, but not really about real life and about real people. We are the whipping boys. And I don't mean occasionally. The number of things said that are in the general sense derogatory about homosexuals on the job, for me, in one day would be in the hundreds. I don't mean five times a day. It's an *obsession*. It's *all the time*! They're jokes that are not even meant to be funny. For instance, one guy said something to me about fucking someone's butt, and I said, 'I wouldn't wanna fuck his butt, he's too fat for me.' In an office that might be the end of it. That won't stop a grip. That's just the *start* of the conversation. Now it's into territory like, 'What kind of butt *do* you fuck, if you did want to?' Then he says, 'You probably would prefer mine.' So I looked down at his butt and said, right in front of people, 'Well, yes, I'd much prefer yours.' It was an honest response. I honestly really would prefer to fuck his butt than the other guy's. He knew it was true, too. He was aware of his sexual attraction. I'm not saying he's in the closet. I'm not saying he's gay. I was just being honest. But it's a whole *deal* with these guys.

"To be subordinate to someone else in a job is to be a 'bitch.' So if you're in the sewing room where you sew the big cloths and flags together, you're 'stitch bitch.' It's a really good job. Some skill is involved and most of the guys do it. But you're a stitch bitch. It doesn't mean that you're gay. You should see some of the stitch bitches. In fact, I don't know any gay person that does it. So we all laugh about the term. Maybe at not every single opportunity, but some of the time. At the same level, if a male co-worker is in the way, you might say, 'Come on, honey.' It's not fag baiting. It's a kind of universal male thing in blue-collar or physical occupations. When you're touching and doing things together, and you work very close, it's full of sexual innuendo. That's why most of us don't drink together. There's kind of sexual banter, some of it fun, when men work together in close physical proximity. What we usually do is we all start laughing. But sometimes it goes way too far.

"There's a guy I know. He has a wife, and he's heterosexual, but he respects gay people. He's definitely a little rough around the edges. So he's talking, and among other things, he brings up transvestites. To him that's a big fascination. He once told me about having dinner with some 'European muckety-muck fags' that were production designers. He *had* to tell me they were gay. What did it have to do with the story? Nothing, really. It was like he had crossed some kind of line because he was socializing with known homosexuals. He brought it all up, but it's like he felt a little embarrassed. He knew that he *should* have dinner with those guys. And I doubt it was all business.

"He has a buddy," Dornbusch continues, "who's *really* rough around the edges. Looks like he just got out of prison—and did. A very likable guy. And they're friends and drinking buddies. We call them boyfriends, because one was in prison and the other is European. They don't really give a fuck. And no one really thinks they're gay. They just play along with it. So I'll say, 'Have you seen your boyfriend lately?' And he'll just smile. In fact, he once went on and on and on about how he admired Liberace. I thought that was fascinating. He just thought that Liberace had lived his own life. Gotten really rich, made people happy. He just really liked Liberace!

"[There's] a TV show that most of us have worked on that's got like a—I don't know what the sex of this person is—post-op or pre-op transsexual, maybe. More or less a drag queen for sure. The writers for this show are real flaming queens. And I noticed that the grips just *knew* that they had to cool it; that they couldn't fag-bait these people 'cause they're the show. The comments were quieter. No one was going to be spoken about really loud, and the drag queen was not going to be talked about *at all,* rather than all the time. It was kind of like a truce based on business. There was a certain level of discomfort, but it wasn't intense. That was sort of interesting. There's one queen who works on that show, and no one gives him a hard time because he's very established with people that matter. He's older, and not seen as a sexual threat. He's just really nice and quiet and plays the passive queen role. And obviously he's done this for a lifetime. His occupation has a lot of gays in it, so it's not shocking. It's to be expected. And he works with a bunch of women. So people can deal with him. It's just like he's 'tradition.' No disrespect intended, but I probably have nothing in common with him at all other than being gay."[38]

One of the things you realize is that in the past ten years American culture as a whole has become comfortable with the concept of gay people and straight people living side by side," says producer Alan Poul. "Gay people date, and marry and fight, and have sex, and do funky things just like straight people do. That has emerged gradually. Even though I know that a film set is not a microcosm of American society, it's a lot straighter than you would think, because most of the people you're dealing with are trained professional craftsmen who have wives and homes and boats up in canyon country somewhere. They are not bohemian. It's very different from working in the theater in that way.

"When I first started out in show business, people were not comfortable with someone being openly, aggressively homosexual," says Poul, whose credits encompass productions as diverse as Paul Schrader's *Mishima* and the television miniseries *Tales of the City.* "You were expected to tone it down. I'm not talking about flamboyance. You wouldn't say, 'Yeah, I was talking to my boyfriend about that last night, and he felt the same way that you do.' It would get a

reaction. Now it wouldn't. In the past it would be considered an attempt to rub it in someone's face to provoke a reaction. Today it would
be, 'Isn't it nice how at ease he is with himself?' So in that context, I
wasn't out until 1990.

"On the Schrader films I was definitely not 'out.' There were
people who knew and there were people who didn't know. But I certainly did manage that sort of 'discretion in the workplace' kind of
thing, which is the same as it was when I was working with the Japan
Society years ago. I would never walk around saying, 'I'm a big homo.'
People who get it, get it, and people who don't don't seem to notice.
It was a different time. You certainly wouldn't put pinups of guys in
your desk cubicle, because it would be considered a confrontational
act. It was pretty much the same thing in the movie industry. Film
crews are notoriously straight—not always as straight as they appear,
but generally it's a very straight ethic that's going on. Now, on most
crews, even grips and gaffers are comfortable working with gay men
and lesbians. But that wasn't the case in '84, '85, '86."[39]

What this comfort level portends for gays and lesbians themselves, however, is still being sorted out.

"The fact of the matter is, gay people are just like everyone
else," says David Geffen. "Some are happy, some are unhappy, some
drink and some don't drink, some take drugs and some don't take
drugs, some have legitimately quiet and introspective lives, and other
people go and take crystal and dance their lives away. So what?

"There's a grand selection of people who happen to be gay.
That's frightening to some people—particularly to some gay people.
In some way or another they're the ones who seem most upset by it
all. I think being gay is becoming less of an issue in motion pictures
and television, and I think that's probably a good thing. It makes it
easier for young gay people for that reason. There are role models
now. I never had anybody that I could look at when I was a kid. Now
I think it's a lot better.

"On the other hand," Geffen observes, "I think what troubles
everyone about gay people most is that they all seem to take drugs
and dance a lot. It seems to me the most consistent thing. I've done
a lot of partying in my time, and it seems to be what most gay people

do. They go to gay bars and dances and discos and take crystal meth. It's not a very good thing."[40]

And for some gays and lesbians the notion of role models is seen as being not a very good thing.

"You know who my heroes are?" asks activist/answer man Dan Savage in his weekly "Savage Love" advice column in the *Chicago Reader*. "Teenagers all over this country who are coming out, starting gay-straight student alliances, and demanding that their parents deal and chill. A couple of weeks ago, I met a fifteen-year-old who lives in motherfuckin' Mormon freak-show Idaho, and he's out of the closet at his high school. That's heroic. *He* ought to be on the cover of *Time*, not Ellen DeGeneres."[41]

EIGHT

RUNNING FOR

MAYOR

—

W HAT YOU'VE TOLD US IS ALMOST too good to be true," the gay rights activist tells the trio of film producers. "We've seen too many Hollywood movies not to know we can't take what you're saying at face value. We've seen too many situations where promises were made that in the end turned out to be simply empty. Why do you believe that Warner Bros. wants to make this picture?"

The question is the most important asked this evening in May of 1992 at the Women's Building in San Francisco. A public forum is being held to discuss the making of *The Mayor of Castro Street,* a proposed film version of Randy Shilts's biography of Harvey Milk, the gay activist and city supervisor whose 1978 assassination galvanized the gay and lesbian community, both in San Francisco and nation-wide, in the years just prior to the onset of the AIDS epidemic. Pro-ducers Craig Zadan, Neil Meron, and Janet Yang have come to address an audience of over one hundred people from all walks of gay and lesbian life. And what they have to say *does* seem too good to be true. For Gus Van Sant, the celebrated gay independent film maker, is planning to make *Mayor* his first major studio effort. It will be a large-budget project, and Robin Williams has been approached to star as Harvey Milk.

While Milk's life has already been the subject of an Oscar-winning 1984 documentary, *The Times of Harvey Milk,* this new film intends to be quite different. For dramatic fiction can open doors to both character and historic circumstance that documentary cannot help leaving shut. If properly done, *The Mayor of Castro Street* could put moviegoers, both gay and straight, right inside Harvey Milk's head—and those of the many people who loved and hated him.

"This is something we are passionate about," says Zadan, whose producing credits include *Footloose.* "We want to do it correctly, and that's why we're here at this town meeting talking to you tonight. We want to make a movie where a kid who's in high school now in, say, Iowa, goes to the theater and sees it and says, 'It's okay that I'm gay.' We feel that this could be a watershed film. If it's successful, it will open up the floodgates on films with gay themes."

The "town meeting" participants, several of whom knew Harvey Milk personally, are for the most part happy to hear about all of this. They respond favorably when told that the screenplay will attempt to involve every aspect of the Milk story: from his early years as a stock-broker, to his dropping out of straight society into the world of sixties hippiedom, to his rebirth as a gay activist, to his rise as a leader in city politics, to his assassination and its aftermath. Moreover, the producers promise that *Mayor* won't shy away from depicting the more freewheeling aspects of gay and lesbian sexuality of the 1970s. But while enthusiastic and supportive overall, San Franciscans in the auditorium this evening are taking everything they hear with a rather large grain of salt. Craig Zadan and Neil Meron are gay. So is Bob Brassell, the Warner Bros. executive overseeing the project. Still, no one at the studio has any comment to make about a work that is still in "preproduction." Consequently, the activist's question remains hanging in midair. Why *does* Warner Bros. want to make a film version of *The Mayor of Castro Street*? And more to the point, why now?

The "town meeting" comes as the climax to a year in which Hollywood's long-standing negative treatment of gays and lesbians has come under fire as never before. Activist groups have launched a series of protests against an industry in which many gays and lesbians thrive professionally, yet which continues to provide demonizing depictions of their lives and selves in many heavily touted, high-profile releases. As gay bashing rises nationwide, and the AIDS epidemic continues unabated in the face of widespread state and public indifference, gays and lesbians both within and without the industry have come to find Hollywood's image-making status quo inexcusable. The spring of 1992 has seen organizations as diverse as the negotiation-oriented GLAAD and the in-your-face Queer Nation stage protests against Tri-Star Pictures' lesbian-icepick-slasher thriller *Basic Instinct* in several major cities. The Oscar ceremonies, where two other films that raised activist ire—*The Silence of the Lambs* and *JFK*—were up for major awards, also became a protest focal point. When the smoke cleared, *Basic Instinct* had become one of the year's biggest box-office hits, and the threat of on-air Oscar protests failed to materialize as *The Silence of the Lambs* garnered the Academy's Best Picture, Actor, Actress, Director, and Screenplay awards. Still, activists ire didn't go entirely unheeded, as the industry's treatment of gays and lesbians—onscreen and off—was the talk of the town. AIDS discrimination and homophobia quickly became the center of industry attention as gays and lesbians in positions of authority, many of whom had never thought of protesting anything before, began to speak out.

Meanwhile, the filmmakers cited by protestors for gay and lesbian misdeeds quickly moved to make amends. *Basic Instinct* scriptwriter Joe Eszterhas informed the press that his next project, *Layers of Skin,* would be a thriller about an "openly gay" police detective. Jonathan Demme, director of *The Silence of the Lambs,* chose as his next film *Philadelphia,* a courtroom drama about a straight lawyer defending a gay, HIV-positive client. However, the most eye-catching announcement of all came from *JFK* writer-director Oliver Stone, who—just prior to the Academy Awards—stated he would *not* direct *The Mayor of Castro Street.*

Craig Zadan and Neil Meron had worked for six years to get *The Mayor of Castro Street* off the ground when in the fall of 1991 Stone agreed to come aboard as executive producer. (Having worked as a liaison between Stone and the two producers, Janet Yang joined the project as co-producer.) Overnight a film that everyone in town thought would suffer the same fate as the oft-promised but never produced *The Front Runner* became a real moviemaking possibility. Industry insider speculation had it that rather than just co-produce, Stone (who had succeeded Stanley Kramer as the town's voice of "liberal" social consciousness) would also direct. But in the wake of *JFK,* with its factually questionable depiction of businessman Clay Shaw, many in the gay press questioned the wisdom of Stone's directing a film about Harvey Milk.[1] Then, in an interview in the *Advocate* (in which he compared Queer Nation to the Nazis), Stone disclosed that he had decided against directing *Mayor,* acknowledging the "inescapable controversy" that would result otherwise.

"It's really an unfortunate situation," Craig Zadan remarked at the time of Stone's announcement. "The truth of the matter is, the *only* reason the picture got bought by Warner Bros. was because of Oliver. I don't believe that Oliver is homophobic. I had every confidence in him because I spent the last year behind closed doors with him. I knew how he was going to direct this movie. He talked to lots of gay people, and spent a lot of time in San Francisco interviewing the people involved in Harvey's life. He has been aggressively trying to get a major director to replace him, because without a major director we won't keep Robin Williams."

The "major director" they found was Gus Van Sant.

A moviemaking maverick whose works first saw the light of day at gay and lesbian film festivals, Van Sant's career took off when his prize-winning 1986 feature, *Mala Noche*—a tale of a gay liquor-store clerk hopelessly in love with a Mexican teenager—led in 1989 to his directing the critically acclaimed study of seventies-era junkie street life, *Drugstore Cowboy*. Nineteen ninety-one saw Van Sant gain further glory with *My Own Private Idaho,* his recasting of Shakespeare's *Henry IV* as a tale of unrequited love between youthful street hustlers in the Pacific Northwest. Van Sant offered the *Mayor* team a chance to kill two birds with one (Oliver) Stone. Van Sant's presence would quell activist upset at the film's famous executive producer, while at the same time his being "openly gay" ("Couldn't I just say I'm 'casually gay'?" he famously remarked to his publicist—and *My Own Private Idaho* featured player—Mickey Cottrell) would constitute a Hollywood "first."

"The only analogy that I can think of," producer Neil Meron tells the "town meeting" audience, "is with David Lynch and *The Elephant Man*. There is no one more idiosyncratic than David Lynch. Yet he was able to make that film without compromising his own artistic sensibility. I believe that Gus can work with us that way— tackling this material in his own style, and yet reach a broader audience." The analogy is apt. But what makes Meron feel the film's further-reach potential is possible is due to another factor—Robin Williams. Williams's success in both comedy and drama (*Good Morning, Vietnam; Dead Poets Society; Awakenings*) would, to some, make him an ideal choice to play the tragicomic Milk.

Some of those present at the "town meeting," however, feel otherwise. "When I heard about Robin Williams," one man recalls, "my reaction was one of annoyance. He has a long history of doing derogatory characterizations. He comes out of a 'progressive comedian' type of thing, with all his work for various causes. But his act is very homophobic. It's like, 'Oh, I'm just doing a little effeminate bit here, but it's no big deal.' "

"Finally we're going to have a positive gay image onscreen," says another "town meeting" attendee, "and we have it played by someone who is not an enemy exactly, but certainly not a great friend. That's a bit of a slap in the face."

"I'm waiting to read the interviews where he says he had to go deep within and find the gay person inside of him to do the part," remarks another man derisively. "He'll be wearing his little red AIDS-awareness ribbon and talk about what a great opportunity he had playing a gay person. He isn't your only choice, you know. You have thousands of people in Hollywood. If you dangled in front of them the same salary you're offering Robin Williams you'd have people running out of the closet so fast!"

"Robin is a very sensitive human being," an unflappable Craig Zadan replies. "He brought up to us at a dinner we had with him early in his career that he had done some comedy that might be misconstrued as being questionable. It really hurt him deeply that people were offended by what he had done. He said that it was very important to him that the gay and lesbian community embraced him."

"Listen," says longtime San Francisco activist David Robinson heatedly, "to waffle on how something Robin Williams did in the past may be perceived—that's bullshit. He may not have meant it maliciously, but that's part of homophobia—*people don't think!* And it wasn't just a few things he did at the beginning. He did it on Johnny Carson's last TV show just the other night!

"It's a privilege and and honor for *him* to do this movie," Robinson continues. "He's not doing us any favors, and neither is Oliver Stone. It's a privilege for *him* to do this movie too. This is the easiest gay movie for Hollywood to make—the story of a dead martyr. And it's a measure of how intensely homophobic Hollywood is that it's having so much trouble."

"Hollywood is absolutely homophobic," says Zadan matter-of-factly. "What we are doing is breaking down that homophobia with this movie."

*   *   *

Did you see *Newsies*?" Gus Van Sant asks gleefully. "You really missed something. Boy, was that great. Now I know this sounds strange, but I want *The Mayor of Castro Street* to be just like *Newsies*, only without the singing and dancing. "I'm serious. Print that!"

It is the Monday after the San Francisco "town meeting," and I'm talking with Van Sant about it in his room at the Chateau Marmont Hotel in Los Angeles. He is in town to discuss his next project: a long-planned adaptation of Tom Robbins's sixties-era tale of a free-wheeling, large-thumbed, free-spirited hitchhiker, *Even Cowgirls Get the Blues*. Tri-Star Pictures, originally set to back the project, has "put it into turnaround"—Hollywoodese for cancellation. Now Van Sant is going to get it set up with New Line Cinema. Still, as involved as he is with *Cowgirls*, the writer-director hasn't forgotten about the preparations being made for *Mayor*. And while there's a marked element of "camp" in his enthusiasm for one of the Disney studio's greatest flops, there's another level on which Van Sant means every word he's saying.

"*Newsies* has this really great element in it in that there are these kids that sell newspapers for about half a cent apiece," he explains excitedly. "Essentially they're street trash. It's child labor and they stand up and strike—like in those old John Garfield movies. You know—the workingman stands up against the system, and mirrored in back of him is the populace saying, 'You can't do this to us because *we are the people!*' Then you get all these heroic extras shot from below. Well, believe it or not, *The Mayor of Castro Street* is a lot like that!'

"Look," Van Sant continues in a somewhat more serious tone. "The types that Harvey Milk was involved with were considered street trash. These were people who had never been asked to do anything by anyone. These were the people that the establishment ignored. That's why I see this picture as a chance to construct a history of gay radicalism. San Francisco has this great gay history stretching all the way back to the turn of the century. There were things that went on that were different examples of the same things that went on in the 1970s with Harvey."

Van Sant is somewhat surprised to hear about the intensity of opposition expressed at the "town meeting" to Robin Williams, who according to Neil Meron won't remain on the film if Van Sant doesn't approve. "I met with him about the film just the other day. He's very interested because he lived in that neighborhood at one time and knows it real well. I talked with him about the script. He understands what we're trying to do.

"Harvey was such an identifiable character. Whenever he talked you just sat up and listened. You see, this is a film about people adopting a new sort of society—a new home, new types of families. All that stuff interests me. It's also about that whole shift that came when the hippie era melted away and suddenly it was all gay culture! Now Oliver, he's not really interested in that. He wants to do a film about inner-city politics. He wants to do a film about how a board of supervisors works. He's not really all that involved in the social politics of Castro Street. That's the movie *I* want to make."

But is it the movie Warner Bros. wants to make?

"I *hope* it's the movie Warner Bros. wants to make," Van Sant replies, chuckling.[2]

The Mayor of Castro Street did not continue as planned. David Franzoni was replaced as scriptwriter by Becky Johnston, and Gus Van Sant left the project. In the 1994 edition of director John Boorman's annual film journal, *Projections 3,* Van Sant discussed his leaving *Mayor* in an à clef piece unsurprisingly entitled "The Hollywood Way." "I had only been a gay pawn to calm the fury of the gay politicos so the studio or the producers wouldn't have any trouble," Van Sant claimed.[3]

But by that time he was having career troubles of his own making. Starring Uma Thurman, and featuring a supporting cast that included John Hurt, Angie Dickinson, Roseanne, Lorraine Bracco, and Keanu Reeves, *Even Cowgirls Get the Blues* (1994) proved to be both a critical and a commercial disaster. The structural looseness that had served him so well in his earlier films wasn't suited to a picaresque tale that was too loose by half to begin with. Neither funny nor touching, its central character failed to come into focus, despite Thurman's best efforts, her love scenes with a less-than-charismatic Rain Phoenix being especially disappointing.

Van Sant managed to bounce back the following year, however, with *To Die For*. Written by Buck Henry, this adaptation of novelist Joyce Maynard's loose retelling of the Pamela Smart case—a high-school teacher who conspired with a pair of students to murder her husband—it was Van Sant's simplest narrative to date. With Nicole Kidman cast as the heroine/villainess (a public-access-television office assistant with aspirations to bigtime broadcast journalism), and a supporting cast including Matt Dillon, Wayne Knight, Illeana Douglas, and Joaquin (formerly Leaf) Phoenix, it had the drive and focus *Cowgirls* lacked. It also sported a playful sense of dark humor recalling such Tuesday Weld classics as *Lord Love a Duck* and *Pretty Poison*. It had, however, nothing gay about it—save for a subplot involving Douglas's character (a lesbian skating champion) that was cut by the studio over Van Sant's objections.

Meanwhile, another Tri-Star release, Jonathan Demme's AIDS drama *Philadelphia*, had scooped *Mayor* to become the first major-studio gay (and AIDS) project, winning Tom Hanks the 1993 Oscar for Best Actor of the year. Hanks's acceptance speech, in which he thanked a gay drama teacher who had inspired him, in turn inspired producer Scott Rudin. What, Rudin wondered to frequent collaborator Paul Rudnick, if an actor thanked a teacher who wasn't yet "out"? And so Rudnick's script for the hit comedy *In and Out* (1997) was born. Starring Kevin Kline as the teacher, Van Sant regular Matt Dillon as the student/Oscar winner, and a once highly litigious Tom Selleck as an openly gay television reporter, *In and Out* found comedy in both the outing phenomenon and Middle America's now nonstop exposure to gay and lesbian issues—both in the news and in the movies.

Mayor, meanwhile, had moved on. In 1993, director Rob Cohen took up where Van Sant had left off and returned to David Franzoni's script. Robin Williams was out of the picture, so Cohen sought a new

Harvey Milk in Daniel Day Lewis—whose portrayal of a gay "punk" in *My Beautiful Laundrette* had launched an international career. But by the following year, which saw the passing of Randy Shilts on the seventeenth of February—Cohen was off the project. In 1995, Brian Gibson came aboard and asked Tony Kushner of *Angels in America* fame to write a new script. But the project stalled again.

While failing to make a film, producers Craig Zadan and Neil Meron found great success in television, with new adaptations of the musical classics *Gypsy* (starring Bette Midler), *Bye Bye Birdie* (Jason Alexander and Vanessa L. Williams), and Rogers and Hammerstein's already twice-telefilmed *Cinderella* (with Brandy, Bernadette Peters, and Whitney Houston).

David Franzoni turned from gay politics to slavery, writing *Amistad* for Steven Spielberg.

Putting *Layers of Skin* to one side, Joe Eszterhas followed *Basic Instinct* with the even more grotesque lesbian sexploitation film *Showgirls*. *Telling Lies in America*, his script about a foreign-born teenager's hero-worship of a fifties-era disc jockey, was an uncharacteristically unhyper Eszterhas project—which is doubtless the explanation for its being a low-budget independent release. But *An Alan Smithee Film: Burn Hollywood Burn* found him back in blustery form, attempting to satirize modern Hollywood—to no effect. An absence of lesbian lust was its most noteworthy feature.

In 1997 Gus Van Sant directed his most "mainstream" and commercially successful film to date, *Good Will Hunting*. Starring Matt Damon and Ben Affleck—who also co-authored the script—this tale of a troubled Boston youth who is found to be a mathematics genius was a great hit with the public, but received mixed reviews from critics, who pegged it a "feel good" melodrama of the sort long associated with its co-star, Robin Williams. Still, there's a clear connection between this new "upbeat" Van Sant and the Gus of *My Own Private Idaho*—right down to the film's *Idaho*-echoing last shot of empty roadway. And that's not to mention the visual attention paid the youthful beauty of Damon and Affleck.

The pair thanked him in accepting their Oscars for Best Original Screenplay of the year, as did Best Supporting Actor winner

Robin Williams. Van Sant, the first openly gay director to be Oscar-nominated, lost (as the whole world knew he would) to James Cameron for *Titanic*. But this "loss" was lessened by the gain of major-studio "bankability" *Good Will Hunting* brought him. By April of 1998 it had become the biggest-grossing film in the history of Miramax Pictures. Keeping faith with the spirit of controversy that has always swirled around him, Van Sant announced in the spring of 1998 that his next project would be a remake of Alfred Hitchcock's *Psycho* to star . . . Anne Heche.

And *then*—as if to renew his "license" for being what the fourth estate continues to call a "practicing homosexual"—Van Sant will direct *Brokeback Mountain*. Based on an Annie Proulx story about two otherwise heterosexual cowboys whose passionate devotion to each other lasts their entire lives, the Scott Rudin production will be shot from a script by novelist Larry McMurtry (*Lonesome Dove, The Last Picture Show, Terms of Endearment*) and Diana Ossana. A *Mala Noche Rides the Range* might well result.

The sense of momentousness that once surrounded *The Mayor of Castro Street* has dissipated as one "mainstream" film after another (*My Best Friend's Wedding, In and Out, As Good as It Gets, The Object of My Affection*) has presented gay characters in a sympathetic light of a sort considered unimaginable only a decade before. *The Mayor of Castro Street* revolves around a historical moment—gay politics in the pre-AIDS era—and Hollywood has never been especially adept at portraying political realities in a specified historical context. And that's not to mention the problems involved in selling such a film to a moviegoing public that has rarely shown any interest in the nuts-and-bolts of social history, particularly as regards minorities.

The Mayor of Castro Street is currently in development as an HBO telefilm. Some of its thunder may have been stolen by *Execution of Justice*, a Showtime telefilm adapted from Emily Mann's play about Milk's assassin, Dan White, with Tim Daly as White and Peter Coyote as Milk. But there's more than enough room for *Mayor*. For even as this period of history fades into the past, the issues and conflicts it raises remain.

NINE

MOVING AND

SHAKING

—

"I HAVE A VISION OF AMERICA, AND YOU'RE part of it," said Bill Clinton.

It was the evening of May 18, 1992, at the Palace, an auditorium-style nightclub in Los Angeles, where an AIDS benefit was being held. The "you" being addressed were the several hundred gay and lesbian film-industry professionals who had gathered there to hear what the former Arkansas governor, and then presidential candidate, might have to say. No one familiar with politics was expecting much—maybe a few vague words about his "hopes" for the country, and his "appreciation" of his many supporters, without specifying who those supporters were. Certainly the crowd wasn't expecting Clinton's ringing endorsement of the notion that gays and lesbians are first-class American citizens worthy of attention and respect by both political candidates and, by extension, the rest of the "general public." But that's exactly what they got.

The speech was, by all accounts, a triumph for Clinton. It marked him as the leading contender in what had up until that point been seen as a crowded, and somewhat rudderless, Democratic race. He had at last, all pundits agreed, "found his voice." It was also the first time that a high-profile politician had sought support—in a direct and unambiguous manner—from a widely despised social constituency. To many, the speech stood as proof that the years of painstaking work that so many had put into both street protests and behind-the-scenes discussion were finally beginning to pay off. For Clinton, it would be the first of many overtures that he and the Democratic party would make toward gays and lesbians nationwide—until the whole process crashed and burned in the gays-in-the-military debacle.

Clinton had pledged to lift the ban on gays and lesbians in the armed services, a grotesque and nonsensical prohibition that had led to costly witch hunts, ruining the lives of otherwise well-qualified men and women who had been forced to hide and lie about themselves in order to keep their jobs. But Clinton had never served in the military, and apparently had no notion of the firestorm of opposition an otherwise unremarkable, and perfectly legal, executive order would create. And so he backtracked. The "Don't ask, don't tell" policy, which enshrined lying as an "honorable compromise," was put in its place—leading to more witch hunts and expulsions than had existed in the past. And that reversal was followed a few years later by Clinton's signing of the so-called Defense of Marriage Act, which—in order to fight efforts to extend legal marriage to same-sex couples—enshrines the ceremony as a legal right to be recognized by the state only when the persons involved are of different genders.

In a way, no one should really have expected more from Bill Clinton. He was, after all, a politician. Ending the ban on gays and lesbians in the military was just a campaign promise—to be fulfilled if possible, but to be ignored at the first sign of trouble. But the process he started that evening at the Palace wouldn't end with a presidency that, for gays and lesbians, has offered more in the way of symbolic gestures than concrete action. For whether Bill Clinton was aware of it or not, the message of his Palace speech had begun to reverberate into areas well beyond those traveled by an ambitious professional politician. Bill Clinton had inadvertently awakened the sleeping giant of gay Hollywood.

I was not at the Palace that night," producer Bruce Cohen recalls. "I was on location doing a film. But I got an invitation to go, and I remember realizing when I got it, it came with a letter in which Clinton outlined his desire to get the gay vote, and why he thought he deserved it. This light went off in my head, because there was this hitherto nonexistent connection between politics—which had been an interest and a passion of mine, because I'd always been very, very involved in the Democratic Party—and my homosexuality. Here was a chance to connect those two things on a really profound level. I read the letter, and when I finished I said to myself, He is my candidate, and I am voting for him. What more personal reason could I possibly have to cast my vote than my sexuality, which is such a political issue as well as a personal one? That changed my life in that way. It was by all accounts an incredible, historic evening. It was the beginning of Bill Clinton's national political life. It was also the beginning, I think, of this new generation of gays and lesbians in Hollywood. Even if you weren't there, it was the moment people got involved in the campaign as out gay entertainment industry people, because that was how they were invited to join the campaign.

"Everyone started realizing who we all were," Cohen continues.

"It was a reason to come out en masse together without it specifically being about being out. It was quite wonderful the way that worked. Because if someone had said like they do on National Coming Out Day to 'show up at eleven A.M. at this place and announce that you're out,' no one would ever do it. Instead, it was 'If you're gay and you're out in the entertainment industry, come and work for Clinton.' Suddenly all these people started showing up, and we realized who we were, and how many of us there were. It was a wonderful group of people: lawyers, agents, managers, screenwriters, directors, producers, studio executives. It was amazing. Some actors were there too—not a lot; that's a whole separate issue. Still, a lot of stuff began from that period."

What happened had little to do with the shrouded socializing of the past, where gay and lesbian cliques circulated for off-hours pleasures and nothing more. Likewise, this was something other than a mass "coming out," as the Hollywood professionals at the Palace had "been there, done that" already. The next step came as they began to look at themselves in new ways and reconsider lives that in the past had been rigidly separated into "personal" and "private" spheres.

"At that point I had been in the business about eight to ten years," Cohen recalls. "I had worked at Warner Bros. in a staff position for about a year. Then I got into the Directors Guild trainee program to learn how to be an assistant director. From 1984 on I'd begun to work on movies, first as a trainee, then as an assistant director, eventually as a producer. I was out to my friends. I had a lot of friends on the movies I had worked on who knew I was out. But in retrospect I'd realized I was not really out at work, and there was no real mechanism to come out, or reason to be out. Save for getting up at lunch on a film set and announcing it to everyone, there was no way it would have happened."

"It's interesting," producer Nina Jacobson chimes in, "because even though we ended up in the same place as partners, for me the coming-out experience has been from almost the opposite trajectory. When I was at Universal, that's really where I came out. It wasn't that I was rabidly closeted prior to that. It wasn't that I was creating huge cover stories and taking a 'beard' to events. I just wasn't talking about it. I came to Universal in 1990, and after I had been there about six months I had told a couple of my friends who I worked with about my life. I was out with a senior person at the company who I hadn't told, and I decided to work it into a conversation so he would know. I asked him, 'Do you think that the head of the studio knows? And do they care? And do they think there'll be a problem?' And he said, 'You know, at this point I think it's safe to assume that everybody knows.' That was like the best news I had received."

"Sid Sheinberg hadn't started up Hollywood Supports yet," Cohen notes. "But he was probably already very involved in APLA, and I think had maybe already gotten his Commitment to Life award, because he was one of the very first recipients."

"Sid wasn't really in my life at that point," says Jacobson. "I was a junior executive in the movie division. Eventually I had a very nice relationship with Sid. But at this point I was twenty-five years old, and I was worried about whether my bosses were going to be freaked out by my sexuality. Then to find out six months in that they all knew and it was like 'Okay, I don't have a problem,' I had no excuse *not* to be out. From that point on I was very out. I brought my girlfriend to all the functions. They started to issue invitations that said, 'Bring your spouse or spousal equivalent.' The insurance plan was instituted. I spoke to Sid at my first senior management meeting after I'd been promoted to vice-president and I told him how proud I was to work at a company that had such policies. It was all happening at once.

"For years that seemed to me to be what it meant to be leading a political life—just to be out. The personal was political. That was enough, and I could sort of hold my head up high. Then I was being interviewed for a *Hollywood Reporter* article. It was one of those great 'ageist' articles that they do all the time: 'Up-and-Coming People Under 30.' They had a thing in it about 'career milestones.' I said mine was working on what had been my favorite movie up to that point, *Dragon: The Bruce Lee Story*. Then I realized that that wasn't my career milestone at all. It was a great experience to see something I loved get made, but for me success was really tied to my coming out, because things were better and better for me from that point on.

So the story ran in the trades—and I realized that I still had a lot of internalized homophobia to deal with. Right up until the time the piece came out I kept thinking, Should I call them back and put a movie in there instead? What will people think? Every time somebody comes into my office, that'll be the first thing they know. I couldn't sleep at night. But I decided, no. It *was* my career milestone, it *was* the most important thing I'd done, it *is* the most important accomplishment that I can really point to. Then when it came out and I faced fear again, I realized that it's not enough to be out in the workplace. You have to be out to yourself."

"That article had a major impact," Cohen recalls. "It came out at a time when people under thirty had never had as much power and as much influence in the industry. So every single person under thirty in the entertainment industry, who were the people who this article was about, read that special issue, and read those bios sentence by sentence. First to find out 'Am I in it? which is a silly question. Then to find out 'Should I be in it?' People had never seen anything like that."

"I was friendly with a journalist from the *Reporter* at that time, who wasn't doing the article," notes Jacobson. "She said to me, 'Are you *sure* you want to go with that?' She gave me an out. It was a strange moment. My girlfriend and I were talking about the fact that now, when we knew friends who seemed like they were on the verge of maybe realizing that they were gay, that no matter how much the political climate changes, people are rarely happy for that person. Instead there's this ambivalence from straight and gay people alike. But for me, people were incredibly supportive, and I started to feel like a politically inspired person, which I hadn't felt really since college. At that time my politics were very general leftist loud-mouthing. But I always felt, 'Why couldn't I have been a part of the civil rights movement, or a Parisian student in May '68, or protesting Vietnam?' I'd just missed my turn. Then, because of coming out, I realized I could really make some noise. This is a civil rights movement of its own, which is winnable.

"There was this interview on NPR with Jerry Falwell," Jacobson continues, "in which they played back this tape of him saying interracial marriage was an abomination against God, and he said, 'Well, I didn't really feel that way, it was just the political times.' They said, 'So a few years from now you won't feel this way about gay couples and it was just the political times?' And he said, 'Oh that's different, that's completely different.' That's why it's something I believe we could completely change: from the sort of shrouded second-class citizens that we are, not only in Hollywood but the rest of the world. Just because we have the privilege of being out in this environment, that's not enough of a political act for me. I want to take it to another level to find out what we can do with that privilege.

"I must add that even though I was out to my parents, I never showed them the article. When I was in *Out* magazine I didn't show it to them, either. There's still that sense of shame: I'm out but I don't have to rub their nose in it. That's my thing to work on now. My girlfriend says, 'It's not enough that they should love us, they should be proud of you.' We don't ask for pride. We ask for acceptance, but we don't ask for pride. I can get pride from my parents—and I do. My mom goes to events with me now, and she's a PFLAG [Parents and Friends of Lesbians and Gays] member. But we're still sort of apologizing for who we are.

"My analogy for coming out is that you rarely see people with power wearing a toupee," says Jacobson, brightening at the prospect of the metaphorical. "The toupee indicates that there's a part of yourself that you cannot accept, that you loathe, that's unbecoming, and that you're going to try to pull one over on people."

"Which still has the effect of looking absurd," a greatly amused Cohen adds.

"Right," says Jacobson, "because everyone knows you've got it on. It's an indication of a lack of self-acceptance. And to me you can't have any kind of power without self-acceptance. Name a power person who wears a toupee. Michael Milken. And look what happened to him!"

"I think there's also something all gay people experience, which is universal," says Cohen. "It's that moment when someone has asked you a question, and you know the real answer to that question, and you don't know if you want to answer it. It's right in the middle of the day, always when you least expect it, and you say to yourself, Oh shit! Now in this very moment I either have to give it up or lie. Are you going to say what the person expects you to say when they ask, 'Do you have a girlfriend?' You're forced to either give the safe, unthreatening yes-or-no answer—which in either case is going to be a total lie—or you need to answer that question truthfully, and it's going to be a big deal. To me those are the great defining moments. And the thrill and excitement of rising to the occasion and giving the true answer and getting to watch—sometimes almost with glee—the deck of cards that falls out at that moment when you come out with the right statement: to me that's what life's all about. One of the great joys of being gay is to have those moments in your life.

"A friend of mine," Cohen continues, "told me he was at his sister's wedding this weekend. His parents know he's gay. He didn't realize that the rest of his family didn't. He was sitting with a bridesmaid, who he had just met that weekend and really liked a lot. So his uncle came up to him, right in the middle of the reception, and said, 'So, Paul, are you next? When are you getting married?' And the bridesmaid looked up and said, 'Oh, the President hasn't signed that bill yet!' And *that's* how the uncle found out."

"I think that what Bruce and I realized when we were going to do this," says Jacobson of their support group, Out There, "was we both had an appetite to do something proactive with our outness. The act of writing checks and going to dinners—which is pretty much all that's been expected of you as a sort of PC gay person in Hollywood— wasn't enough. You go and eat the rubber chicken a couple of times a year, and often it isn't even your money that you're donating. Your company buys a table for a function and goes and asks the gay people if they want to go, and that's it. That doesn't feel very empowering. We started talking about it, and called a bunch of people and said, 'Let's get together and talk about the National Gay and Lesbian Task Force and the Human Rights Campaign.'"

"There was a nice kind of coincidence," says Cohen, "because on the same day, both organizations had called both of us and asked us to help them. The national gay and lesbian organizations in '92, '93, and '94 were just beginning to identify the fact that the out gay and lesbian community in Hollywood had a lot of stuff that they needed. We had money, power, celebrities. So there was this chaotic scramble, which continues to this day, by all these different organizations, trying to get to the same relatively small group of people. There are a couple of people who were doing wonderful work in our community. Alan Hergott [film industry lawyer and independent production financier] is one we both know. In '92 they were saying, 'Alan, you must do it.' By '94 they said, 'You must be tired of our calling you. So instead of asking you, who can we call?' So Alan had given both groups both our names. Nina and I met under that guise. If we're two of the people who are going to be called over and over again, maybe there's a way to organize this better."

"We didn't even know each other," laughs Jacobson. "We also felt a little bit panicked. We'd been targeted. What would the money go for? What are we supposed to do about feeling conflicted over which group to give the money to? What was our agenda? How could we be proactive by disseminating information about major organizations that do things locally and nationally? How can we offer support to those who are fighting the fight and know more than we do?

"So we gathered our friends together. I was certain no one would come."

"We had an overflow crowd," Cohen recalls. "It was pretty exciting. The Human Rights Campaign, the National Gay and Lesbian Task Force, and the Gay and Lesbian Center here in Los Angeles all sent their executive directors. That's how strongly they felt we could help them. What came out of that meeting and the ones that followed was that with Out There we would take no money ourselves, but would ask for $110 a year from members. For that people would automatically join NGLTF, the HRC, GLAAD—all the national organizations—and the Center. The idea was not to exclusively support those four, but by joining you were saying you were an out gay or lesbian member of the entertainment industry. We had the word 'out' right in our mission statement, which is highly unusual. It was very controversial, because it was saying that if you're not out you can't be a member of the organization. If you're out, you should at the very least know what's going on nationally. Rather than spending any of our time or resources on doing stuff that was already done, we decided to make sure that our members are receiving all the information and all the mailings. Between those four organizations it's amazing to see what you get in the mail. They do a phenomenal intersecting job, giving you a detailed picture of everything that's going on, all the issues facing the gay and lesbian community in the country. If something goes down, you hear about it right away. Our original thought was, Won't that be enough? We'll provide the information, and people will of course march off to save the world and we will have been the conduit. The reality is, what is most effective is to marshal your members to do specific projects, and not to sit there and hope people are doing things on their own."

"And we realized, too, we're the ultimate novices," says Jacobson. "We have no infrastructure, no staff, no budget. We are literally flying by the seat of our pants."

"And our steering committee," notes Cohen proudly, "are literally the fifteen busiest people in town."[1]

While Nina Jacobson and Bruce Cohen might be said to represent the face of gay and lesbian Hollywood professionals today in a way those within the industry understand, the story that has most consumed press and public attention relates less to an individual than to an entire company—Walt Disney. Though same-sex spousal benefits have become a reality for gays and lesbians working in every major company in Hollywood, only its institution at the Walt Disney Company has raised widespread fourth-estate attention. Part of the reason for this has to do with the vocal opposition of the Southern Baptist Convention, who even before Ellen's "Yep" had targeted the company as the embodiment of all the social ills that so upset them. Same-sexuality was, needless to say, high atop the Baptists' hit list. And few know the meaning of their attack better than Robert L. Williams, president of the gay and lesbian Disney employees group, League.

"If I were to say I was from Universal or Paramount and talking about gay rights, nobody would expect anything unusual. But when you put the words 'Disney' and 'gay' together, people think 'child molester': sex and children, or sex and 'innocence.' What they don't understand is, just because someone's homosexual doesn't mean they're not innocent. A lot of the American Family Association people will blast Disney about things that they've done, lumping gay people into a molester framework. They don't understand that I have just as much of a family as they do, and I'm not the one that puts a dirty connotation on it. Disney knows its base, and generally keeps silent on it. They've been very supportive of League in their policies because it's been *business*. People know that boycotts don't really work.

"A group of people got together about the time Universal had granted domestic partner benefits and talked about wanting to put a club together at Disney, because there was an African-American club and a few other clubs," recalls the thirtysomething, decidedly non-flamboyant Williams. "Originally we were told it wasn't in the charter to have a 'dating club' or 'social club.' We explained that that wasn't what the intent was. Finally we fought for it and it was granted. We sent out a flyer and it caused a lot of controversy. The group started meeting. It didn't really come to any sort of strong leadership until Garrett Hicks and Lee Schaeffer took over and set things up, having regular meetings with guest speakers and mentors. They put together what they called 'The ABC's of DBP's'—which was domestic partner benefits. They were really fighting, along with Hollywood Supports, to get one drawn up. They drew up this document and put all the information on it to answer every question. It was presented to Michael Eisner, and they kind of sat on it. Over time, through a lot of intervention and whatever, he finally agreed in 1996 to participate. It polarized a lot of people. I took over from Garrett after that happened.

"The next step of what League is about is education when it comes to gays in the workplace. Most companies really do need a liaison between gay and lesbian employees and management. These employees need a safe place where they can go and get information in a confidential way, because the majority of people are still very closeted about it. Secondly, it's a good sort of checkpoint for when any issue comes up and we can sort of go about it or investigate it or look into it as a group, and question it and get the information out there.

"For example," Williams explains, "if someone has an issue of their being discriminated against because a straight person gets something and they don't, we'll check it out. Usually it's not the case that it has anything to do with sexuality; but if it is the case we can straighten it out. For example, take the credit union. Your brother can join it, you can *say* someone's your brother, you can *say* someone's your wife, but you can't say someone's your lover. They will not recognize that. That's one of the things we're changing. We've also tried to create an environment for people to hear other people's stories about coming out and their career path. And the funny thing that's consistent was, being gay never hurt anyone. A lot of the people we have are producers and actors and directors. The one thing that they talk about is most of them got fired from jobs because they spoke up about something and that threatened someone in authority. So they started other jobs. But when they came out—both men and women— it was never really an issue. Most of them have said it was the most important thing they ever did, because it gives people less they can hold against you. A lot of people feel if they can trust you on this, then they can trust you on something else. So that's where League is right now—why we're trying to keep it in existence. Also, we're a very big company. The message doesn't always get out."

Williams is both amused and annoyed at the way the Southern Baptists have exploited Disney's "family" image to their own ends, especially as regards the so-called Gay Days at the company's theme parks.

"Disney does *not* have an official Gay Day," Williams declares flatly. "If everyone named Fred said they wanted to meet at Disney World at a certain date, Disney's not going to turn them away. Anybody can meet and go to Disneyland or Disney World on a particular day. Sometimes, as with Disneyland, anybody can go inside the park after hours—and it's very expensive—as long as they observe the code. The funny thing about the American Family Association is they were saying all this 'gay behavior' was going on—men hugging men, women hugging women, leering at straight people and upsetting the families and all that stuff. A lot of things that they spread are so petty. How many people do they come in contact with who are gay? If gay people were to no longer service them, their whole world would stop. And it's not that we're the best or anything, either. But one of the letters I had seen said, 'What do you do after they leave? Do you burn the place? How do we know we're not going to get diseases?' To me that's where their head is. I think that people who subject themselves to those sorts of organizations don't know how to think for themselves. They want to have someone else tell them how to think.

"I'm from the Deep South—Mississippi," Williams continues. "A year ago my partner and I went home. My mother put us up in a room together—knowingly. It was not a big issue. But that came through education. I would daresay five years ago that wouldn't have happened. She didn't hate a *thing*, because I'm not a *thing*. I'm a person. So, for any hate mongers in the American Family Association—*I have a family*. Just as much. We're very middle-class, and kind of boring. But they want to harp on the most excessive sort of behavior in the gay world. I don't go around wanting to harp on the most excessive sort of behavior in the straight world. I recognize individuals. I think the Baptists put Disney in a sort of uncomfortable position. But I think they're smart. They're not saying anything. That's the best thing, 'cause it'll straighten itself out.

"In the short time I've been involved with League, which is about three years, there's been the most change for gays and lesbians in the entertainment industry. I hadn't come out here to do this. I'm a writer, with an acting background. But I sort of became an accidental activist. I don't even like using the word 'activist.' All that I wanted was to be able to be out at my job. This is the first job I've really been out at. I had a little bit of kidding around by people that I didn't know how to handle. Once I was out, the only thing they saw me as was a sex person, not a regular person. Especially the men. Men are the worst. Women are okay. Straight men think it's all just about sex. If you talk to them they think you're hitting on them or whatever. I had to do a lot of work educating people because of that.

"I didn't realize how much I'd hidden and buried until I came out at work. I realized how easy it was. Later on it was okay to be introduced to people as being from League or whatever. My boyfriend, Sean, and I were at a park and I was giving him a hug and there was this little—'Oh!' "

Still, for all the positive aspects of his experiences, and those of other gays and lesbians in the industry, the struggle for acceptance is far from over.

"There's more visibility now, *and* I think there's been more people going into the closet. I think that the people that are going to come out are okay with it, but without more visibility I think there are people who are in a situation that I totally respect, who feel that they would function better not having anybody know. I think that people start living in fear because somebody might be more powerful than them and they want to get ahead, and they think, 'If I don't rock the boat and make my life known, it'll be better for me.' I know two very powerful people who were sort of visible and then went right back into the closet because they think that it's threatening. I think it has to do with the climate of bottom line. Companies can get rid of you like *that* for no reason, because it's 'good business' or whatever. That's their perception. I'm not saying that's the case. It's a strange thing, but there are some people who say, 'I look like a duck, I walk like a duck, I act like a duck—but don't you *dare* call me a duck.' Some of them tend to be older, but there's still a younger group. I know that element. The reason I know it is because I am very visible and have had opportunities to talk to them. They got burned. They felt it was okay, and then got hauled into the boss's office and got their ass chewed out. But you know, it's not their problem. It's perception. I know these people have got an education. Even if they've got education they're not going to change. But the majority—most people—have been open, have been very supportive.

"One of the things, too, I've been wanting to do with League is to move out of this suffering-hero complex that gay people are taking on—like with the AIDS Walk. The Walk naturally started in the gay community because they were being hit the hardest, but I'm asked all the time to do AIDS this and AIDS that. What I'd like to do is sort of diversify and spread our time into other things, because I think that now with everybody doing an AIDS benefit that other sort of important issues aren't being addressed as much. It's, 'I did the AIDS Walk last year, so I'm cool.' "

Williams is also keenly aware of the fact that the Disney Company's attitude toward its gay and lesbian employees proceeded less from moral principles than from business ones. This is especially true in regards to the fact that as a consequence of Disney's success with feature-length animated films, major studios like Universal, 20th Century–Fox, and the new DreamWorks company have been setting up animation units. As many of Disney's leading animators (such as Andreas Deja) are gay, it would be a disastrous business decision for the company to decline to offer the spousal benefits its competitors were quite willing to supply.

"Businesses are business. They are not benefactors," says Williams simply, "The bottom line is, 'Will my actions create something that will hurt me when it comes time to talk to the stockbrokers?' I had somebody infer to me, 'Why do we need League? You already got your domestic partner benefits. We were nice enough to give them to you.' Nice? I didn't *ask* you to do it. I didn't *make* you do it. This came from a good business decision. And you *knew* it. 'Cause they were saying things about the boycott and 'See, you're drawing attention' and whatever. *You* made the decision to trust us. You cannot have it both ways. It is about business and people have to really understand that. It's about making employee packages attractive.

"There are misconceptions about spousal benefits," Williams continues. "The American Family Association is so funny. They say, 'You give them to gay people living together, but straight people living together don't get 'em.' Well, first of all, wouldn't they condemn someone for living together outside of marriage? It's not about casual boyfriends living together. It's about two people in a committed relationship over the years—coexisting. This is about people who have joint bank accounts. They act in every way, shape, and form that if they could get married they would. But they can't, and straight people can. That's why these benefits aren't offered to straight couples. 'Why can't I get my boyfriend on this?' *Because you can get married!* The other thing they don't understand is that for married couples benefits are tax deductible. It isn't for me. So there are these misconceptions about what same-sex spousal benefits really mean.

"We have really cool events at League," says Williams, turning to the group's other educational activities. "People sometimes think it's like a baseball league, so we have to explain it to them. David Lee, the producer of *Frasier,* came and spoke once. A woman came with her husband. She didn't know what League was. She just wanted to meet David Lee—and give him a script. She said, 'What are you? A writers' group?' 'No, actually we're a gay and lesbian organization.' 'Oh!' she said. I told her we're not like *exclusive*—that any Disney employee can come. And she was, 'Okay—bye!' "

M organ Rumpf has had a ringside seat to observe Hollywood's gay and lesbian "mainstreaming." For Outfest, which began its life in the late 1980s as a small-scale showcase at UCLA, has grown into one of the city's most important exhibition venues for independent and foreign films, regardless of the fact that all the films involved reflect gay or lesbian life in some way. And as a result of that, major Hollywood movers and shakers have come in recent years to keep a watchful eye over what Outfest has to offer.

"The industry is made up of different folks from all levels of the universe," says Rumpf, whose presentation of self is indistinguishable from that of other serious Hollywood professionals. "What I think is important to note is the fact that we have more gays and lesbians who are openly gay in all different levels of the industry, and really percolated to the top. We all know the *top* top: David Geffen, Sandy Gallin, and everybody else at that level. They're not the people who actually note what's going on with us. There are, however, working for them, a lot of other people we're corresponding with. We're communicating to that vice-president level, that development director level, that kind of staffing level that has influence over the decisions that are made, but are not necessarily the ones making those decisions. They're the people telling their bosses what to do. Informing Sherry Lansing that Paramount should be supporting the festival this year, for instance. Nan Morales is on our board of directors. She's head of production for Paramount. She's able to place calls to the powers-that-be at the company, and they listen to her. They believe that she has a valuable and important opinion, and because she says this festival is a valuable thing, they're willing to support it. That level of change is where we are right now.

"There are scattered individuals at the top as well. David Geffen has been supportive of this festival for the last five years, and we appreciate and really value him. But has he ever been to the festival? No. That's not something that he needs to do in his daily life, to validate himself in the industry. Nor does he need to come to screenings for his personal edification. Many people from his company come, however, and represent him. I in no way want to represent that he's not interested, but frankly he's at a level where he wouldn't come to the Los Angeles Independent Film Festival or the AFI Film Festival either. It's not a gay or lesbian issue; it's more about the placement of where you are in the industry. If he needs to see a film, there's someone to shuttle a print over to him. We've tried to provide access to that film for him—either a print or a tape. But because he's the CEO of a major corporation, he's asking Bruce Cohen, who's chairman of our board, who's a producer at DreamWorks, about what we're doing. Bruce is going to be the one to bring to David's attention the things he needs to know.

"Just as the straight CEOs have their minions, gays and lesbians do as well. That's how films like *Kiss Me Guido* go from the Sundance Film Festival to being released by Paramount Pictures. Our festival is not intended to be the sole universe for gay and lesbian film. We don't want it to be. We want gay and lesbian films to be at New York, at Venice, at Sundance, at Cannes."

Still, for all that's new about gay Hollywood, some of the old, Rumpf declares, remains.

"There are so many people who are out. There are still one or two people in the closet in the industry behind the scenes, and the question is, why? We made a list of people in the industry we wanted to know about the festival. We circulated the list here at work and it was like, 'Oh, he's not out yet.' 'What do you mean he's not out yet?

He comes to such-and-such.' 'I know, but he's not *out* yet.' So we can't put him on the list. And we're all sitting around and wondering, why? It's not an issue. Grow up. Because we have had so many people who are successful in the industry there's no need for it behind the scenes. It's not like we're outing people anymore. It's just that we're so disgusted and tired with it, and all the old excuses of why you had to stay 'in' are really not relevant to this industry at this time—unless you're on-camera talent. And then there are some real things to address. There's a difference between 'nudge-nudge, wink-wink, *we* know' and having everybody have the same level of knowledge that this person is a gay man or woman."[3]

Chastity Bono knows about what's known and what isn't. The daughter of sixties-era pop duo Sonny and Cher spent much of her childhood before television cameras. In her early adult years, however, the less-welcome intrusion of tabloid paparazzi brought her out of the closet in a way she hadn't welcomed. But In the 1990s she managed to bounce back, by lending both her name and "insider" expertise to the Gay and Lesbian Alliance Against Defamation. As its media director (a post she resigned in the summer of 1998 to write a book about gays and lesbians and their parents) she has become in a few years' time GLAAD's most visible force. Frequently seen on television, where's she's almost invariably paired in Ping-Pong left/right opposition to the likes of the Reverends Jerry Falwell and Lou Sheldon, Bono has always managed to keep her cool while delineating issues ranging from the problems faced by gay and lesbian teenagers to the media frenzy over Ellen DeGeneres.

"I think overall there's a general consensus that GLAAD needs to change with the times and to start focusing its work on more of a proactive nature than reactive," Bono observes. "I think the days of the massive GLAAD protests are pretty much over. I can't think of an incident that would prod us to do that. It would have to be absolutely terrible—a situation in which nobody involved would pick up the phone and talk to us. There's definitely more of a consciousness in Hollywood. There are more out gay people now, in all different areas. There's definitely a consciousness of that, and also a willingness to talk about it. I don't find myself being stonewalled at all. In fact, it's been quite the opposite, which is really nice. If there's a problem I can make a call, get somebody on the phone, and have them talk about it. In general, nobody wants to offend any group of people. More and more when it does happen, it's more an instance of ignorance than blatant homophobia—not that there aren't still isolated incidents of that. But more and more my experience has been that if somebody was in a film and portrayed a certain way, or the storyline was inaccurate, it's usually from their lack of understanding about the gay and lesbian community rather than wanting to defame us. I can't think of anyone within the entertainment industry who has spoken out negatively against gays and lesbians."

Bono is well aware that this situation is in sharp contrast to the ones that brought about GLAAD's creation in the late 1980s.

"I think Mel Gibson's a really good example of somebody who's been targeted or labeled homophobic when that isn't necessarily the case. In my interactions with him I did not get that impression at all. At the very worst my impression is that he's a Catholic man and probably hasn't been exposed to the gay and lesbian community very much, and the gay and lesbian people that are in his life are probably not always telling it like it is because he's Mel Gibson. That was really the feeling I got from him. If anything it's coming from ignorance. There was never any intention to offend."[4]

The "offense" Bono was mentioning arose in 1992 over an interview the actor gave that was printed in the Spanish newspaper *El País* in which the actor, when questioned about his feelings about homosexuals, replied, 'They take it up the ass,' pointed to his own posterior, and added, 'This is only for taking a shit.' In addition, Gibson "admitted to being baffled and angered at being, on occasion, thought of as gay because he's an actor. 'Do I sound like a homosexual? Do I talk like them? Do I move like them?' "[5] Reports of the interview in the gay and lesbian press startled many, who hadn't imagined that Gibson harbored any hostile feelings toward gays. The release of his medieval-Scottish battle epic, *Braveheart,* made things worse, due to a scene in which the lover of Edward II is casually tossed out the window of a castle tower by Edward I, almost in the spirit of a "sight gag." Many laughed—but few gays joined in. Protests were made, but not of the sort that came in the wake of the likes of *Cruising* or *Basic Instinct*. Moreover, Bono didn't join in them.

"The whole thing with *Braveheart*, which I thought personally was a wonderful movie, and I was not offended by at all," says Bono, "was that nobody involved had any idea that would be the audience's reaction to that scene. It wasn't to say, 'Oh, we threw a faggot out the window.' It was to show the brutality of the king who would just chuck somebody out the window because he didn't like what he was saying. I think it was kind of a snowball effect for Mel with his saying some kind of derogatory comment—or as he characterized it, 'making a bad joke' to a reporter in Spain. Who knows what got lost in the translation? And then this thing in *Braveheart* happened. I truly think had *he* not made the film people would not really have batted an eye over that scene."

It is a measure of how times have changed in Hollywood that rather than pull back and assume a defensive posture, Gibson tried to make amends through GLAAD by bringing a group of young gay and lesbian filmmakers onto the set of the film *Conspiracy Theory*.

"It was basically set up as a film seminar," notes Bono. "It was his spending a day on the set with these very promising gay and lesbian filmmakers, all of whom have made films, but very low budget independent films. See this big-budget Hollywood film being made and then sit down with Mel Gibson and have a no-holds-barred discussion. And at that point a number of issues were addressed. I also think it was an opportunity for Mel to get to see different gay people. The fact that they were filmmakers gave them something in common. It was the bridge that connected everybody together, and allowed them to talk about other situations. He could see what normal, everyday gay people are today—not the few gay people he probably knows in Hollywood, who might be closeted, but proud gay artists. That was really important."

Still, while Hollywood itself poses few problems for GLAAD, contending with an increasingly multifaceted mass media is a full-time job. And the reason for this, Bono feels, is that the line that used to exist between sensational tabloids and the so-called legitimate press has been almost completely erased. Gays and lesbians, traditionally viewed in sensationalist terms, have consequently suffered as substantive issues aren't being taken seriously.

"We had an incident yesterday where we were quoted in the 'Drudge Report' about this Bruce Willis film *The Jackal*. Somebody no longer associated with GLAAD gave a quote to them under our name criticizing the film. We've been having to run around and tell people about this, and the different people we've been having to talk to run the gamut from the *Enquirer* to *Entertainment Tonight,* all around. All the press is going to cover it."[6]

Producer Alan Poul, who has been on GLAAD's board of directors for many years, agrees with Bono that the situation in Hollywood has changed in ways that organizations like GLAAD can profit from.

"I think there's a huge opportunity now for GLAAD as an organization. For years it's been relegated to the outside, and being the barking watchdog on the fringes of the entertainment industry. Complain, complain, complain. It's all changed, because the industry's not afraid of gays and lesbians anymore. It's very willing to have some kind of collaborative, cooperative relationship, and is just as eager to be praised for doing good. The GLAAD Media Awards have become a big deal. It's a very star-studded lineup. The awards are highly prized. It's a commendation people want to receive. We're getting much better results with the carrot than the stick now. Sometimes the carrot is necessary. But there's an opportunity now for GLAAD to have a collaborative relationship with the entertainment industry.

"Now that there are openly gay and lesbian executives at every level at every company, GLAAD should be running a very active database on all projects with gay and lesbian images, just keep track of them, and register a note of concern if something seems wrong, out of kilter or potentially offensive. It's not about being the Politically Correct Police. It's about making sure things are fair and accurate. It's not about never having a gay character be the butt of a joke. Of course they can. But when you and I know the underlying context is 'stupid sissy' it's different. The whole thing about offensive stuff is, you know it when you see it. And with gay images sometimes you don't know.

"One of the interesting things with GLAAD and the community that was really divisive a couple of years ago was 'Men on Film' on the *In Living Color* show," Poul recalls. "Some people thought it was really funny, some were really offended. And when you put it in context of some of the others things Damon Wayans has done it's even more complicated.

"Still, at this point," Poul observes, "the straight audience is ahead of the studios on this. They know what's going on and they get it. Gay material doesn't have to be soft-pedaled or fagged up in order to get across to that audience."[7]

Getting the "establishment" to respond to the requests of a minority is one thing. When you're part of that minority and working in the "establishment," the situation is rather different. The "independent" and "mainstream" filmmakers assembled at Outfest '97 for a panel discussion reflect the genuine sense of responsibility felt by those in the driver's seat, while underscoring the fact that there are no knee-jerk solutions to dealing with gay and lesbian life in either the mass or fringe media.

"My first response has always been 'First do no harm,' " says Todd Holland, whose television work has led to a theatrical feature, *Krippendorf's Tribe*. "I just got through reading two feature scripts. In both of them the villains were vaguely homosexual. The women were lesbians and they were the villains, and the man was very feminine. And there was another project for DreamWorks where the villains were maybe homosexual as well. Unless you say something about this—'Hey, guys, the villains are all homosexual'—that's the first concern I feel: not to associate yourself with negative portrayals. Once you get into it . . . I spend most of my time in the do-no-harm category, because I do mainstream things. I don't generate the stories myself.

"On *Larry Sanders* we've done numerous gay episodes. On one, Hank's secretary, Darlene, used the idea of being lesbian as an excuse not to go out with Jon Lovitz. But the whole context of the humor was lesbian rumors trickling down about her to the other characters, and them being outraged. I kept bringing up that the whole context of the comedy was being outraged if you were accused of being lesbian. So we started shaving away at it, changing the jokes, and it's only because I personally mentioned it. We've got Scott Thompson on our show, and we have a lot of straight writers struggling to write stuff that isn't about him being gay all the time. But that one [with the Darlene character] was difficult. I had to go to the actors individually and say, 'I'm offended by this.' I had to convince them that it should be changed. That was the first time I'd ever taken it that far. Normally you just bring something up and the machine changes the rest of it on its own. But that one was difficult."

"Well, I just finished doing a thriller, a courtroom drama with Melanie Griffith and Tom Berenger," says director Randal Kleiser. "There was a surprise ending to the script in which the killer was a woman who was supposedly straight but turns out to have had an affair with the victim, thinking that would explain the crime. I encouraged them to shift it to another person who was an unlikely candidate."

"One of the questions we have to deal with as a community is, Are we going to allow ourselves to create characters who have flaws or modulate our characters so they'll be palatable to a straight audience—or even our own audiences?" notes writer-director Nicole Conn. "It's very difficult to represent gays and lesbians, because we're all so different. And what may be a positive representation to, say, one group of women in Kansas City is not the same to a group of militant dykes in San Francisco."

"I'd add to that, that because I make horror movies I *have* to offend people," Clive Barker declares. "That's my responsibility—to kill as many people as possible. There was a gentleman interviewing me before for the radio who was going after the idea that because I make horror movies 'you're setting up metaphors for betrayal anyway.' I think with certain story elements there's a sense of 'I mustn't do that—that's my politics.' That's a bad way to act as an artist. There's some politics involved that you have to be aware of, but your first responsibility has got to be to you. You have to think about why you wanted to do it in the first place. I always think when I'm starting a project that it's going to be a year of my life, okay? And it had better be as truthful as I know I can make it. And some of that truth may not be particularly palatable to anybody. My *responsibility* is not to give a fuck about that. My *responsibility* is not to care. I've done stuff that an activist would be very happy with, and some stuff of which I'd say, 'That's a really rotten thing to have done.'

"One thing on this," Barker continues, "is I got a whole lot of shit from the S&M community when I did *Hellraiser*. Apparently it was a terrible thing to do to the S&M community. My first thought was that it wasn't meant that way—I wasn't making an anti-S&M movie. Then I got a great review in *Skin2* magazine—which I only get for the crosswords. They said, 'This is an okay movie, but it will give you great ideas for your dungeon.' This gets to the heart of this whole conversation. Because on the one hand this is a horror movie in which all these individuals are demonized, and on the other they have sex. So let's be aware as artists that there are ambiguities inherent in everything you do and that I don't think you can apologize for. In fact the only thing we should apologize for is not being honest with ourselves."

"But it's another thing when you're a buffering line—interpreting other people's words," says director Paris Barclay, whose credits range from episodes of the deadly serious *ER* to the sophisticated comedy of *The Larry Sanders Show* to the Wayans brothers' knockabout spoof *Don't Be a Menace to South Central While Drinkin' Your Juice in the 'Hood*. "Even with the best of intentions when our writers try to write for Scott Thompson they can just fail utterly. Then Scott's offended, and our producer is gay, and I'm gay, and we all disagree. We can't even find consensus amongst ourselves about where the lines should be. Movies are a different world from television, which is truly a mass medium. Because it's free, television has a totally different responsibility. And we're not in control, as directors of television, as we are of film. The television world is really run by the writer-producers.

"On *ER* we had a script where we have a lesbian character having a sort of flirtatious conversation with Noah Wyle. He's asking her whether she would become 'un-lesbian' for a night. So I'm reading this and I say, 'Oh my God, I've got to run up to see [producer] John Wells really fast.' So I go to his office, and there are already two producers standing in line—who aren't even gay—who are talking about that scene, and how offensive they found it, and how confusing it is to dealing with what lesbianism is all about. So even before I got to the door there were already people complaining about it. And that's the kind of sensitivity shown towards a show they know one in six Americans will watch that really matters. They *do* take a higher standard of scrutiny. Such storylines go through a lot of conversation before it gets on the air. Finally the scene came out great. He turns to her and says, 'Do you think you might perhaps consider—' and she says, 'Not a chance.' And we loved that. That's what she would say. That's who she is. Even though it's Noah Wyle—cute though he may be—it's not gonna work. Everyone was very happy with it in the end."

"In the realm I work in, which is lower-budgeted films for cable," says Sam Irvin, "it's not the same as working for the networks, but it also has its own set of problems. There are a million development executives who at every point along the line are asking the question 'Why is this character gay? Can we change him to a straight character?' My job in taking on a script is to try to preserve the integrity of the original material. If for some reason it becomes offensive to me, the way they want things portrayed, or cast, I may opt to let them change it to a straight character. I don't want it to be something I'm uncomfortable with. I think it's very hard, because it's a business, with so many financial partners, and foreign sales, and whatever, it becomes very hard to do any personal gay portrayal."

"Oh yes," says Paul Bartel. "There's been a tremendous change. My first feature film was in 1972. It was a low-budget horror film called *Private Parts*. Not my choice of title, by the way. Jim Aubrey—'the Smiling Cobra'—who was at that time head of MGM, changed the title from *Blood Relations*, which was more *apropos*. The story was shot at the King Edward Hotel downtown. It would never have occurred to me at that time to introduce any gay material into the script. But there was a secondary character—one of the odd characters who lived at the hotel—a retired reverend, who I decided to make gay just by slightly coloring him. A few little glances, a few little 'um-hmms' when an attractive male character with better billing than his would come onto the scene. The film was a financial and commercial disaster because neither the producer, who was Roger Corman's brother Gene, nor I realized that horror films had to be directed towards a family audience. They had to be watchable by children, because children constitute most of the audience for horror films. And if you make a horror film that has scenes that are so kinky, even though not gay, that children may not be permitted to see them, then you're in big trouble. MGM took its name off the film. I got a very interesting insight as to how producers think, because about a year after the film had crashed and burned Gene Corman said to me, 'You know that gay character? If we hadn't put that gay character in the picture, it would have made a lot of money.' Now the gay character had *nothing* to do with the failure of the film, but I thought it was interesting that he felt that was the problem. Now I didn't write the script of *Private Parts,* but since then I have tried to introduce more and more . . . not perhaps a totally gay sensibility, but gay subject matter, gay characters who were more audience-friendly. They could be accepted by a straight audience, and their sexual interests and proclivities could be seen as attractive. I don't know to what extent I've succeeded."

"About scripts that are 'straight-friendly,' " notes Clive Barker, "I don't know how that works, because it seems to me that I think straight audiences might have the same problems as gay audiences. In New York you might find a very sophisticated response to a gay character or a gay subtext, whereas if you showed an audience in, say, Tucson, Arizona, a picture like *Dead Ringers*—where I sat with an audience of *seven*—they were appalled. And this was at the same time audiences on the East or West Coast might be having fun with that picture. So it comes back to the problem of 'Well, who are you making it for?' If you project the idea of this audience onto the process, one of the things you lose is the need to disturb or shock yourself. I think we should be careful *not* to be so careful. There's a need sometimes to do things that make even you feel uncomfortable. It's an interesting area—who I want to make this movie for. I want to do something that will affect *me*. So I certainly can't make it 'straight-safe,' 'cause I don't even want to make it 'gay-safe.' You see what I mean?

"My movies are filled with with images of violence that no one objects to," Barker continues. "But the kissing stuff—oh my God! Terrifying! I'm producing right now a picture about James Whale, the gay director who made *Frankenstein*—which is a masterpiece. We had on the call sheet yesterday, 'Background extras.' Two of them walked out because it was a gay movie. I guess they weren't being asked to do anything indecent, were they?"

"It was a pool party scene where there were to be a few extras who were nude," says Sam Irvin, who's serving as associate producer on the film. "There were several who stayed who objected—which was really the fault of the extras casting director, who should have let them know more what the content of the scene was. But even *that* brings up a point. A lot of leading actors—even if they're not afraid of playing a gay character—have problems. Having already 'done one,' is Tom Hanks going to play a gay leading character in the next two, three, four, or five movies? Do we have any openly gay actors like Sir Ian McKellen or Rupert Everett who are going to be happy always playing gay characters? No, because they're also going to want to play a variety of roles and not be pigeonholed. And so we do run into that problem, which is a double-edged sword."

"Having a gay character is always seen as a problem," says Todd Holland. "When *Alien* came out it was a shock when Tom Skerritt died in that movie. We never once thought Sigourney Weaver would rise up and become the heroine. It was terrifying because when he died, *anybody* could die. It broke all the rules. You latch on to him as a hero character and bond with him, and he gets killed. So you were willing to follow a woman to the end of that movie when she picks up a flamethrower. The question is, why can't a gay character rise up in a mainstream movie and pick up that flamethrower? Why can't we have the same act, so the audience is given no choice? You either don't get out of that movie alive or you follow that gay character all the way through."

But getting the "mainstream" in gear to deal with gay or lesbian characters in such an in-depth manner is hard when they're content to play with surface and atmosphere alone.

"*Batman and Robin* is so *blatant*," says Barker of the homo-eroticism of the Warner Bros. megaflop, "but it's also curiously un-fulfilling. Is it about anything other than a few plastic-abs shots? It's almost nudity without nudity. And Batgirl does not have nipples, ei-ther. It's not even equal-opportunity fake nudity!"

"Curiously," note Sam Irvin, "you have in *Batman and Robin* a filmmaker, Joel Schumacher, who's very careful of how he'll present himself to the press. He'll talk ad-infinitum about his past as a drug user, ad-infinitum about everything *except* about being gay. He will not utter those words. His latest quote is, 'Well, how can I talk about being gay when I don't have any sex at all?' I find that personally offensive, but I think it's reflected in the film. There's titillation, but there's a shame about it."

"I agree," says Barker. "With Disney—maybe it was Howard Ashman's influence—there's a lot of campiness, and a Broadway quality to the animated features. I'm going to see *The Hunchback of Notre Dame* with my lover and his daughter and we'll find out how much of it she gets—sitting with two gay men who really wish they were holding hands. But I absolutely take Sam's point. The *Batman and Robin* thing really annoys me because we're being played with in all the wrong ways. It's there but it's *not* there. It's plain, but it's not really *about* anything. It's just surface. And I guess all movies are surface now, especially big movies. I read the *People* interview with Schumacher. It's impossible. This man can get any kind of gig he wants and he won't say a word about his homosexuality."

"Especially now," notes Irvin. "Even Chris O'Donnell was quoted in some interview as saying, 'In this film I'm not going to wear the earring. But they are still making me have the nipples.' It was like—why the shame?"

"So awful for Chris to have nipples," says Barker, brushing away an invisible tear. "It's terrible!"[8]

It is indeed odd to read Schumacher in a *Newsweek* interview speak of being "a 'big star' in the fashion world" who was "sleeping

with half the planet" and abusing drugs, yet pull back from from
saying anything that would put it into some perspective.

"It's hard to talk about your sexuality when you're not having
any sex," Schumacher complains to Mark Miller. "I don't really know
how to have a private life yet, to be really honest. I damaged that part
of my life to such a ridiculous degree that I'm not sure what a private
life means to me anymore. I'm not in love. And sometimes those who
are bad at relationships should do everybody a favor and stop."

"But you're not ashamed of who you are," Miller offers helpfully.

"I'm not ashamed of my life," Schumacher offers, "but I certainly am ashamed of some of my behavior. I mean, how can you be
a drug addict and an alcoholic for most of your life and not be ashamed
of some of your behavior? I'm ashamed for stuff I can't even remember."[9]

A nd for a Hollywood professional of his generation, that's about
as far as Joel Schumacher is willing to go. Today, however, there
are those willing to go much farther—not just in terms of their own
lives, but in order to make contact with other gays and lesbians in
the culture at large. Producer Alan Poul is an example of this, as were
any number of others involved in making the celebrated miniseries
Tales of the City and its sequel. But even the commitment of many
can be hamstrung by the resistance of a single individual.

"*Tales of the City* is very broad in its appeal," says Poul. "Armistead Maupin's book was groundbreaking in its time in the way it
intermingled straight and gay characters who took their sexuality
matter-of-factly. That was the important thing. We were not going to
flinch. We were going to present the sexuality as casually as it had
been presented in the books. By American standards, if you do a TV
movie about homosexuality, then homosexuality is the issue—or it
was that way until fairly recently. A character didn't just show up and
be gay. So this was pretty much the first time characters didn't have
to talk about why they became gay. Nobody had to discuss their being

gay. It was just the way it was. The Brits were insistent we adapt it faithfully and not have to make a message out of it. We did a very faithful adaptation, which is always a concern because of the casual, episodic nature of it. It wasn't structured into a taut two-hour drama. It wouldn't stay afloat that way.

"Everyone knows that Armistead has been openly and vociferously gay for a long time. And his lover at the time, Terry Anderson, was also very politically active. In fact, sometimes when you asked him what he did, he'd say 'gay activist.' So very early on, one of the first meetings where we were discussing cast, they said, 'Now we don't want any of this bullshit about closeted gay actors in this show.' It was a very sore point. I argued that, as much as I'm out and I want everyone to be out, and I think that it's the willingness of people to come out that has made a more tolerant atmosphere for gay people in the workplace in the country as a whole: when people find out, they change, it's that simple—however, I myself make an exception for actors, because I know that the rule is no one should feel obligated to martyr themselves on the horns of society, and an actor who comes out, if he is not already successful, is going to find himself very limited in the roles he's going to be offered to play. Granted, talent is still more important than your sexual orientation. And a brilliant gay actor is going to get better roles than a bad straight actor. But it's still limiting, because there's still an education process that is ongoing. So I said to them that I would not make a rule. It's okay for a straight actor to play a gay role on *Tales of the City*, but it's not okay for an actor who's actually gay to play a gay role in the series and not announce that he's gay. That to me is wrong and hypocritical. So we had this argument, and finally what it came down to was that because this was going to be so high-profile, that at least for the major gay roles it would be very bad to have a closeted actor. It would be okay to have a straight actor, but if you have a gay actor as a gay character he should be out. We thought that would make sense. Well, wouldn't you know it, that was exactly what we got!

"I had heard he was gay," says Poul of the performer, whose name he declines to mention—more out of anger than anything else. "I met him. I talked with him. I didn't even bring up the subject. He was gay, and everybody seemed to know he was gay. It didn't seem to be a problem. In talking with him he was very flirtatious. You see, this is a case of somebody who was having a very active gay sexual life that was known to me and everyone in the community. And so here he was playing this high-profile gay character on *Tales of the City*. Suddenly we discovered—to our horror—that he was maintaining this insistence on his heterosexuality in all public statements. Armistead just saw red. It was not pleasant. Especially because if you're going to keep your private life private, then be discreet. Don't spend three hours in the steamroom at the Athletic Club!

"On the last night of shooting, the next-to-the-last setup, it came to blows," Poul recalls. "There were Armistead and Terry and *this actor* screaming at each other on the street. It was tears and the whole thing, and I had to pick up the pieces. There was literally only one more scene to get before we were done with the whole six hours. It was the first time I found myself in the middle of an issue that came from being gay and being in the entertainment business. In general I side with actors, because an actor has the right to keep his sexuality confidential so that he can do the best work possible. But in the particulars of this situation, I had very, very little sympathy, because this guy had hoisted himself on his own petard.

"There's a new generation," says Poul, turning to happier matters. "I'm certainly not just talking about the entertainment industry. They're totally out and involved in the system. It's not a 'defiant' stand. It's just being who you are and being involved in the causes that are closest to home—like Jewish charities. It's not at all considered confrontational to be out and support gay and lesbian causes. But there's an older generation in the same business who are still not out at work. Some aren't even out socially, and they look kind of pathetic.

"I think what's interesting is the whole issue of gay marriage even coming up and being discussed. What has happened is with people being more out in the workplace it's *not* 'the love that dare not speak its name.' So there's much more of a tendency to mimic heterosexual roles and institutions, so than in, say, Hollywood, the hierarchy, if you're invited to a dinner party, you should have a boyfriend or significant other to show up with or to take as your date for the Emmy Awards or whatever. So there is much more of a social structure that reinforces stability, romance, fidelity, or at least the appearances of such as in the heterosexual world, whereas in the previous generation with the so-called Gay Mafia, if you went to a public function you went with a beard—Diane Von Furstenberg or whoever—it was not about having lasting relationships. It was really about having sexual relationships, whether they were fleeting or more ongoing. Therefore, the heterosexual institution that was being aped wasn't marriage but prostitution. The predominant sexual model was *transactional*. And that means a lot in Hollywood when you're dealing with people who are businessmen or whatever. It's ultimately flesh for money that becomes the prevailing metaphor. There's some sort of barter going on.

"In the seventies, when these people had 'boy parties,' " Poul explains, "there were *the boys,* who were all young and pretty and in one way or another ambitious, and then there were *the men,* the 'daddies,' who weren't really trading on looks, but looks were the predominant dynamic. Now you have a class of middle-aged 'marrieds'—the whole gay-couple kind of hierarchy. I'm not making a value judgment, but it's become much more *seemly*. There are a lot of couples who have been around for a long, long time. So it's interesting that people being out today is kind of a conservative thing.

"Also, it needs to be pointed out," Poul continues, taking a sharper tone, "that I have *never* seen straight people having such 'gay' relationships as in the entertainment industry today. I see straight people who are relentlessly sexually driven and compulsive—driven to a large part by physical desire and physical attractiveness or what-I-can-get-out-of-it. Changing partners and using sexuality to climb the ladder, and all that kind of stuff that people associate with gay men in a negative light. We wouldn't get tarred with that brush if there weren't some truth to it. But it's something I never associated with heterosexual society."[10]

Producer Howard Rosenman, on the other hand, finds a lot to like as he looks across the "New Hollywood" horizon. And in his view, the assimilation of gay and lesbian professionals has played a pivotal role in these changes.

"I see something really incredible coming. Chris Lee, who's the head of Tri-Star, threw a party celebrating his ascendancy. I was just shocked. Gigantically. Normally, in the past, when I would go to a Hollywood party it would all be white Jewish guys. At this party there were African-Americans; many many Asians; many, many lesbians; many, many gay guys—and a smattering of straight white guys. To me, *this* was the future. It was overwhelming—such a gigantic shift. Because in 1974, when I took [producer] Suzanne DePasse, who is very light-skinned, to Mike Medavoy's party, celebrating his becoming the head of United Artists after he was an agent at ICM, she was the *only* person of color in the room! Mike Medavoy's father walked up to her. He was a short Jewish man who fled Europe during the Holocaust, when Mike was born. He said to her, "Tell me, beautiful girl, are you Tahitian?' It was impossible for him to think that a black woman would be at a party like that. And here we are, twenty-three years later, and it's not only a matter of course, *it was the majority!* I see a generalized admixture of formerly ghettoized people gaining power. It will take another ten to fifteen years to express itself on an ownership power level. But it's *there*."[11]

TEN

HAIR COLOR

—

"PULA, WHO IS KNOWN AS AN OUT-spoken, occasionally outrageous, but highly creative executive, will be an interesting match for the more buttoned-down Warner Bros. types," *Daily Variety* noted in 1996 when Chris Pula, the former head of marketing and publicity for New Line Cinema, assumed the same duties for one of the biggest and most established studios in Hollywood. Going on to question how Pula, "who usually rides a bi-cycle to work, showing up in jeans and T-shirts, will mesh with the corporate style of Warner co-chairmen Bob Daly and Terry Semel," the entertainment-industry trade paper went so far as to ask the mar-keting executive whether he'd wear a suit to work.

"Well, I have *one*," Pula told them dryly. "I'll have to check if it's still in style. Is Nehru still around? It's not like I'm going to walk in there in a gingham dress."[1]

"The gingham dress?" Pula laughs, recalling the interview sev-eral months later. "Yeah, and I got sent *seven* of them because of that line! I should have asked for Versace."

What the paper was trying, rather awkwardly, to signal to its readership was the fact that Chris Pula is gay. The gingham dress line was Pula's way of informing *Variety* that they could have asked him the question point-blank to begin with. For he's part of the new gay Hollywood in which being out has replaced coming out.

"Everyone's been tremendously accepting about my gayness," says Pula of his dealings with the button-down corporate "suits." "That's because I've made it like . . . *hair color*. It's a nonissue. But I don't shy away from bringing it up when it's natural. Like, 'Whoa, that Luke Wilson is cute!'—just like they would say, 'Look at the tits on her!' Five years ago they might have been disgusted by me, but now it's, 'Hey, this is cool.' The most difficult part is when I'm in a room or on the executive plane with a group of guys and I have *nothing* to say about sports. But it's gotten to the point where everybody's so cool they'll make fun of me over that. After all, I'm not afforded any level of anonymity, because I *am* a big queen."

Chris Pula is indeed a "big queen"—but not in the gingham-dress–wearing way. He's not over-the-top effeminate *à la* Nathan Lane in *The Birdcage*, nor is he a *soigné* aesthete in the Rupert Everett mold. He's trim and athletic, and his fast-moving and faster-talking manner is that of a cooly self-mocking urban tough guy—part Tony Curtis in *Sweet Smell of Success*, part Robert DeNiro in *Mean Streets*. Not about to fade into the background like a standard-issue "company man," or pop forward only for a campy aside or two like a gay "side-kick" or court jester, Pula is as driven and competitive as anyone who has ever worked in the movie business.

"Even though I recognize I've traveled up the corporate ladder, I started fairly high," notes Pula. "I am in a fairly gay-friendly business, and I started in the creative side of a gay-friendly business. I represent, for better or worse, the new wave of marketers. You can't just be some flack/friend of the studio chief any longer. You need to have some marketing background and packaged goods experience. I have an MBA as well as packaged goods experience.

"I started out in this business at Grey Advertising in New York, which had a small entertainment division. I came out here in '88 to Fox Film Corporation, then I went to Fox Broadcasting. I was creative and account supervisor for ABC movies, miniseries, and prime-time series. It was back when Barry Diller and Brandon Stoddard headed up the entertainment division—back when TV movies were good. Like *Something About Amelia* and *The Day After*. Actually, TV movies are still good—they're just being done at TNT, Showtime, and HBO."

It was when Pula became part of the marketing team that made *Home Alone* a megahit that his career really caught fire.

"With *Home Alone*, if we hadn't done a lot of homework we wouldn't have realized the film had a big credibility problem in terms of selling it. One: how could a woman forget her own child? Two: once forgotten, how good a mother could she possibly be? Three: is the child okay? So there are three 'pods' of Catherine O'Hara throughout the trailer, desperately trying to get back to the kid. You had to make certain the mothers who brought their kids to the movie knew this wasn't about an abused child or a horrible mother."

Pula next moved to New Line Cinema, where he handled product as varied as the Jim Carrey smashes *Dumb and Dumber* and *The Mask*, the surprise-hit horror-mystery thriller *Seven*, and the black female urban action film *Set It Off*. The success of such films, in tandem with their long-established *Nightmare on Elm Street* series, quickly moved the company from "independent" to "mini-major" status. It was Pula's ability to "counterprogram" against the majors—

finding audiences "where no one had bothered to look before," for offbeat, non-star-driven fare—that won him the attention of Warner Bros.

"When you've been in the trenches for five years and you don't have big budgets, you don't have big stars, and you don't have big directors, you've got to ferret out consumers in places you're not used to looking," notes Pula. "I'll give you an example: young black men read voraciously. They have something like fourteen different hip-hop publications: *The Source, Rapstyle, Hype Hair, YSB, Upscale.* You can really reach an audience that way. And I'm talking *young.* You can reach young white women through *Seventeen, Sassy,* and *Tiger Beat.* Young black women watch *Oprah.* Young white boys? *They don't read!* Sure, they subscribe to *Sports Illustrated,* but that's a magazine for everyone. The black teenager is the most primed moviegoer out there. They want to be on top of everything. They want to be there— first in line, the very first day for the new hot film. They'll even buy bad pirate copies of films made with cheap video cameras—shot from theater seats, so you'll actually see someone's head in front of the image. You know what that is? That's a marketing tool! If your movie's *not* being sold on the street, you've got to wonder why. Because these same kids who'll buy the pirate video will *still* pay to watch it on the big screen! *And* buy the real video later on.

"My job is extraordinarily stressful," Pula continues, "and I know it's not just *my* job. I'm at the end of the food chain in a motion picture's life. The theatrical release is the caboose of the whole train. The movie is a baby by the time it gets to me. I represent the last chance, and the cold slap of reality: 'Is there a consumer out there in America that wants to see this damn thing?' So you can see by my knuckles that it's a tremendously stressful position. There's hyper-competition and *tonnage* out there. That makes it even *more* stressful. So having alleviated that burden of trying to hide who I am, it's just one of those additional factors that *I don't have.* Anyone who is pretending, or in the closet, or isn't able to bring up their significant other in casual conversation, or always has to find some 'beard' to take on a date—that's just got to be a *ton* of stress, and you really shouldn't afford yourself that sort of stress.

"Just the other day in the middle of a conversation, reading the menu," says Pula of a stress-relieving incident, "I saw there was a pepper ratatouille pasta, and I said, 'What a fabulous drag name— Pepper Ratatouille!' There was a soup spiced with ginger and cilantro and I thought, Ginger Cilantro! Fabulous! 'Ladies and gentlemen! Singing the songs of Diana Ross, Miss Ginger Cilantro! And the Lady Pepper Ratatouille!'

"I don't *force* my sexuality to be the topic of conversation, but whenever people talk about their spouses I always bring up Tom. I think that's everyone's individual battle. That's our job: to make people realize who we are on a day-to-day basis. I know it sounds like I'm candy-coating it, but being gay never *has* been an issue. I don't think there's been a glass ceiling of any sort. I came in at a fairly high level. But I traveled from VP of creative to marketing president in two different places. I don't think that's solely due to being openly gay, but yes, it does have to do with the fact that it helps when you don't give a shit whether they know you're gay or not. You can be *fabulous,* and 'He's so *adorable!*' "

And being "adorable" means Pula doesn't have the familial duties to contend with that often create conflicts for workers in high-pressure, white-collar professions.

"Yeah, I don't have those pesky kids," he says, chuckling before launching into a Lenny Bruce–style riff about the then-in-the-news Louise Woodward trial. "I think that's what they're going to do on Fox next. Instead of *America's Deadliest Swarms,* it'll be *America's Deadliest Nannies.* And after that, it's *Nanny-Cams: Caught on Tape, Part 3; When Au Pairs Attack, Part 4.*"

Still, pressure and the need for corporate teamsmanship haven't stopped Pula from speaking up on gay issues when he sees the need.

"On the first cut of *Dumb and Dumber* there were quite a few homophobic references—gay-bashing type of humor," Pula recalls. "Now I *know* the director, Peter Farrelly. He's a very nice guy. He's not a homophobe. But he's also got a lot of that frat-boy, *Porky's* type humor in him. And I hate it when gay people can't laugh at themselves. I'm so tired of hearing people bitching about *In and Out* and *The Birdcage.* But the reason I got mad about *Dumb and Dumber* was because I knew as the marketer the target audience was twelve- to seventeen-year-old boys and younger. They're not old enough to process that information properly. The film made it look all right to gay-bash. And you know to [New Line Cinema president] Bob Shaye's and Peter Farrelly's credit, they *did* extricate all but one reference. They didn't have to listen to me. It wasn't a marketing issue. I put it in a note. I let 'em read it first. I didn't wrap it in 'trying to preserve some dignity.' I do believe that when there's very few representations of a niche, you should protect those representations. Protest groups have the right to be upset about the overly feminine portrayal of a gay man—even though *I* lost all traces of masculinity years ago. However, I understand the dynamic. Now there's so much on the market. Look at the gay movies and teen black movies. There's so much *tonnage* in each niche that pieces of shit are now not getting business. The dilemma with 'gay' is it's a niche that's differentiated on sex and sex alone. It's easy for everybody to bring it down to that. Yes, we have a lot more going on in our lives than sex, but realistically it's very difficult for nongay people to understand that it's not about our penises—that it's about our being who we are. And there's still, subliminally, this feeling that we could decide to change. Consequently, they think it's all about having sex and nothing else.

"The thing that disappoints me about some stars," Pula continues, "is that they could probably afford to come out the most on many levels. Obviously they have a lot of money, and a lot of self-gratification that they've completed the task of proving themselves. And they've built a brand with the consumer that will probably suffer a little shake-up, but they won't have to start from ground zero. When you're a big star you bring so much baggage to a role anyway. It's 'Tom Cruise in *Mission: Impossible*.' Nobody remembers his character's name, because his persona overwhelms it. A big star can come out on a professional level and be confident that since there's already so much celebrity baggage they're bringing to the role this piece of information is only going to have an *incremental* effect. Whereas if you're a new star with no brand awareness, gayness *could* overwhelm everything else—though I think Anne Heche is going to be okay."

As for gay-and-lesbian-themed movies, Pula is less optimistic.

"Hollywood is so stupid glomming onto things. We're going to have a shitload of slasher movies now because of *Scream*. I hope they're not going to make any gay project they can because of *In and Out*, because that could just as easily kill everything if they don't succeed; [then] it's 'Gay movies do badly!'

"Gay people make me so mad sometimes. I got into a horrible argument the other day with this angry queen—and it was obviously based on the fact that he'd had a horrible coming out with his parents. It centered around the Catholic bishops' letter where they're telling parents not to reject their gay and lesbian kids. He said, 'It's masking the same love-the-sinner-not-the-sin crap!' I said, 'You douche bag! The very fact that they would write this thing using that language— even though it's not basically changing that much—is so *profoundly* big! And you idiots who stand up and scream—you set everybody back.'

"Something's gotta happen," says Pula, nervously returning the conversation to marketing. "Somebody's gonna go under. They can't continue to make movies like this. Movies were already the most shortened shelf life—next to an elected official. The average consumer thinks the 'window' to home video is 2.7 months. The reality is still around six months. So you've got seventy-seven television channels, and five new movie choices a weekend. The average consumer sees only *six* movies a year! And on top of that, we've now got two generations spending an hour a day on the Internet. There's no dearth of entertainment!

"I don't know where I got it, cause my family's so fuckin' sweet, but I'm the most cynical queen there is. And being a cynical queen, I think, has made me a good marketer. I think the consumer looks at every single movie and says, 'Why *should* I see that?' Because they haven't caught up with the five movies of *last* week, or even the five movies from the *previous* weekend. Today one movie doesn't just compete with four others—it competes with a really good episode of *ER* or even an *L.A. Law* rerun on Lifetime!

"You know, it's very *anti-Catholic* for me to talk to you about this," Pula says, his tone darkening as he contemplates Warner Bros. slate of product for 1997: *Father's Day, Batman and Robin, Midnight in the Garden of Good and Evil, Mad City, Conspiracy Theory, The Devil's Advocate,* and *L.A. Confidential*—all of which, by year's end, will be rated financial "disappointments." "We Catholics are not raised to be anything but a martyr. Any sort of pleasure, something's gotta give! I've got a good job: somebody's gonna die. I've had tremendous—I hate to say 'luck,' 'cause I'm well aware of the fact that I'm good at what I do. Do I look horrible now? 'Cause its been a tough year—but for a different reason than the tough years I've had in the past. I realize that my life would be much easier if all of Warner Bros.' movies were hits. It's just that I'm the 'new guy' in this very staid, lifetime employment business.

"The thing is, they've been living not in the seventies but the late eighties, when they released two hundred films a year. It was, 'Just throw a big star into anything and people will come.' The fact is, it's not about big stars anymore. Everybody has big stars. It's about concept. It's about story. Stars can be 'value added.'

"And oh, by the way, there's a whole level of stars they've got to get to know. Billy Crystal and Robin Williams are fabulous, but they're forty-nine years old! And more often than not the demographic on the screen represents the demographic that attends the movies. They wouldn't know any of those *Party of Five* people if they came in and shit on the table! The real story right now isn't Billy Crystal or Robin Williams, it's Jennifer Love Hewitt and Sarah Michelle Gellar. It's embarrassing, 'cause she's in our own *Buffy the Vampire Slayer* series. Or take Jewel—our own singer. *Get to know some younger stars!* They want to do *Lethal Weapon 4.* I said, 'Give me Chris Rock or Bugs Bunny and we'll make it like *Space Jam,* 'cause who the fuck wants to see *Lethal Weapon 4?*' 'We're going to make a new *Superman?* What about Parker Posey as Lois Lane?' *They didn't know who she was!*"

"I've not been here like all those people who've been on board a thousand years and can't talk up because it's like talking up to their dad. Well, I'm very respectful, but it's like, 'Guys, what are you doin' here?' We've got *Mad City, Conspiracy Theory, Devil's Advocate, Father's Day.* They all represent very well-dressed *B movies*! If you look a little too long, it's 'Have I seen this before?' That was the biggest problem with *Mad City*. Guys, get real: it's *Dog Day Afternoon* meets *Ace in the Hole*. Plus we've got the goddamned *Nanny* on TV every night. Welcome to the magical island of Who Gives a Shit! And I *had* to be there that year. So it would be *really* horrible during all of this to have on top of it trying to pretend being a straight boy.

"The yardstick for success is rendered very nebulous now," Pula continues. "We're shitting all over ourselves over twenty-million-dollar openings. We've got movies that normally would have made a hundred million making forty 'cause there are too many movies out there. We're embracing thirty-percent drops as 'legs'! *I Know What You Did Last Summer* is number one for three weeks. Wow. But *Home Alone* was number one for thirteen weeks!

"Your friends call you with the rumors, but your enemies do too. And the one time there was a rumor of me not making it at Warner Bros. was not because of the movies—everybody knows the movies are bad—it's because I was so *bitchy*! It's because of telling them 'Reality check! Reality check!'"[2]

But this "rumor" of Pula's not making it was eventually followed by his dismissal from his Warner Bros. post. Some claim the cumulative effect of the studio's unsuccessful year meant that it was inevitable that Pula would have to take the fall. Others declare it had to do with Pula's occasionally acerbic personal style—in an industry world famous for its coddling of star performers, filmmakers, and studio personnel. Still others cite the failure of *L.A. Confidential* to find a market even in the wake of its clean sweep of critics' association awards for 1997. In fact, an *Entertainment Weekly* article noted this curious state of affairs, citing a "rival studio executive's" claim that Warner Bros. didn't understand the film's "potential," taking exception to its "murky promotional campaign, obscure poster art, and particularly, its release in the no-man's-land of September. Agrees another rival exec: 'I don't think they knew what they had.'

"Warner's response is, uh, blunt. 'They can kiss my ass,' says Chris Pula, the studio's president of theatrical marketing. 'It's easy to piss on someone else's campaign. We've got a brilliant movie—but anyone who thinks it's an easy sell is an idiot.'"[3]

And so the handwriting was on the wall. But gayness had noth-

ing to do with it. Still, Warner Bros. took his advice and hired Chris
Rock for *Lethal Weapon 4*. As for Parker Posey, the new *Superman*
was put into "turnaround."

"Marketing and publicity are now perceived to be vastly more
critical to the success or failure of a motion picture than it was ten
years ago," says entertainment journalist Charles Fleming of Pula's
problems. "These fields have traditionally been viewed as not very
masculine ends of the profession, and therefore these are areas where
women and gays have been welcomed. And one of the side effects of
this of course is that women, seeing an opportunity to take power in
an area where men weren't interested, now dominate publicity. And
many of these women are gay as well.

"I hear all the time about marriages of convenience. More at
Morris and ICM that at CAA—although I've heard it about CAA as
well. Gay is fine. Gay and not single is better. Straight is even better.
Straight and married is even better. And straight and married with
kids is best of all. I don't know how many agents have acted upon
this. Then there's gay man/straight woman and straight man/gay
woman who put aside their differences to have children. I'm sure at
the behind-the-camera-talent level, and certainly at the lower-studio-
executive level, things have changed, but not at the top so much."[4]

Still, in November of 1998, Chris Pula was appointed President
of Marketing for Walt Disney Pictures, world-wide.

I had a meeting with Scott Rudin and he asked me what I was doing,"
says writer-director Andrew Fleming, "and I said to him, 'Well,
I'm living with this guy and his son.' And he said, 'All in the same
house?' And I said, 'Yes, all in the same house.' And he said, 'I want
that movie!' "

That movie would unfold in a relatively modest house in the San
Fernando Valley that the writer-director of the offbeat romantic comedy
Threesome (1994) and the equally offbeat fantasy-thriller *The Craft*
(1996) shares with his lover, Scott Nicolaides, and Nicolaides's son. It
sounds like a far more unusual situation than it actually is. For Fleming, in both his life and his work, isn't an edgy gay radical; he's a

patient, softspoken man in his early thirties. His career began in 1988 with a relatively straightforward thriller, *Bad Dreams,* produced by the very major-league Gale Anne Hurd. The films that followed likewise have little in common with the likes of a Todd Haynes or John Greyson—or even a Gus Van Sant. For Andrew Fleming is already "inside" Hollywood—not an independent struggling to break through. And Nicolaides, a Walt Disney executive whose duties involve the company's dealings with its Miramax subsidiary, is even more "inside" than Fleming. In many ways the Fleming/Nicolaides alliance recalls that of James Whale and David Lewis—a bright, up-and-coming director and an executive with some degree of "clout." The differences, however, mark the changes that have come over gay Hollywood in some seventy years. For while Fleming and Nicolaides live a quiet life, it's not in utter isolation from the rest of Hollywood, gay or straight.

"I had never been *openly* gay, because nobody had ever bothered to ask," says Fleming with great amusement. "My friends all knew I was gay. I had met Scott when I was writing *Threesome.* Suddenly I knew it would be an issue—and it didn't worry me at all. It was sort of inexorable. I had no control over it. I was making this movie about a gay character; everyone's going to ask and I'm going to tell them the truth. I remember one day someone from *The New York Times* calling and saying, 'Are you gay?' and I said, 'Yes.' And they said, 'Okay, thanks.' That was it! I don't even know what the article was for. I was really happy to do it. I would never consider for a second saying, 'No, I'm not gay, I just have this insight into this gay character,' or something. It was this interesting roller-coaster ride."

And a roller-coaster ride it was. For while *Threesome* won mixed notices and moderate box-office returns, its tale of a trio of college roommates—two straight (Lara Flynn Boyle and Stephen Baldwin) and one a just-coming-out gay (Josh Charles)—touched a nerve in a way that made it one of the most-talked-about "small" films in years.

"I was just remembering my aunt had this crazy girlfriend in Malibu," Fleming recalls of his adolescence. "She had a lot of interesting friends, including Christopher Isherwood and Don Bachardy. Just the fact that they existed and were a couple—I didn't realize until much later that I'd always held them in my mind as an example of two guys who lived together, and were public, and were individuals, and weren't weird leather queens or something. It meant a lot to me seeing them. I was literally just introduced. I was very, very young, but I knew who they were. I remember too that my mother had this friend who we all knew was gay. I was brought up in optimal circumstances 'cause they would say things like, 'So-and-so is gay, but that's all right 'cause that's who they are.' I suppose I went through a crisis about being gay when I was twelve or thirteen, but that's when everything horrifies you—*life* horrifies you. I suppose high school was the most hostile environment, 'cause it was all boys. There was this one kid who was very effeminate. Who knows whether he was gay or not— he was very effeminate. And he was *crucified*. At NYU, where I went to college, on the other hand, if you were *normal* they would crucify you.

"I remember these freshmen would come in—very ordinary— and a few months later they'd be smoking and their hair would be all matted. It's the first time you're away from home and you're trying out new things. It didn't happen to me when I was a freshman, but it *happened,* a bit later. I think that's part of the reason I wanted to go to New York, because I knew there was this thing called the West Village. If I stayed here in Los Angeles I was just going to be locked into what my old anxieties were.

"Oh yes, and at NYU," Fleming continues, "there was a teacher there in the school of animation who was gay. And he was just a wonderful guy. He would bring you over to his house and have tea, and there was food. The whole class was over to show their films and he would make dinner. It was wonderful. 'Role model's' a bad word. He was a mentor. It was very sad—he died of AIDS a couple of years after I graduated.

"I remember some reporter trying to get the hot scoop on gay sexual harassment in Hollywood," Fleming relates. "I said, 'As far as I know there is none.' In fact, I found it to be the opposite. There isn't a club or anything, but there is a sense of support from gay producers and directors and whatever. You feel one bit more safe. Maybe it's an illusion. But there is a kind of a bond. The bottom line is, people are with you if they think they can make some money off of you, and if they can't, they're not going to cut you any slack. But there's a sense of familiarity among gay people in Hollywood that makes the whole thing less daunting. If you know there's a gay executive there or a gay producer, it just makes it seem like it isn't all hostile territory, [which] you wouldn't get in, say, the automotive business or somewhere where people might be likely to treat you like a freak. I've never felt like I didn't get a job because I was gay. But I don't get sent a lot of action scripts to begin with.

"I obviously live this very suburban, seemingly normal existence," Fleming continues. "Scott's an executive at Disney, but in his previous life he was a horse trainer. We have horses. I have a baby horsey! We had a foal last year. We go to horse shows, which is a great thing because it's a totally other business. William Shatner does the same thing we do with raising horses, and we see him there at the shows—but it's not show business. It's incredibly therapeutic. It's interesting 'cause Scott's relatively open, I suppose. I don't know how he was before we met, but we knew a lot of the same people, and before we knew it we were just this cuddling gay couple going to dinner parties and screenings. I don't know that many other examples of that. We don't go out that much, but when we do we don't make any bones about it.

"It's sad," says Fleming of less forthright Hollywoodites. "There are people who aren't willing to tell me that they're gay, but they are. With us it's just . . . it hasn't been weird. There's no ugliness. We live together and bought a house together and sleep together and have horses together. But we're at a certain comfort zone where people have to be nice to us.

"It's interesting, though. On *Threesome* I felt that when I had to communicate something about being gay, I was able to blurt it out without worrying about how 'gay' I came off. I could just say whatever the fuck I felt, and I *immediately* became a better director, because there was nothing frightening me anymore. I suppose as a teenager there's always that thing of 'I don't want to come off the wrong way. I'm worried about how people think of me.' And in the years preceding *Threesome* I sometimes just didn't give a fuck. I remember when I told Lara about when I told someone I was gay for the first time, what

it was like. It really helped her do her role. If you can be really open
and honest, it's tonic. Then they feel like you're trusting them. It's a
really weird thing, getting the right moves so people can act. It's the
most fun part, 'cause it's a game you're playing with them. How do
you get it right and communicate it to them? You never know. Everybody's different every day. And if you're not honest, you're just not
going to get anything except anxiety."

Oddly enough, *Threesome* provoked no small degree of anxiety
itself, for both critics and audiences. While on the surface a lightweight comic romance in which a brash-but-sexy goofball (Stephen
Baldwin), a smart, forthright coed (Lara Flynn Boyle), and a shy,
guarded "nice guy" (Josh Charles)—just on the edge of "coming out"
as gay—find themselves assigned to a coed college dorm, *Threesome*
explored sexual territory even independent films hadn't chartered.
The most controversial area dealt with the question of exactly how
close straight and gay might be, as the trio's members found themselves relating to one another in a manner well outside the scope of
traditional sexual-orientation boundaries.

"In *Threesome* Josh plays an incredibly normal guy, much more
reasonable than the guy Stephen plays. We're introduced to him, get
to know him a bit—and then we find out that he's gay. In one sense
it's kind of an intentional manipulation. I remember sitting through
a screening in Tucson, Arizona, at this incredibly white college auditorium where suddenly everybody in the room just bristled. Here
in town or in New York you would never get a reaction like that. In
fact, you might get the opposite: 'This isn't offensive enough.' But it's
really interesting if you veer off the interstate. To me *Threesome* is
the most tame movie—completely nonconfrontational. Lara said to
me one day, 'This movie is just about being *in the moment*.' That's a
real 'actor' sort of thing to say, but it's true. It was designed like one
of those two-character plays where it's just two people on a stage
talking, and that in and of itself is supposed to be interesting enough.
I knew that going in, and knew it should be staged that way. The
locales are sort of generic. There are no culturally specific details in
the movie at all about where these characters are from or what they

do. That's just background. It's all very ordinary, so you see that they're just normal people in this incredibly kinky situation. But it's interesting how different things can play depending on the audience. A lot of people got up and left—didn't even want to bear witness to this. But then you found out that the audience that stayed was with it even more, 'cause they found out you could laugh at it. It was just a human situation. That was the real revelation—that you could deal with the gay character like any other.

"I had written, at first, a script about college that did not have a gay character," Fleming recalls of the project's development. "But looking back on it, there was this blatantly homosexual character in it who never came clean. People sort of liked it. It was an outgrowth of the film I'd done at school about waiting for a home pregnancy test. Then in acting class I was watching this exercise about a girl who was attracted to a guy, and he's gay. It took that for me to realize that that had happened to me a bunch of times. I had been in these situations where I'd thought I'd been pals with these girls, and they were very sexually motivated and I wasn't, and it was very funny and sad and interesting. And that night I just happened to watch *Jules and Jim,* and I remembered that I'd had these two friends in school. This was sort of independent of the relationship with the other girl. We were just friends, but everybody thought we were having some weird kinky thing going on. And then I thought of this other relationship with two people that was much more complicated. It suddenly cohered into these three people, and I knew exactly who these three people were. They were amalgams of various characters, but they were so clear.

"Anyway, it just sort of happened that Josh and Stephen and Lara all knew each other and liked each other and wanted to do it, so it was a package. Josh and Lara had worked together on *Dead Poets Society*. Stephen and Josh were very good friends. I was delirious. We had one rehearsal and I said, 'These are the best people imaginable.' I was like their baby-sitter. They were having fun and giggling and laughing—much to the crew's consternation. But I was hesitant to tell them to shut up, 'cause the hardest thing is to get people to look like they're having fun. So we put it all together and I think people were surprised by what it was. They were expecting a more teenage-type movie. There are like three dissolves in the movie. It's all cuts and very few effects. So the first cut was very presentable. It looked like a finished movie. We had this screening at the Directors Guild for all these acquisitions people, and in this big room it played really, really well. Several people were interested in buying it just on the basis of that, but eventually Tri-Star came through.

"I was really worried because I was afraid it might be castrated by the studio, 'cause there's a lot of language and a few confrontational gay-type things—but not many. I thought they were going to tell me to tone it down, but they did not. Like there's a scene with Stuart, the Stephen Baldwin character, where he brings a girl home and they're mean to her. They were worried that because the characters were being mean the audience may not like them. We ended up not changing that, but just as an example, that's what they were worried about more than the gay thing. They were just not willing to say, 'Maybe it's too gay.'

"People should want to see a movie 'cause it's good. But that's a hard argument to use at a meeting. *Threesome* was 'generating heat,' as they say. I'd met a lot of people, but now it was, 'Oh, Andy's coming and I love him!' I knew all these people when they were assistants, and now they're vice-presidents. That's just the way it is. The movie actually got a rather rocky critical reception—which really shocked me. It wasn't like they were injuring me, it was just, 'You don't get it.' Then there was this horrible 'Generation X' thing, that some people claimed it was about, which became the bane of my existence. It meant *nothing*. I've never had a discussion with anyone about 'Generation X'—except journalists. It was also set up as a 'gay movie,' which creates other expectations of explaining things to people about gayness that they've never heard before."

With *The Craft*, the situation involved something that everyone thought at first they *had* heard before, for it centered on a trio of high-school girls (Neve Campbell, Robin Tunney, and Fairuza Balk) experimenting with witchcraft. But rather than *The Exorcist*, the model for this clever dark comedy is the Tuesday Weld/Anthony Perkins classic *Pretty Poison*. For it was less about the supernatural than about such thoroughly natural phenomena as fear, envy, and competition among teenagers.

"The funny thing is, when the script of *The Craft* was going around, people kept telling me, 'Oh, Andy, it's so *you*.' And I really felt when I went in to talk to the writer I could say, 'You can trust me.' I didn't know too much about witchcraft. I'd known some witches. But it wasn't really about that at that point. And you know, it's kind of a gay movie!

"Don't you know these are all men in drag?" says Fleming, tongue firmly pressed in cheek. "I think the studio didn't know what to expect. It cost about fourteen million, which for them is a relatively small movie. That's a lot of money to me, but to them it was the poor stepchild. But it opened at number one that weekend, so to them it was like 'Hoo-ya!' I thought, Well, that's good. But it really rattled everyone when that happened, 'cause it opened on a weekend where the competition was a Sharon Stone movie and a Damon Wayans movie. The reaction to this was very intense. I'd never gotten so many calls in one day in my life! My phone machine literally gave out. And for me it was like, 'Are you calling me 'cause it's number one or 'cause you liked it?' It was kind of odd. But then two weeks later *Twister* came out and then there we were. But it did well all over the world."

Fleming's future would seem assured, but he's quite cautious about what he'd like to do next.

"I've tried to avoid typecasting myself, and so I get the most off-the-wall things, serious and funny. I've gotten a few gay projects, but there really aren't that many around. It's not like I'm desperately trying to get all these gay movies made. I don't know what there is to say about it. I'm interested in stories that have gay characters in them. The thing I'm working on now has gay characters, but it isn't like making 'a gay movie.' I don't know what the one big statement to make about it is. There are a lot of stories to tell. Whenever you see a gay movie it's usually a marginal movie for the gay subculture— which is fine and fascinating, but it is just that: it's marginal. In a way it's isolating gays from the rest of the world and saying, 'This is for us.' It's a clique. If it's not that, then it's the marginal character in the mainstream movie—the guy next door. I think there's a whole other territory that hasn't been explored: showing gay characters incorporated into the world at large in an intelligent, humanistic way. That's what you don't see now, and that's what I'd like to see."[5]

Producer Laurence Mark would also like to see gay stories that aren't isolated from the rest of the world. And to that end, he's been guiding force behind two of the most notable of them: *As Good As It Gets* and *The Object of My Affection*.

"It's tiny steps, *tiny* steps," says Mark, who began his career as an executive trainee at United Artists before moving on to key publicity and marketing posts at Paramount Pictures, where he rose to vice-president of production, and later at 20th Century–Fox. With a credit list that includes *Terms of Endearment, Broadcast News,* and *Working Girl,* the fortysomething executive is as "inside" Hollywood as it gets. And for that reason he's well aware of just how difficult it is to get a "hot button" issue like same-sex relations onto the screen in a "mainstream" way.

"What makes me so happy about in *As Good As It Gets* is that Greg Kinnear is able to play this gay character in a very straight way. Not ludicrously so, mind you, but he's not something out of *The Birdcage. The Birdcage* is fine, but this is something else. This story is moving in a different direction."

And it is indeed a very different direction for a "mainstream" film, one of whose three leading characters is gay, to present his sexual identity as a simple matter of fact. Written by Mark Andrus and director James L. Brooks, this tale of an outrageously antisocial writer (Jack Nicholson), a single mother (Helen Hunt) working as a waitress while fretting over her sickly son, and a painter whose life is upended when a group of apartment robbers nearly cripple him in a beating (the gay role, played by Greg Kinnear) provides an image of gayness that doesn't ask for special pleading, or supply the distance of bizarre behavior. For the Nicholson character, who in addition to his aggressive unmannerliness suffers from obsessive-compulsive disorder, is about as bizarre as it's possible to get.

"One of the most amusing things that went on with this film

was with the MPAA," Mark relates. "This was the first time they've allowed the use of the word 'fag' in a trailer. It was a *big* deal. But it was really interesting because Jack Valenti took the counsel of Chastity Bono. And Chastity was really smart on it. When the time came, she had two things to say about why she didn't think it was offensive. One, he was an equal-opportunity offender. He hated everyone! And so when Jack said, 'Carol the waitress, meet Simon the fag,' clearly he was being a jerk. Part two is that in the trailer—forget the movie— by the end of the *trailer* he's redeemed. We have the scene where Greg says 'I love you' and Jack says, 'Buddy, if that did it for me I'd be the luckiest guy alive.' So we were not glorifying this fellow who's free with the word 'fag.' But it was rather amazing—slightly mind-boggling—that they would be so protective of that word.

"You know," Mark continues, "that's part of the Lenny Bruce thing I've always been fascinated by: if you just keep saying the word it loses its negative connotation. We didn't test this with audiences, but our backup for 'fag' was 'queer,' because 'queer studies' programs exist, and therefore [it] wouldn't be so offensive. But 'queer' is not as funny a word as 'fag.' My hunch is that if you stopped a guy on the street in Peoria and asked which was the more offensive, he'd say, 'Equally.'

"Being gay in this business doesn't seem to matter," says Mark, who has been in it long enough to know. "I really don't think that for directors or producers or writers or executives it matters. I don't think doors slam. In some cases doors open. On *As Good As It Gets* I was the unofficial 'tentacle consultant.' People wanted my opinion, and I offered it too. Like when Greg did that little flounce with his head in one scene. I was the one who said, 'Leave that flounce in! Love that flounce!'

"The next step in all this, I think, which happens in *The Object of My Affection*, actually, is to allow the Greg Kinnear character—in this case the Paul Rudd character—to have a sex life. An erotic attachment or two. Not that it has to be *in our face*, mind you. Just the *existence* of it. *In our face* is *way* down the line, I'll tell you that. The thing is this. Studios do make movies to make money. And one of the key factors in making money is *relatability*. This is simply the truth of it. The more people that can relate to your movie, the bigger hit you will have. Yes, a smaller movie can get made that's not as relatable, but because it's smaller and doesn't cost as much, it's worth making.

"In *The Object of My Affection* we come at the story from the straight woman's point of view. Stephen McCauley's book comes at it from the gay guy's point of view. Wendy Wasserstein's script comes at it through Jennifer Aniston, which for the audience is more relatable. And one other thing which we hope will work a little bit—'cause this is never going to be *Liar Liar*—but what we hope is, and it's true of course, that everyone has at some point in their lives, often generally more than once, fallen in love with the wrong person. For whatever reason: he's married; he's got an obsessive-compulsive disorder; he's gay. In *Ghost* he's dead. So everybody can hopefully relate to it. It's a *little* step."

Mark is encouraged by the success of *My Best Friend's Wedding;* its depiction of a friendship between a gay man and a straight woman smoothed the way for *The Object of My Affection.* And that way has been far from smooth. Mark purchased the rights to Stephen McCauley's novel about a woman who wants her gay best friend to help her raise her child, rather than its actual father, in 1987. The decade it's taken to bring the film to the screen has brought with it any number of changes in the lives of gays and lesbians. And those changes have affected Hollywood as well. For Mark had to fight to keep his film faithful to the spirit of McCauley's novel, instead of going with a conventional Hollywood flow that would have the hero turn heterosexual in the last reel.

"That wasn't what the story was about," Mark explains. "It was like that line Helen Hunt has in *As Good As It Gets:* 'It wasn't about sex. What I needed he gave me great.' You see, we can all find sex. But for someone to understand, someone to connect with me, care about me—that's something else. The other thing in *As Good As It Gets* and *My Best Friend's Wedding* is that the revelation that he's gay is not 'Oh my God! The sky is falling!' As a matter of fact, we got a tad nervous in *The Object of My Affection* where there's a very funny scene where she mentions he's gay and an old guy says, 'Oh, every-body's gay.' "

In *As Good As It Gets* the fact that Greg Kinnear's Simon doesn't exist in a hermetically sealed "gay world" goes a long way toward making him more "relatable." Where the film takes chances is with the character of his art-dealer friend, played by Cuba Gooding, Jr., for some critics have "read" him as being Simon's lover. And this fascinates Mark no end.

"It's deliberately ambiguous," the producer remarks brightly. "The backstory that Cuba was working on—purely backstory, and never, ever does it come front and center in the film—was that they had been lovers at one point. For a moment, two moments—we never know how long—but for a moment in time they had their moment. That was the backstory he was playing off of. So I'm happy that people are getting something of that. Once again this is very Jim Brooks, because the truth is, he's all about real life. It's not like in soap operas where it's—just in case you missed the last three months—a woman answers the phone and says, 'Is this about the man who raped my daughter who became a nun?' Jim doesn't do that, because it doesn't happen. Helen Hunt's character would not be talking about the child's father all the time."

But "gay," as Mark is well aware, is always a "backstory." And one of the more unusual things about the film is how nonchalant it is about dealing with it—even when offered the opportunity by the plot, which involves an aborted trip to meet the gay character's parents.

"We got a bit of Simon's growing up in the scene in the car, where he talks about them," Mark notes. "But that wasn't about his being gay. So we never get the Freudian cliché of the henpecked husband, the domineering mother, and all of that, This is something totally different. In the past if a character was gay that was a big deal. Eyebrows were raised. You had to explain it. The nice news now is that it can be presented as not a big deal at all. That's lovely. It's also nice that the characters no longer need to be 'camp' to be believable. And now, hopefully, we'll be able to move just a little *tad* more and they will be allowed to have boyfriends, or lesbians will be allowed to have girlfriends. But that has never, for whatever reason, ever been as threatening as two fellows. For some women—gay or straight—they couldn't care less about it. Straight guys get turned on by two women. Whereas with two gay guys, women were less upset at it, but straight guys got *really* upset."

Mark feels that independent film has led the way toward dealing with gay and lesbian material. "I guess I should go to more of those offerings at Outfest, but every time I go I'm disappointed. The bottom line is, gay audiences actually have taste. So sure, they might be able to rustle up a crowd for the film festival, but to actually go to the movies in droves for any length of time, it actually has to be good. I'm really interested in Todd Haynes's work, though. And I'll be interested to see what goes on with Rupert Everett. The project he's developing now with Julia Roberts—*Martha and Arthur*—about two movie stars who have a marriage of convenience, and who end up falling in love, by the way—that's really interesting. It's more of that straight woman/gay man thing.

"That's what's so fascinating to me about the Cole Porter story," says Mark excitedly. "Yes, he was gay, and no, they didn't have sex, but they had one of the best marriages in the world. They loved each other deeply. Because often when you say of it, 'Oh no, it was an arranged marriage,' it's like there's something wrong with it. But their situation was so far from that. They were *desperately* in love with one another and had the best time together. When she died he was bereft. His muse had vanished. It was one of the best marriages of all time—and it had *nothing* to do with sex. It's a fascinating relationship that you really could explore today. You would think it was the sort of thing that was not meant to work. But of course it worked.

"Yes," says Mark. "I'm really thinking about that story a lot."[6]

E L E V E N

"NOT THAT
THERE'S ANYTHING
WRONG WITH
THAT!"

———

FALL 1995. LOS ANGELES, CALIFORNIA.
Thursday morning at Paramount Studios; the set of the hit
NBC sitcom *Frasier*. The cast is rehearsing an episode that is five
days away from filming, so no cameras are present, and the bleachers
overlooking the stage are empty. Jane Leeves (Daphne) is ballroom-

dancing with David Hyde Pierce (Niles). She extends one leg high into the air, then lowers it gently onto his shoulder. He can't resist pulling her sensuously toward him. Nearby, standing halfway between the sets of *Frasier*'s living-room set and his radio station, watching the actors intently, is Kelsey Grammer, the show's star and—of this episode, at least—its director. On a movie set, the director is all-powerful; but here in television, the real power lies with the eleven writers standing off to one side, pens and pads in hand. When questions arise about a line or a piece of business, all eyes invariably turn toward them. In response to Grammer's suggestion that a particular punch line needs adjustment, one writer assures him, 'We're already working on it." When Pierce asks to trim a speech, he seeks a nod of approval from the scribes. In short, sitcoms are a writers' medium.

The cast prepares to run through the show's opening scene. Grammer sits behind the console of the radio-station set and starts right in from the top. "I think we have time for one call," he says, pushing a button on the telephone console, perfectly in character as radio therapist Frasier Crane. "Hello, Marianne, I'm listening."

"Okay, here it is, Dr. Crane," says a script assistant over a studio speaker. (When the show airs, the caller's voice will be performed by special guest voice Jodie Foster.) "If my husband and I don't have sex in the next two days I'm going to a department store to pick up a stranger."

Grammer's eyebrows rise a fraction of an inch, but before he can respond, the caller gasps. "Oh Timmy, look who's here—Nana and Pop-Pop. I'll call you back, Dr. Crane," she quickly blurts out before hanging up.

"To all you Mariannes out there," Grammer says after a long, poker-faced pause, "sex with a stranger is never the answer. Better pack the kids off with Nana and Pop-Pop, lead your husband to a sturdy kitchen table, and let the postman ring twice."

It's one of the best lines in the script. And while sitcom writing is always a group effort, it's not surprising that many suspect the line's most likely author to be Joe Keenan. "Joe is our Preston Sturges," says fellow writer Anne Flett-Giordano. "He always seems to come up with the best lines."

Before coming to California to write for *Frasier,* Keenan was an up-and-coming New York comic novelist. His dramatic aspirations were toward the Broadway musical stage, not TV. But two summers ago, *Frasier* executive producer David Lloyd found himself at a beach on Martha's Vineyard, laughing helplessly while reading Keenan's novel *Blue Heaven.* "I'd seen a blurb in *The New York Times,*" recalls Lloyd, whose credits include *The Mary Tyler Moore Show, Taxi,* and *Cheers.* "They said it was as if P. G. Wodehouse had written a 'Gay Mafia' novel—so I just had to read it." An admitted heterosexual, Lloyd sensed that Keenan had the right style for a show like *Frasier.*

Keenan was hired, and this year he won a Writers Guild Award for an episode in which Grammer is mistaken for gay by a romantically inclined male co-worker. "Joe is terrifically talented, a marvel of good taste," says Grammer. "In the gay community, it's acceptable to be very entertaining and charming and witty and urbane. I think everybody should be doing it more often. There are so many dull straight men. They don't seem to want to state an opinion." And to keep such opinions flowing, Grammer recently optioned the film rights to *The Only Thing Worse You Could Have Told Me . . . ,* the one-man show about gay life by *Frasier* regular Dan Butler, who plays the show's aggressively heterosexual jock, Bob "Bulldog" Briscoe.

There is nothing out of the ordinary about hiring a gay writer to write a straight sitcom. Besides Keenan, the *Frasier* staff boasts David Lee, a *Cheers* veteran and co-creator of *Wings,* and former *Kate & Allie* writer Chuck Ranberg, who was discovered by Lloyd after he saw a staged reading of Ranberg's successful gay comedy *End of the World Party.* There are openly gay and lesbian writers on almost every major prime-time situation comedy you can think of, including *Friends, Seinfeld, Murphy Brown, Roseanne, Mad About You, The Nanny, Wings, The Single Guy, Caroline in the City, Coach, Dave's World, Home Court, High Society, The Crew,* and *Boston Common.* Screenwriter Douglas Carter Beane (*To Wong Foo, Thanks for Everything, Julie Newmar*) is developing a series for the Carsey-Werner company about a straight woman and her gay roommate. The "out" gay writing team of James Berg and Stan Zimmerman (*The Brady Bunch Movie*) has created a new Fox series for Pauly Shore (yes, Pauly

Shore!). And Kelsey Grammer has a sitcom in development. "Part of it takes place in a drag bar," he says, "and I would imagine that some of the drag queens *might* be gay." In short, when it comes to sitcoms, gays rule.

Elsewhere, things haven't changed very much. Sodomy laws remain on the books in more than twenty states, gay-bashing incidents continue to occur with alarming frequency, gay and lesbian teenagers are still tossed to the mercy of the streets by disapproving parents, and antigay diatribes from politicians, pundits, and preachers of every stripe haven't been stilled to any degree. In Hollywood, closeted performers still feel obligated to lie and dissemble, aided by publicists only too happy to bar the press from questioning clients about their "personal lives." Yet in spite of all this, a growing number of talents, unperturbed by their sexual status, have risen through the ranks to dominate sitcoms as never before.

"Gays were always a fact in this industry—a rampant, wonderful, joyous fact," says writer/director/performer and all-round comedy guru Mel Brooks, who began his career writing for the legendary *Your Show of Shows*. "In the past, gay was never out there, never mainstream. Now it's becoming mainstream." This fall 1995 season, *The Crew, High Society, Roseanne, The Larry Sanders Show,* and the fleeting *The Pursuit of Happiness* had recurring gay characters. There were also the much publicized "gay wedding" episodes of *Roseanne* and *Friends*. And one week in the spring of 1995, NBC's entire "Must See TV" lineup—*Friends, Frasier, The Single Guy,* and *Seinfeld*—featured episodes in which straights were mistaken for gays.

But gay-themed episodes and individual gay characters are really beside the point. In a way, *all* the episodes of these shows are gay. Like the Jewish moguls who ran Hollywood in the studio era, gay and lesbian sitcom writers are keen observers of the majority culture that surrounds them. MGM's Andy Hardy series is a perfect example of how the Jews understood the Gentile sensibility better than Gentiles did themselves. But where the studio-era Jews were loath to acknowledge—much less promote—themselves, the gay and lesbian TV writers of today have been pushing the envelope every chance they get. In fact, they're encouraged to do so. Since current comedies are positively obsessed with the intimate sex lives of straight young singles, who better to write them than members of a minority famed for its sexual candor?

"So much of television has to do with the politics of sexual relationships," says Phil Hartman, star of the sex-obsessed *News-Radio* and a veteran of the equally libidinous *Saturday Night Live*. "The gay community has always had a delightful sense of sarcasm about sexual mores. Unfortunately, to a large segment of our society, gay people are viewed as sexual outlaws. God forbid a straight person should acknowledge that there are pleasures associated with their anus. That's a big door that people *don't* want to open."

As a result of the influx of gay writers, even the most hetero-sexual of sitcoms can often be said to possess that most elusive of undertones, the "gay sensibility"—*Frasier* being a case in point.

Frasier's David Lee is sitting with writing partner Joe Keenan in a plush, wood-paneled office at Paramount, speaking proudly of their series of episodes in which Mercedes Ruehl guest-starred as a domineering station manager who clashes with Frasier professionally, only to find herself attracted to him sexually. The icy Kate and the reserved Frasier throw caution to the winds and engage in some pre-cipitous quasi-public sex before coming to their senses. "It was one of the truest arcs of a relationship I've ever seen," Lee declares. "It began with a passion born out of naughtiness, continued with a pas-sion born out of the fear of discovery, then ended with the two finally getting to know one another on their first—and last—date, and finding they had absolutely nothing in common!"

The Kate/Frasier story arc seems like a perfect dramatization of a relationship more associated with gays than straights—particu-larly those gays who regard first-date sex as a matter of course. But Lee shies away from the inference. "I really can't isolate anything about approaches to comedy that is common to gay writers on the show and not the straight ones," he says. "I can't, either," Keenan adds.

"The only thing you *will* notice," continues Lee, starting to laugh, "is when the subject turns to basketball, Joe, Chuck, and I tend to get up and walk out. Likewise, when it turns to Broadway shows, there's a different exodus."

"Except for David Lloyd, of course," says Keenan of his discoverer. "He's the only straight Broadway show queen I know."

Keenan and Lee banter with the sort of easy camaraderie that many gay men—even if they've known each other briefly—fall into almost automatically. They finish each other's sentences and top off each other's jokes. As they sit back in the office's comfortable chairs, they look less like a pair of TV writers on a high-pressure deadline than a couple of gay sophisticates having an afternoon coffee. In truth, they're both. They agree that most gay writers favor playfully malicious dialogue and larger-than-life characters. And they're in sympathy with New York food and culture critic Jeff Weinstein, who famously remarked: "No, there's no such thing as a gay sensibility, and yes, it has an enormous impact on the arts." Still, they see it working a bit differently in sitcoms than elsewhere in the culture.

"I can understand 'camp' as something that's a little nailed down as specifically gay," says Keenan, "but none of the shows on right now really traffic in camp. All sitcom characters have to be taken seriously on some level, and camp isn't serious."

"When you're talking about a gay sensibility," suggests Lee, "you're starting to describe a very urban, very educated—"

"—ironic, detached, iconoclastic attitude," adds Keenan.

"But look," says Lee, "all I have to do is walk down the street to any number of bars, and I can show you gay people who don't have a single qualification for a gay sensibility."

Other gays in the industry feel the sensibility question isn't quite so obscure, especially when it comes to *Frasier*, whose decidedly unmacho leads—Grammer and Pierce—frequently recall comic legends Edward Everett Horton and Franklin Pangborn in their 1930s heyday.

"*Frasier* has lucked out in terms of gay sensibility by having two characters who—regardless of what their sexuality may actually be—could be seen as gay," says New World Pictures vice-president of casting Joel Thurm, who recently turned film producer with *It's My Party*.

"Frasier could easily be an elegant queen," he continues, a playful grin broadening across his features as he peers over the scripts piled on the desk of his Westside office. "So could Niles. It's a lot like it was with *The Golden Girls*. As far as I'm concerned, Blanche was gay. And I know for a fact that I'm not the only gay man who feels this way. Blanche spoke frankly and openly about sex the way many gay men do. In fact, *I* identify with Blanche, especially now that I'm getting older   and hornier."

Jamie Wooten and Marc Cherry, co-creators of *The Crew*, joined the staff of *The Golden Girls* midway through that show's eight-year run. And they view the show the same way Thurm does. But they were in for a shock when they arrived at the writers' table.

"*The Golden Girls* had always been our favorite show," Wooten recalls. "When we got the job, we thought, 'Oh, how fun, we're going to meet so many gay people!' We were stunned. We were the only gay writers at the table."

Things are considerably different at the production offices of *The Crew*. "We have eleven writers on our staff this year—eight of them gay," says Wooten. "This wasn't out of any plan on our part; we didn't know they were gay when we hired them. In fact, two of them came out for the first time because they felt so comfortable working with us."

Wooten and Cherry agree that this high ratio is still unusual for sitcom staffs. But they don't think the openly gay character they've created for *The Crew* is in any way offbeat. "It's a show about flight attendants, for goodness' sake!" says Wooten, laughing behind his desk in a toy-strewn office at KTLA Studios in Hollywood. "To write a show about flight attendants and *not* have one of them be gay would be . . . a sin!"

"Our theory about gay characters on TV," says Cherry, "is that to the average housewife, talk shows have gotten so sleazy that a gay man on a sitcom is at least ten freaks removed from the norm."

"Sitcom writing isn't something just any child in America is brought up to want to do," says Wooten. "I'm from poor white North Carolina trash. There is absolutely no excuse for my being here. Mark is from California, right out of 'Behind the Orange Curtain' Republican land. We're from opposite sides of the country, yet we've led parallel lives. We were the children who didn't play outside, didn't play games, but were glued to the TV. So when we made our plans to break into show business—"

"—we just had to do sitcoms!" Cherry chimes in from the couch. "We were made for this sort of thing—"

"—because of our painful childhoods."

"Yeah, don't you love it?" Cherry asks, totally deadpan. "My painful childhood has paid for my new Lexus."

R obert Horn and Daniel Margosis, who wrote for *Designing Women* and *Living Single* before creating *High Society* for CBS, have found a comfort level similar to Wooten and Cherry's. Their show, about a pair of fast-lane New York women (Jean Smart and Mary McDonnell), is right up there with *Frasier* and *The Golden Girls* on the "gay sensibility" meter.

"There are times when we have done things on our show and been told, 'Only West Hollywood is going to get that,' " Horn says in the show's art-deco-trimmed offices at Gower Studios. "My feeling is, a lot of that attitude will stay that way. But look at a show like *Home Improvement*. There's a dynamic there that caters to a certain group I'm not part of. I'm not out there doing carpentry work. But is it written broad enough and funny enough for everybody to enjoy? Yes. So why can't that be true for characters written from a gay point of view— whatever that may be?"

"It's not like we get up in the morning, look at ourselves in the mirror, and say, 'We're gay men, and that's how we've got to approach everything we do,' " adds Margosis. He bounces gleefully in his chair as he thinks up his next line: "It's not like we're pushing a gay agenda—though we would if it got us more dates!"

Still, Horn and Margosis, like Wooten and Cherry, are well aware of how far they can—and can't—go. "The network is always scared if you do a lot of gay stuff," says Wooten, " 'People not into that will turn away,' which is probably a fair assessment—you can't force-feed America.

"You know, it's funny," he adds. We were watching the promo for the *Friends* lesbian wedding episode the other night, and my boyfriend said to me, 'You're in big trouble.' I asked why, and he said, 'There's going to be a backlash. It's too much.' I said, 'You're kidding.' I thought the show was fine, but we talked about it all weekend. He said, 'They're shoving it down people's throats.' "

Friends' co-creators, David Crane and Marta Kauffman, don't agree. Before unleashing their sitcom supernova, they had worked together for years—from off-Broadway musicals co-written with Kauffman's composer husband, Michael Skloff, to unsuccessful sitcoms like *The Powers That Be* and *Family Album*. They've become a close-knit team, and they feel their show is on the right track.

"*Friends* is a nine o'clock show that's on at eight," says Kauffman, curled up in a chair alongside Crane in the show's Warner Bros. offices. "I can understand those people who don't want to let their kids watch it. That's part of being a parent—deciding what's appropriate for your kids to see. So when people say, 'These shows should not be on at eight,' fine. Change the channel."

"It's really NBC's call," Crane declares. "They know what this show is."

Kauffman seems almost protective of her writing partner, glancing in his direction whenever he speaks, ready to lend support. "It's not a family show, but I think our characters are in many ways a family," she says. "*Friends* is very much like it was for David and I when we were in our twenties and living in New York. We took care of each other, kept each other in line. It's a nonfamily family."

Gays and lesbians, more than anyone else, know about "nonfamily" families, which is why so many of them have been burning up the Internet about *Friends'* ostensibly straight Joey and Chandler (Matt LeBlanc and Matthew Perry), whose emotional interplay is indistinguishable from that of a gay couple. When Joey moved out of Chandler's apartment this winter, it took the form of a full-blown romantic breakup along the lines of *The Way We Were*.

Crane and Kaufman don't see it that way. "I don't think there's a specifically gay dimension to this show," says Crane. "So much of writing is just a matter of empathy. Certainly, a gay writer is going to bring certain life experiences to the table. But I don't think friends-as-family is in any way the exclusive domain of gays. I've read scripts by gay writers that don't reflect any knowledge of gay life. On this show, I'm not sure how my being gay fits into the picture."

There are millions of gays and lesbians watching his show every week who could tell Crane in exhaustive detail how same-sexuality "fits into" *Friends*. But Crane sticks to his guns—although not without a trace of ambivalence.

"Inasmuch as I am the sum of my parts," he says, "I don't think there's a . . . I don't know. I hate to define myself. I've been reading a lot of things where I've been called David-Crane-openly-gay-producer. It's virtually become one word!"

"I have to assume," says Kaufman, breaking in on her slightly exasperated partner, "that there are, in the life experience of a gay person, certain things brought to the table, but I don't know that I could tell you what they are or generalize in any way."

"I certainly can't," says Crane firmly. "I mean, I'm the only gay person in our room."

"That we know of," says Kaufman evenly.

"Yes, that we know of," concedes Crane, starting to smile.

When you sit down and think about it, it's really remarkable what's happened over the past few years," says industry veteran Joel Thurm, who has done everything from casting a Broadway production of *Hello, Dolly!* to playing a casting director in the film *I'll Do Anything*. "When I was with *The Bob Newhart Show*, I never met a gay writer or any other gay person, except maybe in makeup or wardrobe. Same with *The Mary Tyler Moore Show*. I think there were a couple of gay people backstage, but none of the writers were gay. It was very much a boys' club. Not homophobic, mind you, but a real football-watching crowd."

"Still," he adds, "they did one thing somewhere in the middle years of *Mary* with a wonderful actor-director named Bob Moore, who's dead now. He directed the original production of *The Boys in the Band*. He played Phyllis's brother. Remember that episode where he kept dating Rhoda and driving Phyllis crazy because she hated Rhoda so much? Then Rhoda told her that the brother was gay, and Phyllis said, "Thank God!' That was one of the first gay-themed episodes on television. After that show Bob directed regularly for MTM. But he was the only person around in those days. You might say he was the Rosa Parks of *The Mary Tyler Moore Show*.

"There's definitely a generational thing going on," Thurm says. "The younger gays aren't as closeted. Their mentality is: if your writing is good, it doesn't matter. Still, it's not okay for anybody to be gay unless they're good at what they do. In fact, you have to be better than anybody else. If you are, then everything's fine."

"There's a pattern within the industry of self-identified liberals who love you when you're a funny queen," says veteran television writer Richard Gollance, (*Beverly Hills 90210*, *Falcon Crest*), who isn't shy about admitting he sometimes fills that bill. "But when you have a serious point to make or are upset about something—which happens with AIDS—they have a lot of trouble shifting gears, because they're not used to taking gay people seriously.

"About two years ago, there was a show I worked on where we did The Gay Episode," Gollance continues, his usually genial features suddenly taking on a very serious air. "And there was this enormous conflict on their part about what to do with me. I was the only openly gay man on the set. When I was first interviewed for the job, a show like this was presented as something they wanted to do. It was what I like to call the *Cry Freedom* school of drama—how straight white people are going to deal with this 'other.' I didn't think it'd get done, but I thought it was a very gracious thing for them to mention it to me. When the episode actually came to be made, they suddenly didn't want me to write it. At the same time, they still wanted me to look at the script and tell them what the gay character would or wouldn't do. I have never had that explained to me in any credible way."

Gollance emphasizes that this incident took place some time ago. But *Roseanne*'s William Lucas Walker recalls a more recent occasion when he was writing for another show he would rather not name.

"I had always heard about how liberal Hollywood was, and I guess I believed it. I was surprised how conservative a town it is in practice, even though they'll say the right things in public. This comedy I worked on was a real straight-boys' club. It reminded me of the high-school locker room, only the guys weren't as cute. I wasn't closeted, but I didn't really talk to anyone about it unless they asked. I thought the jungle drumbeats would get out and everyone would know. They didn't."

The last straw came when a comedian working on another show, whom Walker had considered a friend, dropped by to discuss his recent appearance on *The Tonight Show*, which also featured an appearance by singer-pianist Michael Feinstein. "He was taking about what a 'fag' Feinstein was, and all the writers were joining in. I felt my whole insides imploding in slow motion. It was like walking in on a Ku Klux Klan rally."

Walker's experience is by and large an exception to the rule these days. Gays have planted themselves firmly in the comedy business—with the Jews who came before them setting the pace. "Brash Jewish humor from New York really opened the door for what would have been considered unseemly, bizarre, and untoward material," says Mel Brooks, who first mined such material with Woody Allen, Larry Gelbart, and Neil Simon for the benefit of Sid Caesar. "I think Jews have always been good at comedy, because if people are laughing at you they can't kill you. It was as if to say, 'I don't know what you've heard about Jews, but we're not monsters. We don't have horns, and we're neither the wild, kill-crazy Communists nor the conspiracy of bankers you've heard so much about. We're *amusants*.'

"That same approach was taken by black comedians like Richard Pryor," he adds. "He talks about his family, and I'm thinking, Hey, they could be Jews! He made it universal. And now, in the same way, homophobia is being broken to pieces by these really smart gay comedy writers. I can see a gay sitcom being done on the networks probably sooner than later."

"I helped start *The Nanny*," says Joe Voci, one of the smart gay comedy writers Brooks is talking about. "Fran Drescher is playing this very New York Jewish girl, and audiences just love her."

"It's the same with *Seinfeld*," says *High Society*'s Robert Horn. "That show has touched a nerve in all sorts of people. But if you did a show today where the humor was as specific in its gayness as that show is in terms of its Jewishness, I don't think it would get on the air."

Not now, but soon. "Jews and gays are very close in sensibility," Jamie Wooten notes. "It's just a chromosome away, really."

Mel Brooks laughs when told of Wooten's remark. "A chromosome away? I like that. That's true. In the past, a show like *Seinfeld* or *The Nanny* would have been considered too ethnic. Woody Allen and I wouldn't have made it in show business with a name like Seinfeld at the time we came along. Woody could not have used his real name, Konigsberg, and I could not have used mine, Kaminsky. So we kind of falsified our passports, so to speak, by giving ourselves incredibly Anglo-Saxon names: Allen and Brooks. But once we were in the door, we behaved in a very Jewish manner.

"I think Mel is right," says *Roseanne*'s Walker. "But does that mean gay people should think about changing their names to DiMaggio and Namath?"

Perhaps such drastic measures needn't be taken, if the example of *Seinfeld* is followed. Its writers—gay and straight—have managed to come up with some of the most bizarre comic material ever presented on television. No, not the "gay episode," in which—thanks to a prank of Elaine's—George and Jerry are mistaken for a gay couple ("Not that there's anything wrong with that!" they invariably add). What truly sets *Seinfeld* apart is the episode in which it's revealed that the father of George's fiancée, Susan (whose brief lesbian love affair figured in an earlier episode), has a brace of love letters written to him by the late novelist John Cheever.

"Could anything be more arcane?" raves Brooks, breathless with admiration. "Imagine—referring to John Cheever's bisexuality on a mass-market TV show. Amazing!"

"That's the show everybody talked about?" asks a surprised Peter Mehlman when told the news. "Gee, really? Hmmm. The Cheever thing was [series co-creator] Larry David's idea," says Mehlman, who, like David, is a writer-producer of the television phenom—and straight. "I love—and everybody on the show loves—testing the limits of comedy. The Cheever letters had just come out, and we'd heard they had all this stuff about his sex life. When Larry brought up the idea of using the letters as a gag, we all just laughed so hard, we couldn't resist it."

As for *Seinfeld*'s Jewish content, Mehlman feels much like David Crane regarding the possible "gay sensibility" of *Friends*: guarded. "Although the show has a Jewish lead, it's not really a Jewish show," he says haltingly. "We have plenty of non-Jewish writers. We're not making a statement about being Jewish—or about anything, for that matter."

So what of Brooks's notion of a gay sitcom being the next step? "I think you can have a gay character leading a show," says Mehlman, "but for it to be truly accepted, the sensibility of its leading character—whether they're gay or Jewish or whatever—has to be that of . . ." It takes him a moment to come up with the word he's looking for. ". . . of a citizen of the world. That's it. A citizen of the world. You got that? I think that's the best thing I've said this entire interview."[1]

Spring 1998. Los Angeles, California. *The Crew* and *High Society* are gone. So are *Wings, Coach, The Single Guy, Dave's World, Home Court,* and *Boston Common.* Phil Hartman died at the hands of his wife, Brynne, who took her own life shortly afterward. *The Larry Sanders Show* has come to an end, on the orders of its star, Garry

Shandling. But the *Sanders* finale is as nothing compared to the end of *Seinfeld*. Provoking media coverage of a sort more associated with a papal succession or the fall of a monarchy, *Seinfeld*'s finale brought with it a mass reconsideration of not only sitcom but television itself. *Frasier* and *Friends,* meanwhile, have continued as successfully as ever (with William Lucas Walker joining the former's writing staff), though the sitcom market has become more competitive as networks lose audience share they had counted on in the past to cable, video, the Internet, and all other manner of diversion. In sitcoms, secondary gay characters and casual references to gay and lesbian life have become common in such shows as *Suddenly Susan, Working,* and *Veronica's Closet.* "Special" gay episodes are rare. In fact, *Just Shoot Me* offered what amounted to a parody of one, in which David Spade's Dennis was mistaken by for gay by a father (played by Brian Dennehy) all too eager to declare he's "proud of my gay son!"

And then there was *Ellen*.

And *then* there was Ellen.

In one sense, it was Mel Brooks's prediction come true, a lot sooner than he had expected. After struggling along for several seasons as a heroine who didn't appear to have a love life, Ellen Morgan got one. She came out as a lesbian. But once the hoopla of her coming out had subsided, the show, its staff, and its star faced real trouble. Just how do you go about creating a situation comedy about a lesbian, starring an openly lesbian performer? It had never been done before. There was no guidebook or map to reach a secret cache of buried lesbian comedy treasure—just a nervous network whose attitude toward the show seemed to change from hour to hour, and a star who seemed to have switched from anything-to-please "nice girl" to lesbian activist overnight. And that wasn't to mention the impact of nonstop press attention to DeGeneres and her lover, Anne Heche, who for much of 1997 appeared to spend the bulk of their time at parties and premieres. Both, however, were working nonetheless.

Ellen soldiered on, trying to fit "prelesbian" cast members into a new plot arc involving Ellen's budding love affair with Laurie, a single mother played by actress Lisa Darr. This new character was in every way a serious one—neither the butt of jokes nor their generator. Ordinarily this wouldn't be a problem. Shows like *Roseanne* had always managed to find a way to swing between comedy and drama, not only from show to show but even within individual episodes. But *Roseanne* had a clear identity, which stayed in place right up until its last wildly idiosyncratic season. *Ellen* had never made up its mind about what kind of show it wanted to be. And while a lesbian love story offered a prime opportunity to do so, it was at the expense of whatever comedic material might be involved.

Still, this plot and character insecurity was in many ways beside the point. For the network had begun to slap an "Adult Content" warning label on the top of every show that featured even the most minimal sort of intimacy between women. It was nothing short of a "Keep Away" sign, and it had its effect. From a coming-out all-time high, *Ellen* slipped back to its old middle-of-the-pack rating level in just a few months' time.

Ellen DeGeneres knew very well that this might happen. "I told them [at ABC Television], 'This is my life. *I* am taking the biggest risk here. I am willing to take the risk because that's how much it means to me,' " she related to Diane Sawyer on the night of the coming-out episode, adding, "The main reason I didn't want to do this was because I don't want to become political. I don't want to become some gay activist."[2]

But that is indeed what she became on the night of September 14, 1997, when, picking up her Emmy for the coming-out show's script, DeGeneres told the television audience, "I accept this on the behalf of all of the people and the teenagers, especially, out there who think there's something wrong with them because they're gay. And there's nothing wrong with you. Don't let anybody make you ashamed of who you are."[3] Soon she was protesting the network's "Adult Content" label, complaining on an *Access Hollywood* interview, "It's okay to see somebody die on television. It's okay to see somebody killed. It's okay to see somebody raped. But you can't show affection between people of the same sex, and I think there's something really, really wrong with that."[4]

The show itself was soon taking political potshots, most memorably in an episode in which Emma Thompson guest-starred as a closeted actress (also called Emma Thompson) who decided to follow Ellen's example. "Let's go out and terrify some Baptists!" she said. But the show's best line was given to series regular Joely Fisher's character, Paige, who opined of Hollywood, "Half of this town is gay, the other half pretends it is to suck up to David Geffen."[5]

What the line left out was the part of Hollywood that wasn't sure what to do about gays and lesbians—real or fictional.

"I'm gay, the character's gay and that's the problem everyone has with the show. It's just too controversial. Nobody wants to deal with it," DeGeneres confessed to *Daily Variety* in February of 1998, as the handwriting was on the wall and both *Ellen* and Ellen were on their way out.[6] On April 24, 1998, it all became official, with the show's cancellation supposedly based on declining ratings alone.[7] But in an *Entertainment Weekly* cover story and on-line interview DeGeneres excoriated the network for not supporting her show, and most important of all for scaring viewers away with the "Adult Content" disclaimer.

Citing a promotional spot for *The Drew Carey Show* in which the star is shown kissing another man, DeGeneres complained, "There's no disclaimer on that show at all, because it's two heterosexual men, and they're making fun of heterosexuality." She also pointed to a kiss between Michael J. Fox and Michael Boatman on *Spin City* being disclaimer-free "because neither of them is really gay in real life." As for the disclaimer, its verbal aspect was most distressing to DeGeneres. "It was like this voice like you're entering some kind of radiation center. It was very offensive, and you don't think that's going to affect ratings? Or scare people?"

Pointing to the fact that the ratings for the returning *Spin City* were comparable to those of the canceled *Ellen*, DeGeneres cast herself in the role of any number of gays and lesbians in any number of professions—fired when the boss "found out" and couldn't deal with it: "They'll never say you're fired because you're gay. They're using the excuse that it's ratings. But I was fired basically for being gay."[8]

Ellen and *Ellen* underscored a Hollywood paradox. On a personal level, the town had no problem with DeGeneres, at least not one it would admit. It was on a professional level that the problems arose. There was no precedent for a show about a lesbian. As a one-time-only "event," Ellen's coming out was perfectly in keeping with standard policy. It was a surefire ratings grabber and prize-winner. But you can come out only once, not every week. In many ways the Ellen/*Ellen* situation mirrors the problem the culture as a whole faces with "open" same-sexuality. If it's "in the closet"—which is to say, known to all but never discussed in "polite" conversation—then it's "acceptable," like Oscar Wilde before the fall. Once it's "out," the culture is in the witness box. Who is this gay or lesbian person, and where does he or she fit within the broader social scheme? That question is still in the process of being answered. And in many ways gays and lesbians have as much trouble answering it as straights do.

"*Ellen* is so gay it's excluding a large part of our society," Chastity Bono told *Daily Variety* when asked about the show's problems. "A lot of the stuff on it is somewhat of an inside joke. It's one thing to have a gay lead character, but it's another when every episode deals with pretty specific gay issues."[9] Bono came to regret her words, quickly realizing how a fourth estate hostile to Ellen and *Ellen* from the start would seize on it. In fact, to read some of the coverage of the two-year span of Ellen/*Ellen* events, one might suspect that the simple act of watching a television show constituted some sort of mass referendum on same-sexuality.

It is extremely difficult to create and promote a successful situation comedy. It is even harder to do so when said sitcom revolves around a member of a widely despised minority group. "If the series of corporate decisions reviewed here were in the context of any other program, you would be questioning the business judgment of your senior executives," said an ad supporting *Ellen* placed by GLAAD and the Human Rights Campaign in the hope of encouraging ABC president Robert Iger to change his mind.[10]

It was a nice gesture.

"TV is not the mass medium it once was," Howard Bragman observes. "A huge show may get ten percent of the country watching it. Twenty million is huge. It's not like it used to be, with forty or fifty million people. If the radical right doesn't want to watch your show, you can probably get good numbers without them—particularly in the bigger cities. The right has numbers in the areas where people don't care as much, so they're not the problem."

Bragman's tone darkens as he contemplates the real problem faced by *Ellen,* Ellen, and millions of others.

"I don't know what people want of gays and lesbians in this country. If it's a choice, how many people want to make that choice? Gay people are supposed to have sex fifty times in the afternoon. 'Okay.' I want one lover and I want to be monogamous and have the right to marry. 'No, you can't!' So they don't know what to do about it. They just don't like us. *They just don't like us.*"[11]

TWELVE

TOM CRUISE

—

I N THE END IT ALL COMES DOWN TO TOM
Cruise.

Or maybe the beginning.

The latter would be the case if you count yourself among those

who have skipped the prologue and eleven other chapters of this book because you couldn't *wait* to learn the answer to that all-important, earth-shattering question.

Is Tom Cruise really gay?

Well, of course not.

Sort of.

And . . . well, it depends.

Over the past twelve years "Is Tom Cruise really gay?" has been asked, asked, and asked again by any number of parties, both inside Hollywood and out, across the entire spectrum of sexual orientations. So insistent has this question become that it's often seemed as if its answer were less linked to Cruise in particular than a tool to discover the very meaning of homosexuality itself. But as those of you who *have* read the prologue and eleven other chapters of this book already know, that's just not possible. Even if "the truth" about Tom Cruise were made incontrovertibly available, it would be as nothing compared to the fantasies he's inspired in viewers of every sexual stripe. For Tom Cruise is the embodiment of sexual desire. And sexuality is anarchy.

"I don't know where this whole thing about Tom Cruise being gay got started," says Chastity Bono. "Look, I remember when he was seeing my mother. I mean—I was *there*."[1]

Logically, Bono's "being there" should carry more weight than those who "swear" a certain male escort service has his name on speed dial, or others who claim to "remember" the young Cruise sleeping with all and sundry to get ahead in an acting class. Such idle gossip shouldn't hold sway over observable fact. The problem with sexuality is that occasions to make a verifiable observation of sexual activity are rare. There are no Tab Hunter or George Michael "moments" to be found in Cruise's résumé.

But that's not to say it's free of sexual dalliance. "My former partner, and still business partner, Terry Anderson, used to drive a limo in Atlanta years ago," says novelist Armistead Maupin. "Once he was driving Tom Cruise and Rebecca DeMornay around. They were right there, in the backseat of the limo—fucking!"[2]

Well, that should pretty much settle the matter. Except, of course, for the fact that sexuality is sometimes malleable, and often as not more so among members of the acting profession. On that basis it wouldn't be entirely outside of the realm of human possibility for a Tom Cruise to have known the pleasures of his own sex at one time or another. But that wouldn't, in and of itself, make Tom Cruise gay.

"People are desperate for Tom Cruise to be gay," says supermogul David Geffen. "Well, he's *not*. I've known him since he was a teenager. Finally, I find nothing gay about him. What he is is a very cute guy that lots of guys wish were gay because they'd like to have him as the focus of their romantic fantasy."[3]

Cruise's homoerotic appeal is undeniable. But there's the rub. For the attraction he holds for gays doesn't exist in a same-sex vacuum. Straights are watching as well, and Cruise's erotic power clearly disturbs as it threatens to draw them under his spell. A gay Cruise would be easy to dismiss—he's "one of them," therefore he has "nothing to do with me." Except that Cruise, gay or straight, has something to do with everyone. For that's why he gets the big bucks.

B orn Thomas Mapother, Tom Cruise first came to widespread public attention in *Taps* (1981), a drama about a revolt at an elite military academy. It starred Timothy Hutton and Sean Penn, but Cruise's well-sculpted physique made the greatest impact. For the very same reason, he stood out from the crowd (which included Matt Dillon, Rob Lowe, Ralph Macchio, Patrick Swayze, C. Thomas Howell, and Emilio Estevez) in Francis Ford Coppola's teenagers-in-trouble programmer *The Outsiders* (1983). But it was *Risky Business*, the romantic comedy about a middle-class teenager who stumbles into becoming the pimp of a call girl (played by fellow limousine enthusiast Rebecca DeMornay), that crystallized the young actor's sexual image. The shot of Cruise wearing nothing but sunglasses, a shirt, white socks, and briefs and skidding across a polished wood floor offered him up as a fully eroticized vision the likes of which hadn't been seen since Marilyn Monroe's famous encounter with a subway vent in *The Seven Year Itch*.

Leading men hadn't been sexualized in "mainstream" films

quite this way before. He wasn't an androgyne, like Valentino or Ramon Novarro. He was the boy next door. *Top Gun* only served to reinforce this fact, particularly in the scene where Cruise and his fellow hotshot aviators play volleyball, their pectorals gleaming with sweat. Never had the boy next door seemed so carnal.

Needless to say, Tom Cruise had more in mind for his career than offering a taut tush. His performances in *The Color of Money* (1986), *Rain Man* (1988), *Born on the Fourth of July* (1989), *A Few Good Men* (1992), *Interview with the Vampire* (1994), and *Jerry Maguire* (1997) testify to a commitment to serious acting. Nonetheless, all that many remember of Cruise in these films is his physicality: leaping about a pool table, racing though an office, or even standing calmly in an Armani suit or a frilly eighteenth-century ensemble. For whether he likes it or not, Tom Cruise is an erotic spectacle—a body to be devoured by all eyes. And in a culture still insistent on sexual apartheid—straights over here and gays over there—Cruise's erotic energy is highly problematic, even though the problem he poses resides solely in fantasy.

"I've heard that I'm a misogynist. I'm a homosexual. I'm brainless. How can I be all these things?" Cruise complained to *Vanity Fair* interviewer Kevin Sessums.[4] It is, of course, perfectly possible for Cruise to be all three things at the same time. But such iconic disorder is precisely what Scientology (that self-styled religion whose antipathy to same-sexuality is well documented) was designed to eliminate.

Scientology promises its acolytes a chance for total control over their lives. But, taking no chances, Cruise hired Pat Kingsley anyway. Still, neither religious dogma nor Kingsley's fabled public-relations clout can control the imagination of the moviegoing public. If it wants a gay Tom Cruise, it will have one. This in turn leads to Geffen's claim of finding "nothing gay about him." Knowing Cruise personally as he does (being the producer of both *Risky Business* and *Interview with the Vampire*), Geffen has had a chance to observe him on any number of occasions. But the truth of proximity is different from that of the distance movie images provide. There is obviously "nothing gay" about Cruise the way there *was* something gay about Cary Grant. He's not a light romantic comedy player. Similarly, there's nothing about Cruise remindful of Montgomery Clift or James Dean, icons of another era who could have fit any of his more interesting roles. Yet in their lifetimes both Clift and Dean managed to escape the concerted attention afforded Tom Cruise's sexuality, even though their screen images were far more homoerotically coded than his. And that's not to mention Valentino, of whom a *Chicago Tribune* columnist famously wrote, "When will we be rid of all these effeminate youths, pomaded, powdered, bejeweled and bedizened, in the image of Rudy –that painted pansy?"[5]

That isn't, of course, to say that Cruise has been without his detractors. But their complaints have had more to do with his overall attitude toward the press than anything specifically related to his sexual life. In a scathing article written for *Los Angeles* magazine in 1993, critic Rod Lurie recounts the hoops he was forced to jump through in order to execute what had begun as a straightforward profile. Interested in learning about Clearsound, the Scientology-promoted sound system that Cruise had reportedly insisted on using for the film *Days of Thunder,* as well as other aspects of his burgeoning career, Lurie was met with a brick wall of resistance:

> I was granted a fact-checking-only "interview" with Cruise. It went like this: I had to submit my questions in writing to Kingsley—21 of them—to which the star responded through written answers that were then read to me over the phone by Kingsley, who said she was "in touch with Tom." Meantime, Kingsley herself was conducting her own "interview" with me, calling from Los Angeles, from Paris. No matter how far she went, she was never far from a phone, questioning and, in some cases, even screaming that certain areas we were looking into were none of anyone's business.

Declaring that "for many who know Cruise—and work with him—the boy-next-door image is far from accurate," Lurie spoke of a Cruise whose industry image was "petulant and demanding, some-thing of a control freak who shows flashes of a prodigious ego." Not helping matters, Lurie felt, was the fact that on the press junket for the film *Far and Away* Cruise and his wife and co-star, Nicole Kid-man, "demanded that reporters sign contracts stipulating which publications the stories would appear in and run. Further, the contract stated that anything Cruise said could only be used in conjunction with *Far and Away* and could not be mentioned in regard to any other Cruise article or project. In other words, the content of the interviews would be the sole property of Cruise."[6]

This was well beyond the pale of demands made by most Hol-lywood stars when dealing with the press, a fact noted by many other journalists besides Lurie. Clearly Cruise and Kidman were concerned that words uttered at a junket might make their way into "exposés" published by the dreaded tabloids. But why should the "legitimate" press suffer for tabloid sins? And what could Cruise or Kidman pos-sibly say in the highly controlled atmosphere of a press junket that would work against them in a tabloid context? The strategy only served to fan the gay-rumor fires, which reached a peak at the time of *Interview with the Vampire*.

Cruise's casting had been the subject of much criticism, not the least of which was registered by the book's author, Anne Rice. The consensus was that not only was the all-American Cruise wrong for the role of the ultra-decadent vampire Lestat, but his "control freak" skittishness would be sure to compromise the project in other ways. This impression was confirmed by a *New York Times* article about the film's making, in which critic Janet Maslin noted, "It has been reported that the material's homosexual nuances have been toned down at Mr. Cruise's insistence—Lestat's grief over a dead brother is now mourning for a spouse for instance."[7]

"Rumor has it that Cruise insisted all homoerotic strains be removed from the movie, and refused to do any vampire kisses above the shoulder," claimed writer Mark Ebner in *Spy*.

When *Premiere* confronted him he got very uptight, just as he did when questioned about his sexuality (questions he squirmed around) during an interview in *Vanity Fair* last fall. And recently, Cruise forced *McCall's* to print an apology after it quoted a movie critic who said that CAA initiated his marriage to Nicole Kidman to "squelch the gay stuff." Considering the almighty star power involved, the magazine wisely yielded, and explained in a subsequent issue that it "knows no evidence" that Cruise is homosexual."[8]

The finished film was in no way free of homoeroticism. But it was almost entirely the result of Cruise's co-stars, Brad Pitt and Antonio Banderas, who effectively "stole" the entire project. Clearly, if Cruise was in the closet, then the hinges on his door needed oiling.

"I had a joke last summer," recalls comic Lea DeLaria. "I was holding up that *Vanity Fair* with Tom Cruise on the cover and singing 'I'm not gay, I'm not gay' to the *Mission: Impossible* theme song. People screamed with laughter. It becomes silly."[9] She was, of course, exaggerating. But it was undeniable that the Cruise controversy was beginning to affect the gay community in many different ways.

"I think it angers people if they think someone is gay— which is why this whole Tom Cruise thing has gone on," says Robert L. Williams of League. "I have no knowledge about Tom Cruise whatsoever. I don't think anybody does. People have a lot of internalized homophobia when they feel they can't tell someone about their life, but they can release this sort of frustration and blame someone else. They can blame Tom Cruise for not—allegedly—coming out."[10]

"Unless he sleeps with me he's of absolutely no interest to me," journalist/filmmaker Richard Natale says coolly. "Knowing that he's gay would make me more depressed: not that he likes boys, but that he'd never like me. So what's the point? It doesn't bring him any closer to winding up in bed with me. In fact, I'd have a much better chance with some straight actor who felt like experimenting than I would with Tom Cruise. Because if Tom Cruise is gay, he can have anyone he wants!"[11]

And that, of course, is the beating heart of erotic fantasy—having anyone one could ever possibly want. And so in that sense—reality, for purposes of argument, be damned—Tom Cruise "is" gay.

"Even if it isn't factually true, it becomes part of common knowledge," Don Bachardy observes. "That's what makes it as good as true. It's true *eventually*. And that's why it simply won't go away from Tom Cruise. On the other hand, it seems to have gone away from John Travolta. It's partially because he's made a comeback after having appeared in a string of failures. It's also because of his marriage and their having a kid. And it's partly because—he's no longer attractive! Before all that it was inescapable."[12]

A Scientologist like Cruise, John Travolta flatly denied being homosexual when asked point-blank in a 1983 *Rolling Stone* interview: "That's a notorious rumor. . . . They say that about me, Marlon Brando, every male star, especially the first year you become a star. It wears off after a while, but I've heard it said of just about everybody."[13] This is, of course, a familiar complaint: suggesting that Hollywood is a town without gays, only heterosexuals falsely accused.

Travolta's denial was registered seven years in advance of a *National Enquirer* article in which gay porn performer Paul Baressi claimed "I Was John Travolta's Gay Lover," with a picture of the two of them together, circa 1982, included to supply "proof."

"I would like to apologize to John Travolta and his family but also to the gay community and anyone else I may have offended. I cashed in. If I could do it over again, I wouldn't," Baressi told the *Advocate* in an interview five months later—without formally denying the affair took place.[14] But Baressi, a curious figure who cropped up as a tabloid informant during the 1994 Michael Jackson child-molestation scandal, clearly lacks the "credibility" normally associated with "informed sources" (though the heavily hyped "scandals" surrounding President Clinton may have altered that concept forever). Whatever his relationship with Baressi may or may not have been, John Travolta is married to actress Kelly Preston (another active Scientologist), whom he met while filming *The Experts*, a barely released 1989 comedy made at the lowest point of his career. The couple (who have a son, Jet) are still together. As for Travolta's career, it's been put in such high gear that as the century comes to a close it's harder to think of the films he *isn't* in. And while he's as scrupulous regarding public relations as any other actor in Hollywood, Travolta has shown none of the "control freak" tendencies many have attributed to Cruise. Moreover, his personal charm has made him a welcome television-talk-show presence, even though—as Don Bachardy notes—"he's just not pretty anymore."[15]

Perhaps Cruise's public-relations problems might be accounted for by an aura of blandness that gay rumors—if nothing else—serve to dispel. For even his divorce and remarriage, ordinarily the stuff of reams of press copy, passed as mere blips on the Hollywood radar screen.

In 1987 he wed actress Mimi Rogers, a Scientologist six years his senior. In a *Rolling Stone* interview published in January of 1990, Cruise remarked, "I care about my wife more than anything in the world. She's my best friend."[16] But the very month the interview appeared Cruise filed for divorce. In December of that year Cruise married another Scientologist, actress Nicole Kidman, and in interviews began to refer to her as "best friend" as well. They have adopted two children. Yet when it comes to romance, Kidman has been put well into the shade by Rosie O'Donnell, who has whiled away countless talk-show hours declaring her undying devotion to "my Tommy." Oddly enough, O'Donnell's hyperactive toadying has done more to make Tom Cruise look like a semiordinary mortal than any up-close-and-personal chat with the more sedate likes of Barbara Walters ever could.

Meanwhile, Cruise has, like so many others in Hollywood, found a way to negotiate "gay" through the splashiest of all AIDS charity events, the annual "Commitment to Life" gala. "Halfway through the program," journalist David J. Fox wrote of the 1994 presentation, "Tom Cruise noted the thousands of names of the dead that had been flashing on overhead screens and, in one of the more remarkably touching moments, asked the audience to stand and shout out the names of the friends, lovers, relatives they have lost."[17] Fox would succumb to the disease himself not long after writing those words.

Cruise, for his part, was discovering favorable publicity on another front. "Actor Tom Cruise is being praised as a hero for calling paramedics to help a woman in Santa Monica who was injured in a hit-and-run accident and then paying her hospital bill," the Santa Monica *Outlook* noted in March of 1996.[18] In July of that year, the *Los Angeles Times* noted a repeat performance of sorts:

> Tom Cruise turned on the heroics when he rescued a 7-year-old London boy being crushed in a crowd of fans at the London premiere of *Mission: Impossible*. Cruise, arriving with wife Nicole Kidman Thursday night, rushed to help Laurence Sadler when he saw him being pressed against a barrier..... "It was scary, man. I could see the color draining from the kid's face," Cruise told the press. "After I pulled him out I gave him a hug and he seemed OK." Sadler's mother, Kim, praised the star. "At first I was worried for Laurence but he ended up having the time of his life."[19]

But no sooner had these favorable items registered than (shades of Tom Selleck) Cruise found himself launching a $60 million lawsuit against the German magazine *Bunte* for calling him "a sterile man with a zero sperm count." An article about the suit published in the *Hollywood Reporter* quoted "Cruise's lawyer, Bert Fields, [saying that] the actors' career depends on his fans' 'willingness to believe that he does or could possibly possess the qualities of the characters he plays.' "[20]

It's a breathtakingly bizarre statement. Surely even Cruise's most devoted fan didn't believe that the actor actually propelled his body through a railway tunnel in the shot of *Mission: Impossible* that was then being featured in the trailer run at least once an hour on every television outlet in the known world. Therefore, it was scarcely a surprise when later that month, throwing sperm-count caution to the wind, the *Los Angeles Times* reported that *"Mission: Impossible* star Tom Cruise sprang to action in real life when he helped rescue five people whose yacht caught fire off of Italy's resort island of Capri."[21] It was beginning to be a regular routine.

Still, there was one rescue effort Cruise couldn't make—though that didn't stop him from intervening verbally. For in August of 1997, when Princess Diana met her death in a Paris traffic tunnel, shots of the crushed car being wheeled away, beamed live worldwide by CNN, were accompanied by a live voice-over commentary by . . . Tom Cruise. Putting aside his usual media shyness, the actor solemnly expounded on the murderous appetites of the paparazzi—who, as the world eventually learned, can be said to have played only a marginal role, if any, in what turned out to be a simple drunk-driving accident. When a mere actor can claim such august authority over so ghastly an event, it seems almost churlish of him to object to public interest in his sexuality.

B ut Cruise can't claim to be singled out as a scapegoat of public hysteria over same-sexuality. "For some reason unknown to us, there has been an enormous amount of speculation in Europe lately concerning the state of our marriage," begins the "Personal Statement" by Richard Gere and Cindy Crawford published as a full-page advertisement in the London *Times* on May 6, 1994. "This all stems from a very crude, ignorant and libelous 'article' in a French tabloid," the statement continued, without mentioning the publication in question, *Voici*, by name. "We both feel quite foolish responding to such nonsense, but since it seems to have reached some sort of critical mass, here's our statement to correct the falsehoods and rumours and hope it will alleviate the concerns of our friends and fans."

Voici had claimed that the Gere/Crawford marriage was a sham that was about to end because the actor had decided to come out as a gay man. To the contrary, the Personal Statement insisted, "we got married because we love each other and we decided to make a life together. We are heterosexual and monogamous and take our commitment to each other very seriously. There is not and never has been a pre-nuptial agreement of any kind. Reports of a divorce are totally false. There are no plans, nor have there ever been any plans, for a divorce. We remain very married. We both look forward to having a family. Richard is not abandoning his career. He is starting a film in July with others planned to follow.

"Marriage is hard enough without all this negative speculation," the statement concluded, adding the admonition that "thoughts and words are very powerful, so please be responsible, truthful and kind."[22] As if this were insufficient, Gere's publicist, Pat Kingsley, told the same paper two days later, "All this is totally false. There is no problem. Everything is absolutely fine with them."[23]

However, by that summer Gere and Crawford had divorced.

That Richard Gere would become party to such an awkward PR stunt was a surprise to many. Many of his closest friends—including photographer Herb Ritts and agent Ed Limato—are gay. Gere has never been shy about supporting gay rights and AIDS causes. Like many non-macho-obsessed European stars, he has never been shy about embracing male friends in public in a manner that only the sex-obsessed would call homoerotic. As for more formal erotic display, Gere's career was in many ways jump-started by the portraits Ritts took of him fairly early on—much in the manner of a modern equivalent of the glamour shots of the studio era. And in those portraits, Gere displays none of the sexual skittishness associated with those concerned about their audience's gender.

According to Limato, *Esquire* reported, "the idea for the ad came from Gere's advisers. 'He was talked into it. . . . She [Crawford] agreed to it. He had turned the other cheek for too long.' "[24]

What Gere had "turned the other cheek" to weren't the usual gay rumors, which had circulated ever since his appearance on film in *American Gigolo* and onstage in the play about gay Holocaust victims, *Bent*. For in the wake of the release of *Pretty Woman* (1990), a patently absurd story had begun to circulate—literally nationwide—that Gere had been admitted to the emergency room of Cedars-Sinai Hospital in Los Angeles to remove a gerbil from his rectum.

In an analysis of this "urban legend" published in the *Advocate*, journalist Catherine Seipp traced the gerbil story back beyond Gere, when it was linked to television news anchormen in Philadelphia and Oklahoma in the 1970s. It was revived again at the time of Rock Hudson's passing, as a supposed new fad among the most decadent of gay sophisticates. But it was with Gere that the story, somehow, found a more solid target.

> "I personally first heard the gerbil rumors in 1967, back in junior high," says Sergeant Corl Whetstone, field supervisor for the SPCA's investigation department. "In the last twenty years, I've heard about ten different male celebrities, mentioning four or five different hospitals—and in the stories, they always go to a highly public hospital, never a private doctor.
>
> "About this actor," Whetstone continues, "we've received about 25 different phone calls [from people] who know a friend of a friend who would lose his job if he came forth. This is [a story] that will not die."

But this was not the most fascinating aspect of the gerbil story. For in the course of her investigation Seipp learned that gerbils are banned in California under Fish and Game Code 2118, Section 671, Title 14. In other words, not only was Richard Gere being accused of having carnal knowledge of a gerbil, but one that had been smuggled illegally across state lines.[25]

Gere might have been better advised to follow the example of actor Alec Baldwin, who was cited in Charles Kaiser's *The Gay Metropolis* in a chapter concerning that most egregiously overpublicized of mass-media phenomena, Studio 54, as he had once worked there as a waiter. Thinking he might be upset, the ever-sensitive Liz Smith "called Alec ready for an onslaught. He laughed. 'Liz, the idea that anyone reading this book would take the implication as meaning I am gay makes me absolutely ecstatic. These days it's a compliment. I couldn't be more pleased. . . .' " Kaiser had, in point of fact, discovered this information via Baldwin himself, as the high-spirited actor had several years before in *Interview* magazine recalled with great amusement how many a well-heeled gentleman would tip him generously if he would be so kind as to "fetch" them a pack of cigarettes.[26]

Tom Cruise, too, would be well advised to follow Baldwin's example.

"When you're going to see a film starring Tom Cruise, chances are if you're a man, whether you're straight or gay, you'll identify with him, want to be him, want to be near him, be attracted to something he did or said," says Morgan Rumpf of Outfest. "Like there's that famous quote, I forget from where, of 'I wouldn't kick him out of bed for eating crackers.' If it was that scenario—the desert-island scenario, the elevator-stopping scenario we've all heard a million times—we'd all be thrilled and delighted."

Rumpf sees the current, looser atmosphere as heralding a trend in better relations between the different sexual orientations.

"Just as there were a lot of scripts looked into after *The Birdcage* that were dealing with issues of drag—funny drag characters that 'everybody can respond to and love'—now we're going to see a series of 'gay best friend' movies like *My Best Friend's Wedding*. It's something people feel comfortable in dealing with. It's not the leading character. You don't see his love interest. He has a dinner party in the film where you see his lover there, so you know he has a lover. He's referred to, he's a handsome man, they are together. And they have no interaction in any way that would make the audience uncomfortable. It's funny to have somebody quipping throughout the film and saying fabulous lines that you can laugh *with*. And one thing I will give the film incredible kudos for is that you're laughing *with* this character and not *at* him. He is the savvy, funny character that you want to identify with. It's something that women—and this is a film that's definitely targeted at women—are comfortable with. Here's a nonthreatening character that's truly original and funny. Or maybe he won't be funny. Maybe he'll be used in other ways.

"Tom Cruise can have his life, and whether he's gay or not, I don't care. There will be a person to take advantage of this moment and be the first gay action hero. And maybe it's Rupert Everett."[27]

Indeed, there's every reason to believe that it may very well be Rupert Everett. For while tongues had idly wagged about Cruise allegedly being in the closet, few in the media had noticed someone who was already out—until he captured mass-media attention with his entire-movie-stealing turn in *My Best Friend's Wedding*. And part of the reason for this has to do with the fact that many in the media have no idea about how to talk about him.

"Mr. Everett, one of the few actors to say that he is gay," begins Bernard Weinraub of *The New York Times*, on the actor's sudden (at least as far as Hollywood was concerned) success, observing the editorial etiquette that demands gayness remain invisible unless it is announced formally in quasi-ceremonial fashion.[28] Everett had no such ceremony, being "out" from the very beginning of his career— had any party chosen to inquire. The real story of *My Best Friend's Wedding* was that a performer who had a least a decade's worth of success in low-budget European film and theater behind him was making an unexpected splash in a commercial arena where few would have imagined he'd ever find a home.

Rupert Everett has played a rather wide variety of characters, ranging from a gay university student who becomes a secret agent and deserts England for the Soviet Union (*Another Country*), to a thoroughly heterosexual upper-class twit done in by his barmaid mistress (*Dance with a Stranger*), to a passive thrill-seeker who becomes the unwitting victim of a murderous couple (*The Company of Strangers*), to the feckless womanizing son of a fashion designer (*Ready to Wear*), to a foppish seventeenth-century aristocrat (*The Madness of King George*) and a cartoonish bit player in a family comedy (*Dunston Checks In*). And that's not to mention his two comic novels (*Hello Darling, Are You Working?* and *The Hairdresser of St. Tropez*), or theater work that has encompassed everything from Noël Coward's *The Vortex* to the (formally female) lead in Tennessee Williams's *The Milk Train Doesn't Stop Here Anymore*. "I'm not really in drag because I'm not trying to convince the audience that I'm a woman; I'm trying to convince myself," Everett has said of his stage performance. "I'm a queen with dementia. It's something I've seen happen to people with AIDS, which is a spectre we are trying to raise throughout this part." [29]

But that's a minor act of public-relations "bravery" compared to Everett's confession that *Hello Darling, Are You Working?*, his novel about hustling, was based on personal experience.

"Hustling and acting are the same thing," Everett "snarled" to writer Brad Gooch, "except one you're applauded for and given Oscars and Césars and you can play golf with the president like Kevin Costner. The other you're a reject from society. And they're both equally dangerous. I do admit that being a hustler is the worst thing for your head. But so is being an actor, emotionally. Once you've done that sense-memory thing in front of the camera, where you draw on what for most people is private in public, then that becomes the only way you can do emotion. It's rather like hustlers who can only do sex for money. In fact, that's why a lot of actors have bad marriages."[30]

Whatever "sense memory" resources were required for Everett's performance in *My Best Friend's Wedding*, it not only boosted his career but laid to rest the canard that "mainstream" audiences wouldn't "accept" gay characters—particularly if they were played by "openly gay" performers. For not only did Everett "test well" in the film' early screenings, he proved so popular that the film's makers reshot the ending in order to include him in it.[31]

"I'm being offered a mixture, though I wouldn't mind playing just gay roles," Everett confessed to *People* magazine—in further defiance of the long-held Hollywood belief that gay actors would feel "limited" if only offered gay roles.[32]

"I suppose that's a good sign," says Don Bachardy. "But I still think it's very tricky for an actor like Rupert to declare himself openly and play parts. I'm very interested to see where he goes from here—if he can continue being open in the 'mainstream' movies. He has ambitions to direct, you know. In fact, at one point he came to see me to ask if he could have the rights to a story in *Down There on a Visit*—the 'Ambrose' story. At that point Tony Richardson was still alive and he was ready to produce it and give Everett his first directorial chance. Then they quarreled. I haven't heard from him since."[33]

Everett being Everett, he might very well call Bachardy back. But he has always gone his own way. It would be to Hollywood's everlasting benefit to follow his example. For remembering Rupert Everett is the best possible way to forget all about Tom Cruise.

THE FURTHER

DECAY OF

LYING

—

IF A MAN IS SUFFICIENTLY UNIMAGINA-
tive to produce evidence in support of a lie, he might just as

well speak the truth at once." So wrote Oscar Wilde in "The Decay

of Lying," a critical dialogue first published in 1889. Six years later

the great writer found himself standing in a British court of law, un-

able either to produce evidence to support a lie or to speak the truth
of his sexual identity. Over one hundred years later, those gays and
lesbians in the Hollywood spotlight unwilling to deal honestly with
their same-sexual truth in a public forum are as tongue-tied as Wilde
once was.

No one in Hollywood is standing in the dock these days, facing,
as Wilde did, the prospect of prison and public humiliation. In fact,
as "scandals" go, same-sex orientation (provided it isn't divulged
through what can only be called a George Michael moment) is far
from the biggest PR problem faced by Hollywood stars and their handlers. Drug addiction, prostitution, pedophilia, spousal abuse, and the
curious confluence of crime and celebrity known worldwide by the
letters O and J have resulted in a pile-up of problems even a Pat
Kingsley can't finesse. As a result, same-sex attraction, in and of
itself, seems almost . . . normal.

Hollywood in 1998 is no longer synonymous with sex "scandals" to begin with. As the nation contemplates the curvature of the
presidential penis, pausing every so often to catch the latest variation
of "I Married a Transsexual Lesbian Stripper" on the afternoon television talk shows, it only goes to show that sexuality, of any sort of
variation, is no longer a "private" matter. For those who struggled
through the decades that saw the emergence of the gay and lesbian
civil rights movement, that's as it should be. If nothing else, the movement proved that the "polite" societal declaration that "I don't care
what people do in bed so long as they don't push it in my face" was
a lie—albeit a multifaceted one.

People don't live their lives "in bed." But an insistence on
hiding the fact that same-sex activity goes on there affects every aspect of "out of bed" existence. Unimpressed straights should try nav-
igating a typical day imagining that any mention or circumstantial
indication of heterosexuality (wives, husbands, children, boy- and
girlfriends) was for some arbitrary reason suddenly declared forbid-
den. It should give them an idea of the minefield gays and lesbians
in perfectly ordinary walks of life are forced to trip through daily. Gay
and lesbian performers in Hollywood don't have to go through such a
minefield. They have public-relations representatives to scout the ter-

ritory for them. Logically speaking, there's nothing stopping any performer from pulling his or her sails in and leading a perfectly "private" life, out of the firing range of an increasingly pervasive mass media. But there's a publicity price to be paid for this loss of "exposure." And so the question has become (as was never the case in the past): "Just how 'out' can I afford to be?"

Ellen (and *Ellen*) will doubtless be pointed to (at least in the short run) as an example of dangers risked by becoming "too political." But the cancellation of the ultra-"mainstream" *Dr. Quinn, Medicine Woman* only weeks after DeGeneres's noble experiment came to grief testifies to the fact that there's little safety to be found in "playing it safe" either. Meanwhile, elsewhere in Hollywood, the search for the magic formula that will translate gay and lesbian into box-office magic still goes on—aided by the fact that for a new generation same-sexuality is no longer limited to the ghettos of New York's West Village, San Francisco's Castro, or Los Angeles's West Hollywood. Films have become a vital reflection of this.

You don't have to go to the "sexual underworld" to meet gay people, as was done in the otherwise radically different *Cruising* (1980) and *Victor/Victoria* (1982). As *As Good As It Gets* (1997) shows, the "gay world" is no farther away than a neighbor's apartment. *The Object of My Affection* (1998) is even more radical on this score, in that the hero's emotional character is not made explicable through sexual activity alone. Gays and lesbians are now simply part of the mix. Thanks to Rupert Everett, that mix need not be commercially disconcerting. And thanks to Anne Heche, we're offered the prospect of a world in which sexuality is fluid rather than regimented, and sexual identity inspires thoughtful queries rather than knee-jerk reactions.

We are all—straight and gay, in Hollywood and out—facing a future quite different from the one Proust described in *Sodome et Gomorrhe*, in which he wrote: "When the day has dawned on which they have discovered themselves to be incapable at once of lying to themselves, they go away to live in the country, shunning the society of their own kind (whom they believe to be few in number) from horror of the monstrosity or fear of the temptation, and that of the rest of humanity from shame." This may have been true for some in the fin-de-siècle France Proust knew. And it was certainly true of Proust himself—at least up until the moment that he wrote his book. For in the heat of that moment, and the many moments that came after that as he toiled away in his cork-lined room composing his multivolumed magnum opus, *Proust was lying*.

He would have liked Hollywood.

THE
EPILOGUE
STRIKES
BACK

—

CHARTING THE ROLES OF GAYS AND LES-
bians in the entertainment industry in 1998 is like trying to

publish a map of Eastern Europe as the Soviet Union shattered." So

said journalist Kevin Allman in his *Washington Post* review of the first edition of this book.[1] But in the year since those words were written, it's become painfully clear that as the century turns, charting the roles gays and lesbians are taking on everywhere is an even more daunting task. And the consequences of this cultural realignment, as journalist Joan Biskupic has pointed out in a 1999 "think" piece for that same publication, are more far-reaching than most of us—gay or straight—are yet fully aware of: "From workplace discrimination to child custody, a clear and distinct pattern is emerging as courts, spurred by cultural and political changes across the country, apply the principles of equality to sexual orientation. Just as homosexuality has moved from the fringe to the mainstream of American culture in recent years, gay rights has become a flourishing area of the law."[2]

And a flourishing subject of media attention as well. Back in the early 1970s, activists had to move heaven and earth to get any gay issue into the "mainstream." Today, fourth estate coverage of same-sex American life is practically nonstop. Consider just a small handful of stories that popped up in 1999 alone:

- In a culture that continues to cringe at the sight of the words "Boy Scout" and "homosexual" in the same sentence, former Scout James Dale learned that no less august a body than the New Jersey Supreme Court had ruled in his favor in an antidiscrimination case, demanding the Boy Scouts of America allow the continued participation of stellar—yet openly gay—scouts like himself.[3]

- Then there's Steven May, the Republican state representative from Arizona who stood up for his right to serve in the military reserves in defiance of its "Don't Ask, Don't Tell" policy. While his loss of this battle is a foregone conclusion, May took the opportunity to take on a member of his own party, whose antigay remarks the twenty-seven-year-old congressman characterized as "attacks on my family."[4]

- And then there's David Knight, the estranged gay son of another Republican, California State Senator William "Pete"

Knight, taking issue with a father who has "authored and pushed a number of antigay bills in the legislature," the most recent being a "definition of marriage" initiative designed to exclude same-sex couples. As the younger Knight made plain, there was a decidedly personal level to such actions, not only in regard to his own gayness, but also in regard to his uncle, who died of AIDS.[5]

- But perhaps the most striking 1999 story of all is the saga of Michael Huffington, the multimillionaire who came out of the closet he'd resided in for twenty-seven of his fifty-two years in the wake of both a failed 1994 run for the California Senate (which saw him spend more of his personal fortune on a political campaign than any individual in American history), and his 1997 divorce from omnipresent media pundit Arianna.

According to Huffington's journalistic Father Confessor—self-described "right-wing hit man" David Brock—the couple's children were conceived with the help of some rather unusual visual aids. "She became pregnant after they watched the film *Wings of Desire* at the River Oaks Theater," Brock relates of the Huffingtons' first child, going on to note that their second daughter "was conceived in Houston after the couple watched another film, *Jésus of Montréal*." One can only regret that Brock didn't query the films' respective stars, Bruno Ganz and Lothaire Bluteau, as to their views on being utilized as virtual Viagra. But few in the media would have gone as far as this intriguingly intrepid reporter did in speaking frankly with Huffington about his sexual orientation on any level. Arianna, however, was a different story.

Taking full advantage of the discomfort traditional journalism has had with gay and lesbian matters, always holding them in "mainstream" check (see chapter 7 regarding the reaction to Ellen DeGeneres), the former Mrs. Huffington firmly refused to answer any questions about her curious marriage—despite the fact that her ex-husband's gayness was known to her from the start and, according to

Brock, "made her love him all the more."[6] Instead she has gone on in her columns and numerous television appearances to declare that the "private lives" of politicians should remain off-limits to media scrutiny—even though her *überpundit* status largely sprang from the sport she'd made of President Clinton's judicially disclosed extramarital shenanigans.

Indeed, Oval Office heterosexcapades have only served to place same-sexuality in a far less transgressive, though nonetheless intriguing, light than ever before. Consider the way in which a small, quite unsensational article in the *Miami Herald* about the recently uncloseted life of an obscure, retired Major League center fielder named Billy Bean inspired a larger piece in the *New York Times* and several different television newsmagazine program items. And rather than merely underscoring the novelty of an "openly gay" baseball player, the articles and broadcasts spoke of the happiness Bean had found with his lover, a Miami restaurateur.[7]

But all such stories took a backseat to the continuing reverberations from the death of Matthew Shepard, the gay college student savagely beaten and left to die tied to a fence along a highway in Laramie, Wyoming, in October 1998. Throughout 1999 scores of articles, cover stories, and "prime-time" television broadcasts covered the crime, its victim, its perpetrators, and the calls for hate crimes legislation that came in its wake.

This was all quite without precedent. Matthew Shepard was far from the first—and certainly not the last—gay or lesbian individual to meet such a horridly ignominious end. But none of those who came before or after Shepard made news to this extent. Indeed, most gay murder victims were lucky to win a mention in the back pages of a local paper. Surely Shepard's slight build and boyish, "innocent-looking" features played a large part in his capturing the national fancy. In February 1999 a nondescript thirty-nine-year-old gay man named Billy Jack Gaither was beaten and burned to death in Sylacauga, Alabama—an ugly finish that wasn't granted anywhere near as much attention as was afforded Shepard's passing.[8] Still, had it transpired prior to Shepard's death, Gaither's murder wouldn't have registered as a national news story at all.

"The biggest problem we've got is the primitive, age-old fear and hatred and dehumanization of the other—people who aren't like us," President Clinton told an audience of well-heeled gay and lesbian politicos at a Human Rights Campaign dinner, practically a year to the day after the Shepard killing.[9] His words were more than slightly ironic in that his failure to rescind the military's antigay discrimination policy had resulted in no end of costly and damaging dismissals of otherwise qualified service personnel. Then there was his signing of the so-called Defense of Marriage Act—which banned same-sex marriage even though the practice has no legal standing to begin with—in order to placate congressional homophobes and their fundamentalist Christian allies. Worst of all, a Shepard-like killing occurred on Commander-in-Chief Clinton's watch that summer, as Private First Class Barry Winchell had been beaten to death with a baseball bat by another soldier in his unit while yet another goaded him on. The soldiers had discovered that Winchell was gay, and rather than "ask or "tell" they elected to kill.[10]

Happily, the century's end finds no parallel for this example of "unit cohesion" in Hollywood. The state of same-sex life—both on and off the screen—continues to improve at a steady, if not exactly brisk, pace. And the comings and goings of those who participated in the first edition of *Open Secret*—decidedly less troubled than those going on elsewhere in America—certainly reflect this. Yet one cannot help but think about this roiling background when contemplating such a tranquil Hollywood foreground.

Gods and Monsters (whose production was highlighted in chapter 3) turned out to be not only a fine film, but also a critical sensation, an independent hit, and the winner of the Academy Award for Best Adapted Screenplay of 1998. One of the highlights of the Oscar broadcast was the sight of writer-director Bill Condon beaming down from the podium at his cast—Ian McKellen, Brendan Fraser, and Lynn Redgrave—arms happily intertwined and faces beaming back up at him. It almost served to make up for the fact that McKellen, who had won almost all of the best actor prizes from the film critics' circles that

year was passed over by the Academy in favor of the relentlessly publicized Roberto Begnini. Could it be that Academy voters still harbored the quaint notion that a gay man playing a gay man was simply
"being himself" and not "really acting"? Perhaps. Not that McKellen
should worry about such things, being as much in demand as ever for
films as big budget and "high-concept" as *X-Men*—Bryan Singer's
rendition of the cutting-edge comic book whose gay subtext has been
the subject of much discussion in the world of pop culture.

McKellen has clearly found a route to the "mainstream." But
actress/comedienne/chanteuse Lea DeLaria (chapter 7) continues to
ply its tributaries. Though winning good notices for her role in the
independently made *Edge of Seventeen*, she's not on big-time Hollywood's radar at the moment. Rather she's continued to rock the world
of live theater with performances in productions as diverse as Paul
Rudnick's religious satire *The Most Fabulous Story Ever Told*, to a
revival of Rodgers and Hart's *The Boys from Syracuse*. However, the
"mainstream" seems very much within the grasp of writer-director
Andrew Fleming (chapter 10), who won critical approval for his Watergate satire *Dick*. Though its wit failed to register with audiences
facing far more entertainment choices than they ever have in the past,
it nonetheless solidified his growing reputation as an "up-and-comer."

Jill Abrams (chapters 1 and 7), meanwhile, has left CNN's
Showbiz Today program to become an independent publicist, which
(if you think about it for a moment) is scarcely a radical change. Gay
grip Steven Dornbush (chapters 5 and 7) has gone into the catering
business—which in Hollywood is a similarly lateral move, as it finds
him crossing paths with any number of people for whom he'd worked
in the past. Harry Clein (see chapter 6) enhanced his standing as one
of the smartest people in Hollywood in 1999 by spearheading the
publicity campaign that turned a low-budget horror programmer
called *The Blair Witch Project* into the surprise sensation of the year.
The most active of the *Open Secret* "movers and shakers," however,
remains Chris Pula, whose exit from Warner Bros. (chapter 10) was
followed by an equally intense ten-month stint as head of marketing
for Walt Disney Pictures worldwide. As for his future, he reports, "I'm
planning to decode the Rosetta Stone."[11]

Gus Van Sant (chapter 8) is as much in the Hollywood mix as ever, though his Anne Heche–starring, practically shot-for-shot remake of Alfred Hitchcock's *Psycho* greatly annoyed critics and barely registered with audiences. Much of 1999 saw him being courted by John Travolta (of all people), who wanted him to direct *Standing Room Only*, the life of Mafia-linked singer Jimmy Roselli. But when this pet Travolta project failed to jell financially as a Disney coproduction, it was unceremoniously dropped by the star (and Van Sant's participation along with it) in favor of *Battleship Earth,* an independent film of the posthumously published L. Ron Hubbard science fiction novel about an alien invasion. Still, Van Sant has scarcely been left in any sort of lurch. He has *Brokeback Mountain* in development, as well as *Don't Worry He Won't Get Far on Foot,* the story of paraplegic cartoonist John Callahan, which he expects will reunite him with his *Good Will Hunting* star Robin Williams. And then there's his planned adaptation of Francine du Plessix Gray's *At Home with the Marquis de Sade.*

"The movies have become a different game," the Portland-based auteur observes philosophically, having experienced any number of career highs and lows. "[And] the press is very conservative. I wasn't aware of that."[12]

Ellen DeGeneres surely knows "the game," not to mention the press, in light of the media tsunami of 1997. But in 1999, her featured roles in *Goodbye Lover, Ed TV,* and *The Love Letter* quietly slipped through with only passing comment. Her lover, Anne Heche, meanwhile, continued to carve out a space for herself in the independent arena with a solid turn as the rebellious daughter of a modern saint in *The Third Miracle.* As an off-screen couple, DeGeneres and Heche have continued to lend their services as spokespersons for gay/lesbian causes. Still, DeGeneres hasn't neglected television, appearing in a Heche-directed, lesbian-themed, multipart HBO telefilm, *If These Walls Could Talk 2*—one episode of which casts the comedienne opposite Sharon Stone. Plus there's talk of her possibly doing another sitcom. As for her now-far-from-private life, she's announced that should same-sex marriage come to pass in Vermont, she and Heche would move there in a trice.[13]

Hollywood's most famous "out" lesbians can only have been awestruck by the phenomenon of *Will & Grace,* an "openly gay" sitcom about a male–female platonic friendship, whose success has defied the warnings of media "experts" who claimed that the demise of *Ellen* proved "mainstream" America "wasn't ready" for gay. The reason that America was ready—Rupert Everett—continued to triumph in 1999 both on-screen (in the successful film version of Oscar Wilde's *An Ideal Husband*) and off, via glamorous public appearances on the arms of Julia Roberts and Madonna, whose status as "good pals" carries nothing of the "beard" about them. Taking on a tailor-made lead in *The Next Best Thing,* John Schlesinger's film about a gay man who in a "just one of those things" moment fathers a child by his best female friend (the inescapable Madonna), Everett still has his sights set on playing a gay James Bond–styled secret agent.

"The trouble is one should never talk about things that are in embryo," the soignée superstar declared, "because a lot of stuff happens that you put into development doesn't make it over the first fence, or then the second or the third fence, and it's the end of the race. So that's why it's sometimes better not to talk about it."[14]

"Rupert's Mr. Gay America now," says his friend filmmaker John Maybury, who cast Everett, Derek Jarman muse Tilda Swinton, and gay porn star Aidan Shaw in his prizewinning 1996 avant-garde video *Remembrance of Things Fast.* "You know what he said after the success of *My Best Friend's Wedding*? 'I'm only going to work with these camp, A-list famous women. They love it 'cause they're sick of working with these straight boys. They'll have a great time with me and tell all their girlfriends.' "

Will it work?

"Rupert's the most hopeless strategist known to mankind," says Maybury, laughing, "but she always lands on her high heels!"[15]

Maybury may feel free and easy in talking about his friend, but the "mainstream" media has no idea of how to do so. They seem stunned into silence at the thought of an actor with Everett's increasingly high profile matter-of-factly "admitting" the simple truth about his sexual orientation. Doubtless it's a tad early for *People* cover stories on the order of "Playboy Rupert Finds Paradise for Two in Laurel Canyon Love Nest"; still, it's odd to see the tabloid press chary of tracking Everett's "private life," preferring instead to remain in a fugue state by regarding same-sexuality in Hollywood solely as a "secret" whose "revelation" is feared by one and all. Trying to keep pace with the fact that reader awareness has made gay stories viable, yet proving that old habits die hard, the *National Enquirer* went so far as to confect a cover story, "Travolta Shocker: The Gay Charges & the Truth About His Marriage."[16] The "shock" was just a rehash of decades-old gossip (see chapter 12) with no new information, save for the fact that a lawsuit launched by a disgruntled former Scientology acolyte (who claimed Church officials had told him they'd "cured" Travolta of same-sex attraction and could do the same for him) had been thrown out of court. Richard Gere (see chapter 12) likewise found himself in tabloid fugue state, with the *National Examiner* serving up a "Gay Shocker" story whose supposed "shock" was that anyone would ever consider him gay.[17] Hadn't Pat Kingsley already moved heaven and earth to make sure they wouldn't?

The *National Enquirer*, by contrast, found some actual tabloid news in Kingsley client Jodie Foster (see chapter 5) via a heavily telephoto-lensed piece on her baby, Charles, and her "constant companion," production coordinator Cydney Bernard. "Jodie has tried to downplay her relationship with Cydney," one of the *Enquirer*'s army of unidentified "insiders" reported, letting the visual proximity supplied by the photos speak for themselves—just as had been done in the past with Rosie O'Donnell.[18]

Elsewhere the tabs embroiled themselves in "gay" on the purely superficial level. A calculatedly "provocative" *Rolling Stone* cover of Brad Pitt wearing a dress (and looking about as homoerotic as a dead fish), coupled with an old college days photo of him larking about in women's garb in best frat-boy style, mixed with quotes from a handful of gay magazine editors to the effect that millions of same-sex-oriented men find Pitt attractive ("Well, duh!" as children say nowadays) was all it took for the *National Examiner* to headline "Brat Pitt: Truth About Gay Rumors."[19] Never mind that only a few months before this very same tab was filling its pages with photos of Pitt and then girl-friend Gwyneth Paltrow in the nude. Still, the Flimsy Pretext Grand Prize must go to *The Globe* for its "Prince Charles: 'I'm Gay!' "[20] What was the Di-obsessed periodical blathering about? According to the usual unnamed "sources" the Royal heir was so ill-disposed to con-jugal relations with his wife that he begged off by telling her he pre-ferred men. But as anyone with the slightest acquaintance with the late socialite/land mine expert knows, this announcement would scarcely have dissuaded her any more than it would have . . . Arianna Huffington.

"I'm friends with Diana's stepbrother," John Maybury says, commenting ruefully on the secular sainthood the bulimic fashion plate has received posthumously. "She was camp to the tits, she was! She used to say 'I'm seeing the Girls for dinner tonight.' That would mean Elton John and George Michael!"[21]

Such dinners would have no home in the tabs, where lower-middle-class "family values" rule. But 1999 found ever-so-slightly more adventurous media outlets venturing into uncharted same-sex waters more often. And not on account of anyone's desire to "reveal" a "scandal," but rather due to the increasing candor of the celebrities they had chosen to profile.

"I've acted upon gay situations less than practically every other man I know," Robert Downey Jr. tellingly informed trend-conscious *Detour* magazine.[22] His now formally admitted bisexuality was no sur-prise to anyone so much as half-awake on the Los Angeles club scene. But the far from subtle implication of his remark was that there were more same-sex-related stories in the Naked City of the Angels worth telling—if reporters and their editors were disposed to do so. Clearly, drug abuse, which eventually won Downey prison incarceration, is an infinitely more serious problem in Hollywood than same-sex orien-tation. In fact for some, being gay isn't problematic at all, for 1999 saw several notables bypassing the "Full Oprah" form of coming out, à la Ellen, by simply being out from day one.

Kevin Williamson, the creator of horror franchises *Scream* and

I Know What You Did Last Summer, in addition to the hit television series *Dawson's Creek*, is in charge of adolescent America in a way that no one in Hollywood has been since the heyday of Walt Disney. Yet he has never known "the closet" at any point in his professional life. And as befits the power that has come with Hollywood success, Williamson has inserted a gay character and story line into his series.[23] In some ways, an even more interesting example of "no fuss" outness is Alan Ball, author of the critically acclaimed dark comedy *American Beauty* and the less-acclaimed but nonetheless noted television sitcom *Oh, Grow Up*—both of which feature gay characters.

"In the real Brooklyn household, Ball's being the only gay guy was never an issue, something . . . he duplicates in the series," *Los Angeles Times* reporter Daryl H. Miller notes matter-of-factly of the sitcom's inspiration. "I put the gay character in there because that was one of the realities of the situation in the house I lived in in Brooklyn," Ball remarks. "Also, from a purely practical storytelling point, if you have one of the characters gay and the other two straight, it's going to give you more interesting areas to go than if they're all three straight."[24] No sitcom scribe would take issue with that (see chapter 11). But the most interesting aspect of Ball's success is the fact that *American Beauty* is exactly the sort of satire of middle-class heterosexual domesticity that critic Stanley Kauffmann, in a memorable *New York Times* broadside thirty years ago, claimed that Edward Albee, being gay, had no right to write.[25] But back then being "out" wasn't the option for Albee that it is for Ball today. Moreover, it would be highly unlikely that any contemporary critic would question Ball's "credentials" in the Kauffmann manner. And that's doubtless due to Ball's power position within the Hollywood matrix, and the fact that gays hold the cards in this town in a way they never have before.

"I keep getting asked why *Will & Grace* has done so well," says Max Mutchnick, the gay cocreator (with the openly straight David Kohan) of 1999's most unlikely hit. "I think it's because in a lot of ways what you're seeing in the show is a true dimension of what a regular gay guy is like. We don't run anything we do by anybody. And the day we start doing that is the day we start writing something with an agenda rather than an entertaining half hour."[26]

True, *Will & Grace* has benefited from sharp writing—and great casting—as it charts the relationship of a relatively buttoned-down lawyer (Eric McCormack), his high-spirited female "soul mate" (Debra Messing), and their wacky allies: a demented socialite (Megan Mullally) and a terminally dizzy gay man with no visible means of financial support (Sean Hayes). But what sets it apart from the pack is its lightness of spirit. *Will & Grace* isn't designed to delve all that deeply into the gay man/straight woman bond as *The Object of My Affection* did so interestingly. At the same time, it has avoided the pitfalls of both *Ellen*-style sincerity and the smart-ass freakishness of the short-lived Hollywood satire *Action!*, a show that managed to lampoon Barry Diller and work a male-male oral sex scene past the censors—without any discernible effect on its basement-level ratings.

Will & Grace, James Poniewozik observes in *Time*, wins out by staying within the "fuzzily defined but undeniable limits" that television has set for things gay. In other words, plenty of teasing jokes and tart remarks but no same-sex activity that would raise either the ire or the eyebrows of your aunt Martha. "Gay content and gay characters," Poniewozik notes, "serve as a sort of coolness shorthand, bestowing hipness on their shows and audience, serving as a conduit to cred for the majority group, just as racial minorities have in the past. From Norman Mailer's White Negro we've gone to the Gay Hetero."[27]

Still, for all this seeming ease, the old "Don't Ask, Don't Tell" boundaries reassert themselves when the cameras are off. As writer Karen Baldwin notes of *Will & Grace* costar Sean Hayes (who played a far less flamboyant gay man in the independent comedy *Billy's Hollywood Screen Kiss*), there's a decided disinclination to "address the personal is-he-or-isn't-he speculation that's come with his two out-there roles. 'Right now I'm just starting,' he explains. 'If I was forty and had $8 billion and nothing to worry about, I'd tell people when I go number two on the toilet."[28] In other words, a nonstatement on the order of "Yes—but you don't have my express permission to say so." Nathan Lane (as noted in chapter 5) teetered on this same edge-of-full-disclosure at first, but 1999 found him letting it all hang out in an *Advocate* interview, in which he declared, "this whole thing with

Matthew Shepard happened, and it was like somebody slapped me awake."[29]

Still, some require more than a slap. In 1999 the congenitally "gay-shy" Joel Schumacher (see chapter 9) edged toward the line when presenting a GLAAD award to MTV president Judy Marks, declaring, "I've never been in the closet. My life has been an open book."[30] Apparently, the problem stemmed from the fact that this "book" had been placed on a very high shelf. Schumacher, however, isn't all that anxious to move it down to a more accessible one. In the midst of promoting the release of *Flawless,* the drag-queen-bonds-with-homophobe comedy-drama that he wrote as well as directed, Schumacher pointedly declined to answer the question "Are you openly gay?" when a reporter for the *Toronto Sun* lobbed it at him point-blank. "Why is it always an African-American diplomat or a woman director or a gay actor?" the writer-director (who plans to produce an American version of the controversial British TV series *Queer As Folk*) asked his Canadian questioner. "Are we to assume that everyone in the world is a white heterosexual male Christian?"[31]

Well, as a matter of fact, yes. That's the way this society has always been run, and only the questions raised by its minority members have shaken this status quo. The problem is how to get said minorities to work together for the common good. And that can't be done from the confines of a closet. Or a bookshelf.

The gay bottom line is, as usual, a conflation of the personal with the financial. But it's a line unknown to the likes of actor Roddy McDowall or director Irving Rapper—two "gray eminences" from the Gay Hollywood of yore who passed just prior to the century's close— the latter expiring in its waning days at the exceedingly ripe age of 101. For conventional wisdom still rules Hollywood's upper echelons. That means that coming out is regarded as "killing" a career, in terms of lowering that person's overall financial expectations. Such restructuring has less of an impact on the star in question than it does on the future of those employees the star has hired to keep said career running. And on that front, Pat Kingsley, who had weathered the Ellen/*Ellen* wars, best described the situation in an interview she granted to Bernard Weinraub of the *New York Times* recalling the—

purely professional—role she played in the coming out of former tennis great Billie Jean King back in the 1970s.

"It was so difficult; it was at the end of her career on the courts, and it was going to ruin her ability to make money. She didn't feel she could lie about what happened. She wanted to deal with it in an aggressive way. I said, 'Let's do it here in Los Angeles.' So she gave her statement at this hotel down near the airport. And it was terribly difficult. Her mother and father were there, her family. And it was painful not knowing what the consequences would be. And the things she had signed up to represent went away. And they never came back to this day."[32]

One can easily imagine Kingsley recounting this as a cautionary tale of the risks of letting it all hang out to any number of her clients— same-sex-oriented or not. But one she won't have to lecture is Tom Cruise. After all, his heterosexuality has not only been verbally declared and journalistically tracked (as you have read in chapter 12), but visually elaborated as well in Stanley Kubrick's much-ballyhooed erotic thriller *Eyes Wide Shut*. Yet for all of this, the Cruise camp continues to be bent out of shape by the mere mention of the word "gay" in relation to their star, in almost any context. And what's resulted is an excess of publicity "smoke" that has only served to further suspicions of a gay scandal "fire."

During the summer of 1998, when the first edition of this book was still at the printer, a fairly dramatic exchange erupted between lawyers representing Cruise and those representing William Morrow. Having learned of the existence of chapter 12 through some hyperbolic tabloid headlines, it wasn't surprising that the Cruise camp would fire off an inquiring missive or four.[33] Yet even after Morrow representatives assured him that the chapter did not "defame" Cruise by identifying him as gay or make any remarks connecting such an allegation to his participation in the Church of Scientology, the megastar's legal advisors persisted in demanding a review of the material prior to publication. As that publication was imminent the point was moot. And so Cruise—like Liberace before him—found greener pastures for a lawsuit in England where one was filed against an offending tabloid.

"Cruise and Kidman took the *Express* to court over the paper reporting that their eight-year marriage was a cover for their homosexuality," *Daily Variety* reported of their legal success in the fall of 1998 just as *Open Secret* hit bookshelves.

> The couple have been awarded libel damages at the High Court in London believed to be in excess of $300,000. The money will be donated to charity. The *Express* will also pay legal costs of about $250,000.
>
> Outside the court, Cruise said, "I don't take a whole lot of pleasure in being here today. It is the last recourse against those that published vicious lies about me and my family."
>
> As for the court case, Cruise's lawyer, George Carman, said the *Express* article "recycled a selection of wholly unfounded rumors about the plaintiff of a highly offensive nature. In summary, it alleged that their marriage was a hypocritical sham, entered into as a mere business arrangement, or on orders of the Church of Scientology, or as a cover-up for the homosexuality of one or both of them, and that Tom Cruise was impotent and sterile and that his public denial of this was untrue."[34]

But that wasn't the end of it. For as *People* noted of Cruise in August 1999, "This spring he and Kidman both launched a suit against the US-based tabloid the *Star* for claiming that sex experts had to coach them in the art of lovemaking for *Eyes Wide Shut*, an allegation the couple's attorney, Bert Fields, calls 'absolutely false.' Adds the attorney: 'Tom is not going to let people defame him or his family. He has the means to wage this war.' "[35]

He didn't have to wait that long, for in October the *Star* published the following statement:

> *Star* wishes to apologize to Tom Cruise and Nicole Kidman for an article published in its March 30 1999 edition

about their work in making the acclaimed motion picture
Eyes Wide Shut. Star also regrets any statements made
by anyone questioning Mr. and Mrs. Cruise's motives for
bringing a lawsuit in response to the March 30 article.
Our investigation in the course of that lawsuit and the
information brought to our attention by Mr. and Mrs.
Cruise convinces us that the March 30 article contained
false statements about Mr. and Mrs. Cruise that were
harmful to them, and we apologize for any distress we
may have caused them. We wish to retract any suggestion
that their performances were somehow unsatisfactory to
director Stanley Kubrick, or that Mr. Cruise or Ms. Kidman needed to be coached by sex therapists or anyone
else to improve their performances. To bring this matter
to a positive end, we have agreed to make a substantial
monetary contribution to a worthy charity selected by
Tom and Nicole.[36]

Still it was something of pyrrhic victory. For by then Cruise
and Kidman had crashed and burned in the commercial fiasco of *Eyes
Wide Shut.* While a very interesting study in jealousy and paranoia
surprisingly close to its source (Arthur Schnitzler's turn-of-the-last-
century Vienna-set *Traumnovelle*), *Eyes Wide Shut* wasn't in any way
the boundary-crossing, beyond Bertolucci sextravaganza that everyone had been led to expect. During the lengthy shoot, its maker Stanley Kubrick was—as usual—tight-lipped about its plot and purpose.
But Cruise and Kidman had been operating on a very different track,
using *Eyes Wide Shut* as a vehicle to promulgate their images as the
last word in heterosex. While the film was in post-production Kidman
managed to go so far as to parlay a brief view of her backside in *The
Blue Room* (David Hare's adaptation of Schnitzler's most famous work,
La Ronde) into a Broadway sensation in the tradition of *Oh! Calcutta!*
When Kubrick quite suddenly died of a heart attack right after sub-
mitting his final cut, Cruise and Kidman were left to carry on alone—
and to face the music. For the fears of thinking Cruise gay paled when

viewed in light of something far worse—a public disinclined to think about Cruise at all.

"The publicity for the movie has concentrated obsessively on the fact that Cruise and Kidman are married, with the hint that this can be expected to give their sex scenes some sort of hormonal boost," critic Louis Menard observed in his scathing *New York Review of Books* pan of both *Eyes Wide Shut* and its stars. "In fact they have no sex scenes with each other, apart from a brief kiss, and anyone who has seen them together on television—for example at an awards show—suspects that in real life they have no chemistry. Their marriage may be perfectly happy and sexually fulfilling, or it may be a Hollywood mange blanc. Who cares? It doesn't matter because they have no chemistry in the movie either."[37]

Well, Tom Cruise, Nicole Kidman, and their sundry handlers quite obviously care—a great deal. But it isn't as easy to sue the *New York Review of Books* as it is the *Express*. And that's not to mention an article about the Kubrick swan song by Katherine Rosman in *Brill's Content*, which neatly skewered the couple's on- and off-screen efforts at image management and its effect on *Eyes Wide Shut*'s fortunes, by simply quoting . . . Pat Kingsley.

"So what if it wasn't true? What's the harm? Both the movie and celebrity-obsessed media make out well by playing along," reporter Katherine Rosman noted dryly of the PR disaster before turning to its chief architect—now discovered, quite uncharacteristically, to be at something of a loss. " 'It's all business,' says Kingsley. 'Let it go. Let it go. Let it die. Let the story die. There are far more interesting things for [you] to write about than the marketing campaign on *Eyes Wide Shut*.' "[38]

That may indeed be true. But *Eyes Wide Shut* itself is not without interest—particularly as regards the sexual fastidiousness of the "real" Tom Cruise. For not only is he mistaken for gay by gang or urban toughs and nearly gay-bashed as a result, he's subject to the fey flirtatiousness of an obviously gay hotel clerk, played by the flamboyantly bisexual Alan Cumming.

"This is funny," the actor told reporter Steve Druckman of *Out* magazine. "After the Tony awards, one interviewer talking to me about *Eyes Wide Shut* said, 'So, you're coming out with Tom Cruise on July 16?' First of all, Tom Cruise is not coming out, and if he were, it would definitely not be with me!"[39]

Be that as it may, Kingsley has little to worry about regarding press attention to Cruise, as long as she can stay in the driver's seat. And there she was in October 1999, breathlessly supplying details to the *Daily News* about how Cruise "lost his footing and was hanging by his hands," during the shooting of a stunt for *Mission Impossible 2*, as if *Eyes Wide Shut* was just a half-forgotten bad dream.

"Paramount was concerned it could be a bit risky, Kingsley tells us, but everybody there is happy with the footage," said the *Daily News*.[40] And she is surely happy with respectful fourth estate treatment of this transparent bit of ballyhoo, so wispy as to be unworthy of disbelief. Moreover, she can only be pleased that she's not in charge of negotiating a public image as problematic as that of Kevin Spacey.

When we last left the Academy Award–winning actor (in chapter 4) he was refusing to comment on his sexual orientation one way or the other. But in 1999 Spacey elected to change his story. And who better to help him do so than *Daily Variety*'s Michael Fleming, now serving Spacey much as journalist Sidney Blumenthal did Bill Clinton.

First, Fleming established a sophisticatedly butch atmosphere: "With his baseball cap pulled down low, Kevin Spacey flies through Manhattan traffic on a motor scooter, weaving through bumper-to-bumper taxis, buses, and limousines." But his subject is way ahead of him, getting down to business right out of the gate.

"It's not true, it's a lie," says Spacey of stories which he declines to so much as identify, much less explicate. Still, he offers, "In my industry, I'm surrounded by all types of people. I know gay people, straight people, and people who are bisexual. There are people who haven't figured out what they are."[41]

And when they do, they'll doubtless be sure to tell their publicists about it first thing.

Playwright Tony Kushner wrote a brilliant speech for his Roy Cohn character in *Angels in America: Millennium Approaches*, describing this neo-Cartesian ("I think, therefore I am whatever I'm able to spin") frame of mind:

> I want you to understand. This is not hypocrisy. This is reality. I have sex with men. But unlike nearly every other man of whom this is true, I bring the guy I'm screwing to the White House and President Reagan smiles at us and shakes his hand. Because what I am is defined entirely by who I am. Roy Cohn is not a homosexual. Roy Cohn is a heterosexual man who fucks around with guys.[42]

Ever since its Broadway debut there's been talk of bringing Kushner's prizewinning epic theater piece to the screen. In an industry more geared to the bottom line of profit-making than ever—and in an era that has increasingly come to regard AIDS the tragedy of a previous generation of gay men—a movie version of *Angels in America* has its work cut out for it. But if it ever happens, few would disagree that Roy Cohn would be an ideal role for Kevin Spacey.

Spacey may, however, be otherwise occupied, for as he informs Fleming, "I have been quite open about my hope of having a family." Not that he's chary of playing gay roles because of the *Esquire* affair, he insists. "It's important to make this distinction: It wasn't that I cared if they inferred that I was gay, because I believe people in this country are more advanced than certain members of the media who try to use the medium as a weapon. But I felt betrayed."

But if Spacey didn't care there would be no reason to go to all this trouble. Or would there?

"When I sit down with a journalist he's watching every move I make," Spacey tells Fleming. "They watch where my eyes go. Everybody comes on like they're Sherlock Holmes. I may just be looking around the room, yet they're thinking, Hmmm, aha!"

And thus we're to understand that sexual orientation is nothing more than a form of performance? Hard to say, as Spacey begs off any further inquiry into his acting technique.

"I haven't asked for the public trust. I haven't asked anybody to vote for me. I'm an actor."[43] But there is a vote in Hollywood: the Academy Awards. And as everyone knows, one has yet to be conferred on an openly gay actor. The Fleming interview is, needless to say, part of Spacey's Oscar campaign. And so is a profile of the actor by Jennifer Senior of *New York* magazine, now famous in journalistic circles for this brief but deathless passage: " 'Hell,' he says with gusto, taking a sip of Chablis."

"The problem," Senior goes on to note, "is that the denouement of *American Beauty* turns on the question of Lester Burnham's sexuality—an issue that can't possibly have been lost on Spacey when he took the role. So it seems reasonable to ask: Is he toying with his image? 'I would not manipulate my audiences in that way,' says Spacey, very solemnly."

And Senior finds the film's director striking a similarly solemn chord: "The warmth and tenderness required in this role, adds [Sam] Mendes, wasn't much of a stretch. 'You can see how comfortable he is with women and heterosexuality,' he says, choosing his words very carefully."[44]

Indeed! But wait a minute—isn't Kevin Spacey just an actor? Why should any "comfort level" be involved? Still Spacey's surely far from discomfited that "Page Six" of the *New York Post* saw fit to note his "making out with a brunette model type" atop a table in a London cafe, in an item that appeared simultaneously with the *Playboy* piece, noting that a witness of the incident remarked "Everybody was staring. It was very obvious."[45]

But what was obvious? That was the question for less credulous areas of the media, like Jim Holt's "The Tired Hedonist" column in the *New York Press*:

> Ever since Kevin Spacey made it known a week or so ago
> that he is definitely heterosexual, at least one gay friend
> of mine—I'll call him "Bill," for that is his name—has
> been rather glum. It seems that Bill, a boyish-looking
> blond lawyer, was under the impression that Kevin
> Spacey had picked him up one night in the mid-80s in
> an East Village club called the Boy Bar, and that the two

of them had subsequently shared a tender moment at Bill's apartment. Now Bill knows that this "Kevin Spacey" must have been an imposter, since the real Kevin Spacey is straight. My friend is especially dejected at the thought that he had intimacies with someone who was as physically unattractive as Spacey when that person is not even a star."[46]

Or as Jim Mullen of *Entertainment Weekly*'s "The Hot Sheet" succinctly put Spacey's heterosexual declaration, "If that doesn't work he plans to marry Lisa Marie Presley."[47]

What won't work are incidents like the one reported by "Page Six" on October 10, 1999, in which Spacey walked out of a planned appearance on a Miami radio talk show when he discovered that drag diva RuPaul was the guest host.[48] Did Spacey imagine this playful pop music figure was going to attack him? What a shame, as RuPaul had been trumpeting the actor's performance in *American Beauty* over the greater Miami airwaves even as Spacey was leaving the building. But perhaps this was an isolated incident as, around the same time, Spacey had no problem in speaking to Dotson Radar of *Parade* magazine.[49] Of course he may have felt more at ease in that Radar didn't bring up the *Esquire* story or ask any "personal" questions. The article did, however, feature a photo (uncommented-on in the main text), of the actor with a woman, employed as his production assistant, identified as "longtime girlfriend Diane Dreyer." The photo's caption went on to repeat his *Playboy* declaration about wanting to start a family.

But sometimes it's hard to get information about "long-term" relationships across in the high-pressure world of show business. In its coverage of the "GQ Men of the Year" awards, where he was honored for reviving *The Iceman Cometh*, the *New York Daily News* notes the actor "held hands with a lovely brunette he called his 'date.' "[50] However, it appears this "date" wasn't of the "long-term" variety, as media scribes were quick to note the next day that Spacey was "squiring around Susanna Arvisson, a newly imported Wilhelmina model from Sweden" rather than Ms. Dreyer.[51] But things can get murky in Spaceyland. At a VH-1 event Spacey attended, it was reported that "when he wasn't holding hands with the beauty he brought to last week's GQ award, he was getting to know those cute guys in N'Sync, who livened up the theater's back row with a popcorn fight."[52]

And then there was the item in *New York* magazine's "Intelligencer" column about how the "insistently heterosexual Kevin Spacey was spied enjoying the sight of wafer-thin Ally McBeal costar Lisa Ling and full-figured television cohostess Star Jones having a "lighthearted smooching session" at a party following a Yankees game. "After they kissed, Kevin Spacey was so excited he asked them to do it again. And they did."[53]

Whatever the "truth" about Kevin Spacey may be—holding hands, tossing popcorn, or encouraging same-sex kissing among "celebrity" females—Wilde's "The Decay of Lying" reminds us, "The final revelation is that Lying, the telling of beautiful untruths, is the proper aim of Art. But I think I have spoken of this at sufficient length."

And so have I.

NOTES AND

SOURCES

Prologue: Hypothalamus, Mon Amour

1. Herzer, Manfred, "Kertbeny and the Nameless Love," *Journal of Homosexuality*, volume 12, number 1, fall 1985.

2. Katz, Jonathan Ned, *The Invention of Heterosexuality*, Dutton, 1995.

3. Proust, Marcel, *Remembrance of Things Past: Cities of the Plain*, translated by C. K. Scott Moncrieff and Terence Kilmartin, Random House, 1981.

4. O'Hara, Frank, "Ave Maria," in *Lunch Poems*, City Lights Books, 1964.

5. Isherwood, Christopher, *Christopher and His Kind*, Farrar, Straus & Giroux, 1976.

6. Vidal, Gore, "Sex Is Politics," in *The Second American Revolution and Other Essays, 1976–1982*, Random House, 1982.

7. Barthes, Roland, introduction to *Tricks* by Renaud Camus, St. Martin's Press, 1981.

8. Foucault, Michel, "Sexual Choice, Sexual Act," interview conducted by James O'Higgins, *Salamagundi*, fall/winter 1982–83; reprinted in *Foucault Live, Semiotext(e)*, Foreign Agents series, 1989.

9. Jones, James H., *Alfred Kinsey: A Public/Private Life*, W. W. Norton, 1997.

10. Katz, op. cit.

One: Gay All of a Sudden

1. Cory, Bruce, ". . . 'Disorderly Conduct' Charge Against Tab Hunter," *Confidential*, September 1955.

2. Henry, William A. III, "Forcing Gays Out of the Closet: Homosexual Leaders Seek to Expose Foes of the Movement," *Time*, January 29, 1990.

3. Wilson, Earl, untitled column, *New York Post*, June 26, 1952.

4. Author's interview with Piper Laurie, April 20, 1997.

5. Lambert, Gavin, *On Cukor*, G. P. Putnam's Sons, 1972.

6. Text of contracts for Fred Zinnemann on *High Noon* and George Stevens for Columbia Pictures on file at the Academy of Motion Picture Arts and Sciences.

7. Wilson, op. cit.

8. Hester, Clyde, "How His Marriage Saved Rock Hudson from Double-Scandal," *TV Scandals*, December 1957.

9. Steinmetz, Johanna, " 'The Rock' Stays Dignified—Despite Rumors," *Now!—Chicago Today*, June 27, 1971.

10. Scheetz, Jim, "Setting the Record Straight," *Coronet*, October 1976.

11. Headline in *Sun*, July 24, 1985.

12. Russo, Vito, *The Celluloid Closet*, Harper & Row, 1987.

13. Author's interview with Gavin Lambert, March 24, 1997.

14. Author's interview with James Ellroy, November 29, 1996.

15. Author's interview with Jill Abrams, November 24, 1996.

16. Human Rights Campaign awards dinner, broadcast live on C-Span, November 11, 1997.

17. Bardin, Brantley, "Nathan Lane," *US*, February 1998.

18. Mayne, Judith, *Directed by Dorothy Arzner*, Indiana University Press, 1994.

19. Crowley, Mart, *The Boys in the Band* (1968), in *Three Plays by Mart Crowley*, Alyson Publications, 1996.

20. Stayton, Joanne, letter to *TV Guide*, October 19–25, 1997.

21. Herder, Marjorie, letter to *TV Guide*, November 1–7, 1997.

22. *TV Guide*, March 20, 1997.

23. Remark by unidentified audience member on broadcast of *The Oprah Winfrey Show*, April 30, 1997.

24. Kael, Pauline, "The Glamour of Delinquency," in *I Lost It at the Movies*, Little, Brown and Co., 1965.

25. Dalton, David, *James Dean: The Mutant King*, Straight Arrow Books, 1974.

26. Riese, Randall, *James Dean: His Life and Legacy from A–Z*. Contemporary Books, 1991.

27. Herndon, Venable, *James Dean: A Short Life*. Doubleday, 1974.

28. Riese, op. cit.

29. Corliss, Richard, "Byron Meets Bully Budd," *Time*, August 22, 1994.

30. Peyser, Mark, "The Life of the Party," *Newsweek*, June 23, 1997.

31. Russo, op. cit.

32. Clarke, Gerald, "Cary Grant and Randolph Scott: The Debonair Leading Man and the Western Star in Santa Monica," *Architectural Digest*, April 1996.

33. Harris, Warren G., *Cary Grant: A Touch of Elegance*. Doubleday, 1987.

34. Gill, Brendan, "Pursuer and Pursued," *New Yorker*, June 2, 1997.

35. Timmons, Stuart, *The Trouble with Harry Hay*, Alyson, 1990.

36. Mason, Kiki, "Walk This Way," *Out*, September 1993.

Two: Invisible City

1. Rechy, John, *City of Night*, Grove Press, 1963.

2. Author's interview with John Rechy, December 6, 1996.

3. Isherwood, Christopher, *Diaries, Volume One, 1939–1960*, edited and introduced by Katherine Bucknell, HarperCollins, 1996.

4. Author's interview with Harry Hay, October 20, 1997.

5. Strong, Lester, and David Hanna, "Hollywood Watering Holes,

30's Style," *Harvard Gay and Lesbian Review,* Summer 1996, volume 2, number 3.

6. Author's interview with Kim Garfield, December 23, 1996.

7. Isherwood, op. cit.

8. Author's interview with Ellroy.

9. Author's interview with Harry Clein, September 25, 1996.

10. Banham, Reyner, *Los Angeles: The Architecture of Four Ecologies,* Penguin Books, 1971.

11. Hockney, David, *David Hockney by David Hockney: My Early Years,* Harry N. Abrams, 1976.

12. Morin, Edgar, *Les Stars,* Editions du Seuil, 1960; translated from the French by Richard Howard as *The Stars,* Grove Press, 1961.

13. Author's interview with Lambert.

14. Leff, Leonard J., and Jerome L. Simmons, *The Dame in the Kimono,* Weidenfeld and Nicolson, 1990.

15. Isherwood, op. cit.

16. Author's interview with Hay.

17. Isherwood, op. cit.

18. Author's interview with Hay.

19. Author's interview with Clein.

20. Author's interview with Lea DeLaria, November 4, 1996.

21. Author's interview with Mickey Cottrell, May 27, 1997.

22. Author's interview with Bill Condon, August 18, 1997.

Three: Nobody Said Anything

1. Milne, Tom, "One Man Crazy: James Whale," *Sight and Sound,* volume 42, number 3, Summer 1973.

2. Curtis, James, *James Whale,* Scarecrow Press, 1982 (revised edition, Faber & Faber, 1998).

3. Russo, op. cit.

4. Author's interview with Ian McKellen, July 25, 1997.

5. Author's interview with Christopher Bram, July 23, 1997.

6. Barnhill, Mark, "Mystery Lingers in Filmmaker's Death," Los Angeles *Daily News,* April 12, 1987.

7. Author's interview with Bram.

8. Author's interview with Bill Condon, July 23 and August 18, 1997.

9. Author's interview with Curtis Harrington, August 26, 1997.

10. Author's interview with Gloria Stuart, December 2, 1997.

11. Lanchester, Elsa, *Elsa Lanchester Herself,* St. Martin's Press, 1983.

12. Skal, David J., *The Monster Show,* W. W. Norton and Co., 1993.

13. Lanchester, op. cit.

14. Author's interview with Don Bachardy, July 11, 1997.

15. Author's interview with Lambert.

16. Rechy, op. cit.

17. Author's interview with Lambert.

18. Holland, Larry Lee, "William Haines," *Films in Review,* March 1984.

19. Loos, Anita, *The Talmadge Sisters,* Viking, 1978.

20. Brooks, Louise, *Lulu in Hollywood,* Alfred A. Knopf, 1982.

21. Fox, Christy, "Decorator Is Much Too Busy to Retire," *Los Angeles Times,* December 14, 1969.

22. Goodman, Ezra, "Ringing Up the Curtain on William Haines," *New York Times,* June 8, 1949.

23. McGilligan, Patrick, *George Cukor: A Double Life,* St. Martin's Press, 1991.

Levy, Emmanuel, *George Cukor: Master of Elegance,* William Morrow and Company, 1994.

24. Author's interview with Ellroy.

25. Cukor, George, letters on file at the Academy of Motion Picture Arts and Sciences Library, Los Angeles.

26. Author's interview with Kevin Thomas, June 7, 1997.

27. Cukor, letters on file.

28. Author's interview with Thomas.

29. Author's interview with Lambert.

30. Simone, Lela, "An Oral History with Lela Simone," conducted by Rudy Behlmer, phone interviews 1990–91, Academy of Motion Picture Arts and Sciences Library, Los Angeles, 1994.

Tinkcom, Matthew, "Working Like a Homosexual: Camp Visual Codes and the Labor of Gay Subjects in the MGM Freed Unit," *Film Journal,* volume 35, number 2, 1996.

31. Author's interview with Hank Moonjean, November 7, 1996.

32. Simone, Lela, op. cit.

33. Silverman, Stephen M., *Dancing on the Ceiling: Stanley Donen and His Movies,* Alfred A. Knopf, 1996.

34. Cukor, letters on file.

35. Cherichetti, David, *Hollywood Director,* Curtis Books, 1973.

36. Loney, Glenn, *Unsung Genius: The Passion of Dancer-Choreographer Jack Cole*, Franklin Watts, 1984.

37. Vidal, Gore, *Palimpsest—A Memoir*, Random House, 1995.

38. Author's interview with Lambert.

39. Isherwood, op. cit.

40. Author's interview with Mart Crowley, November 6, 1996.

Four: It's a Scandal!

1. Cory, Bruce, op. cit.

2. Berlin, Brigid, "The One and Only Tab Hunter," *Interview*, volume 4, number 11, 1974.

3. Signorile, Michelangelo, *Queer in America*, Random House, 1993.

4. Author's interview with Lambert.

5. Skolsky, Sidney, "Hollywood Is My Beat," Hollywood *Citizen-News*, May 12, 1955.

6. Winecoff, Charles, *Split Image: The Life of Anthony Perkins*, E. P. Dutton & Co., 1996.

7. Uncredited, "Tab Hunter Seeks Way Out of Confidential Testimony," *Los Angeles Times*, August 9, 1957.

8. Goodman, Ezra, *The Fifty-Year Decline and Fall of Hollywood*, Simon and Schuster, 1961.

9. Gabler, Neal, *Walter Winchell: Gossip, Power and the Culture of Celebrity*, Alfred A. Knopf, 1995.

10. Parsons, Louella, with Bob Thomas, *Tell It to Louella*, G. P. Putnam and Sons, 1961.

11. Lewis, Judy, *Uncommon Knowledge*, Pocket Books, 1994.

12. Author's interview with Hank Moonjean.

13. Author's interview with Thomas.

14. Uncredited film reviews, *Daily Variety*, January 13 and February 15, 1950.

15. Smith, Liz, "A New Maternal Role," *Los Angeles Times*, March 6, 1998.

16. Author's interview with Lambert.

17. Goodman, *Fifty-Year Decline*, op. cit.

18. Bogle, Donald, *Dorothy Dandridge*, Amistad, 1997.

19. Uncredited, "$25 Million Suit Filed by Liberace," *Los Angeles Examiner*, May 15, 1957.

20. Goodman, *Fifty-Year Decline*, op. cit.

21. Whiteside, Jonny, *Cry: The Johnnie Ray Story*, Barricade Books, 1994.

22. Tommasini, Anthony, "Golly Gee, Jimmy Olsen writes Librettos!," *New York Times*, May 15, 1998.

23. Beverly, Al, and Enid Dean, "Homosexuality in Hollywood," *Whisper*, November 1964.

24. Author's interview with Ellroy.

25. Otash, Fred, *Investigation: Hollywood*, Henry Regnery and Co., 1976.

Gates, Phyllis, and Bob Thomas, *My Husband, Rock Hudson*, Doubleday, 1987.

26. Author's interview with Ellroy.

27. Gross, Larry, *Contested Closets*, University of Minnesota Press, 1992.

28. Musto, Michael, "Bold-Faced Lies," *QW*, August 9, 1992.

29. Albright, Diane, "Rosie's Gay Marriage," *Globe*, September 3, 1996.

30. Gibson, Rob, "The Real Rosie," *Globe*, July 8, 1997.

31. Campbell, Laurie, "Meet the Ritzie New Rosie," *National Examiner*, August 5, 1997.

32. Smith, Alan, and Darryl Wrobel, "Rosie's Secret Lover," *National Enquirer*, March 10, 1998.

33. Author's interview with Howard Bragman, March 31, 1997.

34. Lawsuit BC171057, filed May 13, 1997, by Martin Singer and Lynda B. Goldman of Lavely & Singer, 2049 Century Park East, Suite 1400, Los Angeles 90067–2906.

35. Snow, Shauna, "Morning Report," *Los Angeles Times*, May 16, 1997.

36. Smith, Alan, Michael Glynn, Patricia Towle and John Blosser, "Eddie Murphy's Secret Sex Life," *National Enquirer*, May 20, 1977.

37. Snow, Shauna, "Morning Report," *Los Angeles Times*, August 1, 1997.

38. Ebner, Mark, "The Gay Mafia," *Spy*, June 1995.

39. Junod, Tom, "Kevin Spacey Has a Secret," *Esquire*, October 1997.

40. Stockwell, Anne, "Kevin Spacey Confidential," *Advocate*, October 28, 1997.

41. Luscombe, Belinda, "In, Out or None of Your Business," *Time*, September 29, 1997.

42. Fleming, Michael, "Celebs Seeing Red After Mags Go to Bed," *Daily Variety*, September 30, 1997.

43. Author's interview with Michael Fleming; October 2, 1997.

Five: Closet Privileges

1. Uncredited, "Liberace Defends Reputation in Libel Action in London Court," *Los Angeles Times*, June 9, 1959.

2. Foucault, op. cit.

3. "Cassandra" column c. 1956, quoted in *Los Angeles Times*, June 9, 1959.

4. Uncredited, "Libel Denied in Liberace London Case," *Los Angeles Times*, June 11, 1959.

Uncredited, "Liberace Wins Libel Suit, $22,400 Damages," *Los Angeles Times*, June 18, 1959.

5. Oliver, Myrna, "Ex-Chauffeur, 23, Claims He Was Evicted from Penthouse, Lost Job," *Los Angeles Times*, October 15, 1982.

6. Oliver, Myrna, "Suit Over Tabloid Article Names Liberace," *Los Angeles Times*, May 28, 1983.

7. Uncredited, "Liberace Palimony Suit Is Settled for $95,000," *Los Angeles Herald-Examiner*, December 31, 1986.

8. Gaines, James R., "Liberace," *People*, October 1, 1982.

9. Author's interview with Rechy.

10. Parsons, Louella, "Liberace Denies He's Engaged; Not Now, Anyway; Maybe Later," *Los Angeles Examiner*, October 7, 1954.

11. Uncredited, "Girl Friend Tells: My Dates with Liberace," *Los Angeles Mirror*, October 13, 1954.

12. Uncredited, "Liberace Named in $1.5 Mil Libel, Defamation Action," *Hollywood Reporter*, January 16, 1974.

13. Uncredited, "Liberace Manager Sued," *Los Angeles Times*, July 15, 1988.

14. Uncredited, "Liberace's Manager Threatens Libel Suit Over AIDS Report," *Daily Variety*, January 28, 1987.

15. Uncredited, "Liberace Died of AIDS; A Cover-Up Is Alleged," *New York Times*, February 10, 1987.

16. King, Susan, "Carrie Fisher," *Los Angeles Times*, August 13, 1995.

17. Author's interview with Thomas.

18. Goodman, *Fifty-Year Decline*, op. cit.

19. Socol, Gary, "The Golden Rules of Gossip," *Genre*, November 1996.

20. Van Meter, Jonathan, "Sandy Gallin—Mogul Manager," *Out*, November 1994.

21. Greenberg, Abe, "Voice of Hollywood," *Hollywood Citizen News*, April 7, 1967.

22. Uncredited, "Tempo," *Los Angeles Herald-Examiner*, August 2, 1970.

23. Gauguin, Lorraine, "On the Crying Need for a Ross Hunter Film Festival," *Los Angeles*, April 1970.

24. Crono, op. cit.

25. Signorile, Michelangelo, "The Other Side of Malcolm Forbes," *OutWeek*, March 18, 1990.

26. DeGeneres, Ellen, "Ellen DeGeneres Exposes Herself," *US*, May 1994.

27. Seibel, Deborah Stater, "Ellen's Mirror Image," *TV Guide*, November 26, 1994.

28. Soren, Tabitha, "Ellen's New Twist on TV," *USA Weekend*, November 24–26, 1995.

29. Kaufman, Debra, "Ellen's New Beginning," *Producer*, February 1996.

30. Cerone, Daniel Howard, "The Ever-Changing World of Ellen and How She Runs It," *TV Guide*, February 10, 1996.

31. Kronke, David, "Get It Straight," *New Times*, October 24–30, 1996.

32. Stanfill, Francesca, "Jodie Foster: A New Role Puts the Young Veteran Back on Screen and in Lights," *Elle*, March 1987.

33. Wiley, Mason, and Damien Bona, *Inside Oscar*, Ballantine Books, 1993.

34. Musto, Michael, "La Dolce Musto," *Village Voice*, January 31, 1993.

35. Kiley, Sam, "Fatale Attraction," *Sunday Times* (London), May 17, 1991.

36. Shnayerson, Michael, "Pure Jodie," *Vanity Fair*, May 1994.

37. Foster, Buddy, and Leon Wagener, *Foster Child: A Biography of Jodie Foster*, E. P. Dutton and Co., 1997.

38. Schneider, Karen S., and Julie Jordan, Vicki Sheff-Cahan, Amy Brooks, Danielle Morton, Jennifer Longley, "Foster Mom," *People*, March 23, 1998.

Smith, op. cit.

39. Isherwood, *Diaries,* op. cit.

40. Author's interview with Clein.

41. Author's interview with Thomas.

42. Clark, Tom with Dick Kleiner, *Rock Hudson—Friend of Mine,* Pharos Books, 1990.

43. Author's interview with Armistead Maupin, October 20, 1997.

44. Author's interview with Laurie.

45. Author's interview with Maupin.

46. Author's interview with Condon.

47. Author's interview with Bragman.

48. Author's interview with McKellen.

49. Author's interview with Richard Natale, September 10, 1997.

50. Sadownick, Doug, "Gay Hollywood in the Flesh," *LA Weekly,* April 3–9, 1998.

51. Author's interview with Steven Dornbusch, November 4, 1996.

52. Signorile, *Queer in America.*

53. Author's interview with Doug Lindeman, June 9, 1997.

54. Author's interview with Mark Miller, June 3, 1997.

55. Kroll, Jack, "Send in the Clown," *Newsweek,* March 25, 1996.

56. Author's interview with Miller.

57. Blum, David, "Enter Laughing," *Esquire,* May 1996.

58. Musto, Michael, "La Dolce Musto," *Village Voice,* May 21, 1996.

59. Uncredited; "Intelligencer," *New York,* June 2, 1997.

60. Musto, Michael, "La Dolce Musto," *Village Voice,* August 26, 1997.

61. Clark, John, "Let Him Entertain You," *Los Angeles Times,* July 31, 1997.

62. Bardin, op. cit.

63. Author's interview with Miller.

64. Author's interview with Jenny Pizer, November 14, 1996.

65. "Selleck Sues Globe Tabloid, Says Story Depicts Him as Homosexual," *Los Angeles Times,* July 4, 1991.

66. "Selleck, Globe Settle Libel Suit," *Daily Variety,* August 6, 1991.

67. Gross, op. cit.

68. Daly, Steve, "In the Money," *Entertainment Weekly,* October 3, 1997.

69. Galvin, Peter, "Selleck Speaks Out," *Advocate,* September 16, 1997.

70. Weinraub, Bernard, "As the Taboos Fade, More Straight Actors Are Taking Gay Roles," *New York Times,* September 10, 1997.

71. Kasindorf, Jeanie Russell, "Perception, Reality," *New York*, March 13, 1995.

Mead, Rebecca, "Rag Trade," *New Yorker*, May 11, 1998.

72. Socol, op. cit.

Six: Death and Transfiguration

1. Anne Heche on *The Oprah Winfrey Show*, broadcast on ABC Television, April 30, 1997.

2. Rudnick, Paul, "Gaytown U.S.A." *New York*, June 20, 1994.

3. Clark, op. cit.

4. Harmetz, Aljean, "Hollywood Reacts to AIDS Threat," *New York Times*, November 7, 1985.

5. Weinraub, Bernard, "Hollywood Called Hypocritical by Actor Who Died of AIDS," *New York Times*, September 12, 1991.

6. Ryan, James, "Brad Davis Blasts AIDS-Phobia in Hollywood," *Advocate*, October 22, 1991.

7. Murphy, Mary, "The AIDS Scare—What It's Done to Hollywood . . . and the TV You See," *TV Guide*, October 22, 1988.

8. Associated Press, "New Celeb Curse: Outing by Disease," *Hollywood Reporter*, December 10, 1991.

9. Weinraub, Bernard, "Anthony Perkins's Wife Tells of Two Years of Secrecy," *New York Times*, September 16, 1992.

10. Ehrenstein, David, "More Than Friends," *Los Angeles*, May 1996.

Author's interviews with Joel Thurm, Jeff Sagansky, and Joe Voci, February-March 1996.

11. Author's interview with Laurence Mark, January 15, 1998.

12. Author's interview with Bragman.

13. Yarbrough, Jeff, "Fox's Barry Diller," *Advocate*, October 22, 1991.

14. Chunovic, Louis, "Universal's Sid Sheinberg," *Advocate*, October 22, 1991.

15. Author's interview with Rich Jennings, September 15, 1996.

16. Author's interview with Natale.

17. Author's interview with Clein.

18. "Hollywood Supports" panel discussion with Randal Kleiser, Paul Bartel, Nicole Conn, Clive Barker, Sam Irvin, July 16, 1997.

19. Author's interview with Morgan Rumpf, June 24, 1997.

20. Greeley, Andrew M., "A *Nothing Sacred* Episode You Haven't Seen," *New York Times*, March 1, 1998.

Seven: Going Public

1. Author's interview with David Geffen, October 9, 1997.

2. Musto, Michael, "La Dolce Musto," *Village Voice*, May 8, 1990.

3. Signorile, Michelangelo, "Gossip Watch," *OutWeek*, December 26, 1990.

4. Author's interview with Geffen.

5. Author's interview with Natale.

6. Lemon, Brendan, "David Geffen," *Advocate*, #619, December 29, 1992.

7. Citron, Alan, "David Geffen Didn't Take the Money and Run," *Los Angeles Times*, March 7, 1993.

8. Uncredited, "Careless Whispers," *Details*, February 1996.

9. Author's interview with Geffen.

10. Konigsberg, Eric, and Maer Roshan, "Boys on the Side," *New York*, August 18, 1997.

11. Author's interview with Geffen.

12. Author's interview with Bragman.

13. Snow, Shauna, "The Morning Report," *Los Angeles Times*, September 14, 1996.

14. Uncredited, "Cheers and Jeers," *TV Guide*, October 12, 1996.

15. Kronke, David, "Get It Straight," *New Times*, October 24–30, 1996.

16. Bruni, Frank, "It May Be a Closet Door but It's Already Open," *New York Times*, October 13, 1996.

17. Lowry, Brian, "Risks and Benefits Seen for an Out-of-the-Closet *Ellen*," *Los Angeles Times*, February 3, 1997.

18. DeVries, Hillary, "The Queen of All Access," *Los Angeles Times Sunday Magazine*, September 14, 1997.

19. Letter from Gordon Frevel of San Miguel, Baja California, *Los Angeles Times Sunday Magazine*, September 21, 1997.

20. Author's interview with Bragman.

21. Hanania, Joseph, "*Ellen* Takes Back Seat at Talk on Gays' Role in Hollywood," *Los Angeles Times*, October 25, 1996.

22. Author's interview with Nina Jacobson and Bruce Cohen, October 16, 1996.

23. Handy, Bruce, "Roll Over, Ward Cleaver," *Time*, April 14, 1997.

24. Interview of Ellen DeGeneres by Diane Sawyer on *20/20*, ABC Television, April 25, 1997.

25. Interview of Heche by Winfrey, op. cit.

26. Author's interview with Pizer.

27. Dutka, Elaine, "What's Next For Heche?," *Los Angeles Times*, May 3, 1997.

28. Weinraub, Bernard, "Problem For Hollywood: DeGeneres's Companion," *New York Times*, April 28, 1997.

29. Borden, Lizzie, "What's the Problem? Let Her Do Her Job," *Los Angeles Times*, May 5, 1997.

30. Gilbert, Matthew, "Lesbian's Coming Out Leaves Hollywood Waiting," *Boston Globe*, May 7, 1997.

31. Author's interview with Bragman.

32. Author's interview with Miller.

33. Author's interview with Garfield.

34. Author's interview with Abrams.

35. Author's interview with Dan Butler, August 25, 1997.

36. Author's interview with Lea DeLaria, November 4, 1996.

37. Holden, Stephen, "A Tough Comic Comes Out As a Musical Comedy Star," *New York Times*, August 20, 1997.

38. Author's interview with Dornbusch.

39. Author's interview with Alan Poul, October 30, 1996.

40. Author's interview with Geffen.

41. Savage, Dan, "Savage Love," *Chicago Reader*, May 2, 1997.

Eight: Running for Mayor

1. Ehrenstein, David, "JFK—A New Low for Hollywood," *Advocate*, January 14, 1992.

2. Ehrenstein, David, "Homophobia in Hollywood II: The Queer Empire Strikes Back," *Advocate*, April 7, 1992.

Kirkwood, James, *American Grotesque*, Simon and Schuster, 1970; reissued by HarperPerennial, 1992.

Yarbrough, Jeff, "Heart of Stone," *Advocate*, April 7, 1992.

3. Author's interview with Gus Van Sant, June 1, 1992.

4. Van Sant, Gus, "The Hollywood Way," in *Projections 3: Filmmakers on Film-making*, edited by John Boorman and Walter Donohue, Faber and Faber, 1994. Another à clef account of the same events is provided by Van Sant in his novel *Pink*, Doubleday/Nan A. Talese, 1997.

Nine: Moving and Shaking

1. Author's interview with Jacobson and Cohen.

2. Author's interview with Robert L. Williams, April 10, 1997.

3. Author's interview with Rumpf.

4. Author's interview with Chastity Bono, June 12, 1997.

5. Wockner, Rex, "Mel Gibson on Gays," *Outlines News Service*, January 1992.

6. Author's interview with Bono.

7. Author's interview with Poul.

8. Outfest '97 panel.

9. Miller, Mark, "The Mayor of Gotham Speaks," *Newsweek*, June 30, 1997.

10. Author's interview with Poul.

11. Author's interview with Howard Rosenman, August 15, 1997.

Ten: Hair Color

1. Cox, Dan, and Terry Johnson, "Pula Boogies Over to WB," *Daily Variety*, December 5, 1996.

2. Author's interview with Chris Pula, November 8, 1997.

3. Broeske, Pat H., "A 'Confidential' Plan?" *Entertainment Weekly*, December 12, 1997.

4. Author's interview with Charles Fleming, May 15, 1997.

5. Author's interview with Andrew Fleming, April 28, 1997.

6. Author's interview with Mark.

Eleven: "Not That There's Anything Wrong with That!"

1. Ehrenstein, David, "More Than Friends," *Los Angeles*, May 1996. Author's interviews with Mel Brooks, Mark Cherry, David Crane, Ann Fleet-Giordano, Richard Gollance, Kelsey Grammer, Robert Horn, Marta Kaufman, Joe Keenan, David Lee, David Lloyd, Daniel Margolis, Peter Mehlman, Chuck Ranberg, Joel Thurm, Joe Voci, William Lucas Walker, and Jamie Wooten. All interviews done in winter 1995.

2. Interview of DeGeneres by Sawyer, op. cit.

3. Emmy Awards broadcast, September 14, 1997.

4. *Access Hollywood* broadcast, September 24, 1997.

5. *Ellen* broadcast, November 19, 1997.

6. Hontz, Jenny, "DeGeneres Says Her *Ellen* on the Way Out," *Daily Variety*, February 24, 1998.

7. Webb, Cynthia L., "ABC Cancels *Ellen* After 5 Seasons," *Los Angeles Times*, April 24, 1998.

8. Cagle, Jess, "As Gay As It Gets?" *Entertainment Weekly*, May 8, 1998.

Cagle, Jess, "Out Spoken" *EW Special Edition*, posted May 4, 1998.

9. Lovell, Glenn, "*Ellen* Too Gay, Bono Chastises," *Daily Variety*, March 9, 1998.

10. Advertisment paid for by the Human Rights Campaign and the Gay and Lesbian Alliance Against Defamation, "An open letter to Robert Iger, president, ABC television network, regarding *Ellen*," May 4, 1998.

11. Author's interview with Bragman.

Twelve: Tom Cruise

1. Author's interview with Bono.

2. Author's interview with Maupin.

3. Author's interview with Geffen.

4. Sessums, Kevin, "Cruise Control," *Vanity Fair*, October 1984.

5. Katz, Ephraim, *The Film Encyclopedia*, Harper & Row, 1979.

6. Lurie, Rod, "No More Mr. Nice Guy," *Los Angeles*, October 1993.

7. Maslin, Janet, "Meditation on Vampires, by Way of John Milton," *New York Times*, October 28, 1993.

8. Ebner, op. cit.

9. Author's interview with DeLaria.

10. Author's interview with Williams.

11. Author's interview with Natale.

12. Author's interview with Bachardy.

13. Collins, Nancy, "Sex and the Single Star," *Rolling Stone*, August 18, 1983.

14. Brantley, Doug, "Look Who's Apologizing," *Advocate*, November 23, 1990.

15. Author's interview with Bachardy.

16. Gabriel, Trip, "Cruise at the Crossroads," *Rolling Stone*, January 11, 1990.

17. Fox, David J., "A Record $5 Million for AIDS," *Los Angeles Times*, January 29, 1994.

18. Uncredited, "Tom Cruise Is Called a Hero," *Outlook*, March 15, 1996.

19. Snow, Shauna, "The Morning Report," *Los Angeles Times*, July 6, 1996.

20. Uncredited, "Legal Briefs," *Hollywood Reporter*, August 2, 1996.

21. Snow, Shauna, "The Morning Report," *Los Angeles Times*, August 8, 1996.

22. Gere, Richard, and Cindy Crawford, "A Personal Statement," *Times*, (London) May 6, 1994.

23. Driscoll, Margarette, "Happy Ever After," *Sunday Times* (London), May 8, 1994.

24. Gross, Michael, "Even Richard Gere Gets Dumped," *Esquire*, July 1995.

25. Seipp, Catherine, "The Trouble with Gerbils," *Advocate*, July 3, 1990.

26. Smith, Liz, "A Compliment for Alec," *Los Angeles Times*, November 11, 1997.

Kaiser, Charles, "Interview with Alec Baldwin," *Interview*, October 1989.

27. Author's interview with Rumpf.

28. Weinraub, "As the Taboos Fade."

29. O'Kelly, Lisa, "Pretenders to the Drag Queen's Throne," *Observer* (London), November 6, 1994.

30. Gooch, Brad, "Rupert Observed," *Out*, Fall 1992.

31. Goldstein, Patrick, "How One Actor Changes a Movie Before It Even Came Out," *Los Angeles Times*, June 23, 1997.

32. Uncredited, "Rupert Everett (Actor)," *People*, January 5, 1998.

33. Author's interview with Bachardy.

The Epilogue Strikes Back

1. Allman, Kevin, "Hollywood's Changing Closet," *Washington Post*, October 26, 1998.

2. Biskupic, Joan, "For Gays, Tolerance Translates to Rights," *Washington Post*, November 5, 1999.

3. Hanley, Robert, "New Jersey Court Overturns Ouster of Gay Boy Scout," *New York Times*, August 5, 1999.

4. Sterngold, James, "An Unlikely 'Don't Tell' Target: Lawmaker May Face Discharge," *New York Times*, August 26, 1999; Frankel, Bruce, and Jeremy Kammer, "Refusing to Hide," *People*, November 1, 1999.

5. Knight, David, "My Father Is Wrong on Gay Rights," *Los Angeles Times*, October 14, 1999.

6. Brock, David, "The Strange Odyssey of Michael Huffington," *Esquire*, January 1999.

7. Martin, Lydia, "Lunch with Billy Bean," *Miami Herald,* July 25, 1999; Lipsyte, Robert, "A Major League Player's Life of Isolation and Secret Fear," *New York Times,* September 6, 1999.

8. Pedersen, Daniel, "A Quiet Man's Tragic Rendezvous With Hate," *Newsweek,* March 15, 1999.

9. Broder, John M., "Gay and Lesbian Group Offers Thanks to Clinton," *New York Times,* October 4, 1999.

10. Pressley, Sue Anne, "Hate May Have Triggered Fatal Barracks Beating," *Washington Post,* August 11, 1999.

11. Author's interview with Chris Pula, October 15, 1999.

12. Ehrenstein, David, "Van Sant's Seeds of Success," *Los Angeles Times,* July 7, 1999.

13. "Ellen DeGeneres and Anne Heche Want to Marry," Associated Press, October 11, 1999.

14. "Interview with Rupert Everett," *Mr. Showbiz,* August 12, 1999.

15. Author's interview with John Maybury, July 19, 1998.

16. "Travolta Shocker: The Gay Charges & the Truth About His Marriage," *National Enquirer,* October 5, 1999.

17. Camobell, Laurie, "Richard Gere Gay Shocker: The Truth About His Love Life," *National Examiner,* November 30, 1999.

18. Ely, Suzanne, and Marc Cetner, "Jodie Foster's Secret Life," *National Enquirer,* November 23, 1999.

19. Goldfarb, Susan, "Brad Pitt Gay Rumors," *National Examiner,* October 26, 1999.

20. Klinger, Rafe, "Prince Charles: 'I'm Gay!' " *Globe,* October 26, 1999.

21. Author's interview with John Maybury, July 19, 1998.

22. Garbarino, Steve, "Robert Downey's Last Party," *Detour,* February 1999.

23. Epstein, Jeffrey, "Kevin Williamson Unbound," *Advocate,* August 31, 1999.

24. Miller, Daryl H., "A Dreamy Case of Double Exposure," *Los Angeles Times,* September 22, 1999.

25. Kaufmann, Stanley, "Homosexual Drama and Its Disguises," *New York Times,* January 23, 1966.

26. Author's interview with Max Mutchnick, April 22, 1999.

27. Poniewozik, James, "TV's Coming-Out Party," *Time,* October 25, 1999.

28. Baldwin, Karen, "Full Metal Jack," *Entertainment Weekly,* October 23, 1999.

29. Vilanch, Bruce, "Citizen Lane," *Advocate*, February 2, 1999.

30. Weinraub, Bernard, "Gatekeeper to the Stars," *New York Times*, May 3, 1999.

31. "Flawless Film Rings Familiar," *Advocate*, November 23, 1999.

32. Rush & Molloy, "Sheedy's Arms Proliferation," *New York Daily News*, November 1, 1999.

33. "Tom Cruise Battered by Gay Book," *National Examiner*, September 1, 1998; "Hollywood's Gay Secrets," *National Enquirer*, August 25, 1998.

34. Boehm, Erich, "Cruise, Kidman Victorious Over London Tabloid Tattle," *Daily Variety*, October 30, 1998.

35. Tom Gliatto, with Liz Corcoran and Jane Cornwell in London, Julie Jordon, Kelly Carter, and Lyndon Stambler in Los Angeles, "Eye Strain," *People*, August 16, 1999.

36. "An Apology to Tom and Nicole," *Star*, October 26, 1999.

37. Menard, Louis, "Kubrick's Strange Love," *New York Review of Books*, August 12, 1999.

38. Rosman, Katherine, "Why the Media Kept Their Eyes Wide Shut," *Brill's Content*, October, 1999.

39. Drukman, Steven, "Cumming Attraction," *Out*, November 1999.

40. Rush & Molloy, "Daily Dish: Execs Squirm at Cruise Thriller," *New York Daily News*, October 25 1999.

41. Fleming, Michael, "The Playboy Interview: Kevin Spacey," *Playboy*, October 1999.

42. Kushner, Tony, *Angels in America: Millennium Approaches*, Theater Communications Group, 1993.

43. Fleming, Michael, "The Playboy Interview: Kevin Spacey," *Playboy*, October 1999.

44. Senior, Jennifer, "Isn't He Romantic?" *New York*, September 13, 1999.

45. Johnson, Richard, "Page Six: Kevin: Watch This," *New York Post*, September 10, 1999.

46. Holt, Jim, "The Tired Hedonist: Beware of Imitations!" *New York Press*, September 24, 1999.

47. Mullen, Jim, "The Hot Sheet," *Entertainment Weekly*, September 17, 1999.

48. Johnson, Richard, "Page Six: Spacey Won't Share RuPaul Air," *New York Post*, October 10, 1999.

49. Radar, Dotson, "A Glimpse of How Beautiful Life Can Be," *Parade* magazine, October 24, 1999.

50. Rush & Molloy, "Daily Dish: Paltrow's Chosen One," *New York Daily News,* October 25, 1999.

51. Rush & Molloy, "Daily Dish: Itemizing," *New York Daily News,* October 28, 1999.

52. Rush & Molloy, "Daily Dish: White House Happening," *New York Daily News,* October 26, 1999.

53. Keil, Beth Landman, and Deborah Mitchell, "Intelligencer: Lisa Kisses Friends," *New York,* November 15, 1999.

I N D E X